Aortic Diseases: An Issue of Cardiology Clinics

Aortic Diseases: An Issue of Cardiology Clinics

Editor: Erik Hutchinson

AMERICAN
MEDICAL PUBLISHERS
www.americanmedicalpublishers.com

AMERICAN
MEDICAL PUBLISHERS
www.americanmedicalpublishers.com

Cataloging-in-publication Data

Aortic diseases : an issue of cardiology clinics / edited by Erik Hutchinson.
p. cm.
Includes bibliographical references and index.
ISBN 978-1-63927-892-3
1. Aorta--Diseases. 2. Aortic valve--Diseases. 3. Cardiology. I. Hutchinson, Erik.
RC691 .A57 2023
616.13--dc23

American Medical Publishers,
41 Flatbush Avenue,
1st Floor, New York,
NY 11217, USA

ISBN 978-1-63927-892-3 (Hardback)

Contents

Preface ...VII

Part 1 Evolution of Care for Aortic Disease ...1

Chapter 1 Abdominal Aortic Aneurysms: Changing Paradigms in Treatment ...3
Christopher J. Marrocco and Ruth L. Bush

Chapter 2 The Evidence for Management of Abdominal Aortic Aneurysms: Lessons Learned from Randomised Controlled Trials ...27
Reza Mofidi and Stuart A. Suttie

Chapter 3 The Evolution of Aortic Aneurysm Repair: Past Lessons and Future Directions ...45
Ricky Harminder Bhogal and Richard Downing

Part 2 Improvements in the Endovascular and Surgical Management of Aortic Disease ...79

Chapter 4 Endovascular Repair of Ruptured Abdominal Aortic Aneurysms ...81
Cheong J. Lee, Andrew Gonzalez and Mark D. Morasch

Chapter 5 Alternative Surgical Management of Ascending Aorta Aneurysm ...95
Sossio Perrotta and Salvatore Lentini

Chapter 6 Aortic Valve Sparing Operation ...115
Júlia Čanádyová and Aleš Mokráček

Part 3 Anesthetic and Radiation Management in Aortic Surgery ...135

Chapter 7 Endovascular Repair: Radiation Risks ...137
John A. Kalef-Ezra

Chapter 8 Ultrasound-Guided Peripheral Nerve Block in the Anesthetic Considerations for Vascular Surgery - An Alternative Choice for Neuroaxial Anesthesia Techniques ...173
Yusuke Asakura and Hideki Takagi

Part 4 Molecular Management in Aortic Disease ...191

Chapter 9 Nutrition and the Aorto-Iliac Atherosclerotic Disease ...193
Sergio Santana Porbén

Chapter 10 **Role of Cathepsin K, L and S in Blood Vessel Remodeling....................................209**
Andriy O. Samokhin and Dieter Brömme

Permissions

List of Contributors

Index

Preface

Aorta is the biggest artery in the human body. The heart pumps the oxygen-rich blood into the aorta through the aortic valve, which opens and closes with the heartbeat. When aortic valve opens, the blood flows to the rest of the body through smaller arteries that branch out from it. Aortic diseases and conditions usually occur when the aorta or aortic valve of a patient's heart gets damaged or is not able to function normally. Many disorders and ailments can damage the aorta, putting patients at serious risk of death. There are various types of aortic diseases such as aortic aneurysm, aortic dissection, aortic infection, aortic intramural hematoma, aortobronchial fistula (ABF), aortoenteric fistula (AEF), etc. Aortic aneurysm is a condition when a section of aorta becomes enlarged whereas in aortic dissection, a tear appears in the aorta. Such selected concepts that redefine the study of aortic diseases have been presented in this book. It is a collective contribution of a renowned group of international experts. This book will prove to be immensely beneficial to students and researchers in the field of cardiology.

All of the data presented henceforth, was collaborated in the wake of recent advancements in the field. The aim of this book is to present the diversified developments from across the globe in a comprehensible manner. The opinions expressed in each chapter belong solely to the contributing authors. Their interpretations of the topics are the integral part of this book, which I have carefully compiled for a better understanding of the readers.

At the end, I would like to thank all those who dedicated their time and efforts for the successful completion of this book. I also wish to convey my gratitude towards my friends and family who supported me at every step.

Editor

Part 1

Evolution of Care for Aortic Disease

1

Abdominal Aortic Aneurysms: Changing Paradigms in Treatment

Christopher J. Marrocco and Ruth L. Bush
Scott and White Hospital, Texas A & M College of Medicine, Temple, TX USA

1. Introduction

Abdominal aortic aneurysms (AAA) are a well-recognized cause of morbidity and mortality in older persons. The 20th century has lead to many overall advances in surgery and specifically the management of complex and often lethal disease processes. In the early part of last century, advances in anesthesia and critical care allowed for the surgical management of AAA via the open approach, which is to this day still considered by many to remain the gold standard of repair. In the latter part of the last century further advances and innovative thinking led to the minimally invasive endovascular treatment of many AAAs. Endovascular abdominal aortic aneurysm repair (EVAR) has pioneered the treatment of more complex aortic disease and now with greater then 20 years since its début it is in many centers the preferred treatment. There is no longer a feasibility question; these devices have been proven to be safe and efficacious with less perioperative morbidity and mortality than traditional open repair.

In an attempt to improve the world literature and make comparisons more possible amongst the many evolving studies underway globally a need for some commonality in the reporting of results was recognized. The reporting standards for AAA repair, both for endovascular and for open repair have been formulated into guidelines first extended in 1997 and then later updated in 2002. These standards outline the generally measured characteristics touched on by many of the studies reporting on the treatment of aortic aneurismal disease. Included are the common patient characteristics involved in atherosclerotic disease such as tobacco use, hyperlipidemia, hypertension, diabetes mellitus, renal insufficiency, chronic obstructive pulmonary disease, carotid occlusive disease, other associated aneurismal disease and anesthesia risk as outlined by the American Society of Anesthesiology Risk Classification (ASA). These guidelines also address characteristics unique to aneurismal disease known as the anatomical risk factors, such as aortic neck length and angulation as well as access vessels where included with a grading system. Outcome measures of clinical success and the definition of terms such as endotension and endoleak were included. The current devices have gone through several generations of advancement, alteration and modification which has addressed many of the device specific criterions that where offered and for the most part has addressed, and continue to address these limitations as innovation in the field continues.

With further advances and longer length follow up periods many of the earlier unanswered questions are being addressed however in doing so new questions have arisen and the persistent question since the inception of EVAR remains a point of controversy to this day, namely who should undergo endovascular treatment and who should under go standard open repair. A significant hindrance has been the lack of ability to compare these studies head to head and gain useful and usable information from them. The reporting standards conceived by the Society for Vascular Surgery (SVS) were an attempt to make such comparisons more uniform for just this reason.

As well as reporting standards in individual studies being a goal of the SVS reporting standards guidelines the drive for successful management of AAA as well as many other diseases has been taken up by the clinical and administrative bodies of large organizations such as the Veterans Healthcare system and the American Collage of Surgeons based on the VA model. "Soon after introduction of endovascular aneurysm repair (EVAR), with Food and Drug Administration device approval in 1999, robust electronic NSQIP (National Surgical Quality Improvement Program) records immediately began to capture individual facility performances and outcomes for both types of AAA repair. The NSQIP data center provided actual and risk-adjusted analyses for both procedures semiannually. These analyses have been used by its executive board to provide recommendations, often based on site visits, to improve outcomes." [1,2] Data bases like these have been adopted and pioneered by other countries as well and continue to add to the knowledge bases with the goal of efficient, high-quality care [2].

However, in the face of all of the published standards no one accepted method is used and continued publications of standards and measuring techniques can still be found in both the world literature and in the Journal of vascular surgery such as the recently published Validation of a new standardized method to measure proximal aneurysm neck angulation [3] and the recently reported attempt by the French health agency Agence Française de Sécurité Sanitaire des Produits de Santé (AFSSAPS) to determine criteria for the best surgical approach. The high-risk AFSSAPS criteria were however not predictive of postoperative mortality and the authors stated that these should not be used to determine the choice of treatment technique. Other criteria therefore need to be established to determine whether open or EVAR repair should be used. [4]

In the ever evolving field of AAA treatment there has not been an acceptance of the reporting standards, which makes interpretation difficult to a certain extent, but by the common nature of the studies there does tend to be overlap in the reporting making it possible to draw conclusions all be it in a non-standardized fashion from the recently reported studies.

2. EVAR vs open repair: Basic variables in decision making

There are three basic modalities, which are generally accepted and widely available for the management of abdominal aortic aneurysms. These include observation alone, also known as best medical treatment (BMT), Standard or open repair which is the oldest surgical method and for this reason considered by many to be the gold standard, which can be done either by a transperitoneal, or via the retroperitoneal incision, and the endovascular approach (EVAR). There are other options, which are available at some institutions and represent variations on and combinations of the above approaches, these include laparoscopic abdominal aortic repair and hybrid procedures. Of the 3 commonly available and accepted modalities outlined above, EVAR is the newest and most rapidly progressive in terms of technological innovation and industry driven advancements.

The decision on the specific modality for optimal treatment has long been a matter of controversy, and continues to be so to this day. When planning the optimal treatment for

AAA there are 3 commonly considered variables. The first thing to consider is the size of the aneurysm. There is a well-established correlation between rupture risk and the maximal transverse size of the aorta and rupture[5]. Second is the anatomy or morphology of the aorta. All devices have guidelines for use under the Food and Drug Administration (FDA) which where created to assist the clinician in determining anatomical acceptability of the device to ensure the optimal outcome. In the past there has been a 20-60% reported suitability following the information for use guidelines (IFU) [6,7] however with advancing technology the delivery systems for these devices have gotten smaller, with hydrophilic coats and the devices themselves have become larger with different configurations which has greatly expanded the anatomic criteria for the use of these devices. Devices used outside of the FDA-IFU guidelines have been associated with increased complication rates and adherence to these guidelines as much as possible is recommended. [8-11]

The third variable commonly considered is perhaps the most challenging and can impact the other two variables to varying extents when trying to formulate an appropriate operative strategy. This variable is the patient. Multiple considerations on multiple levels often cloud ones judgment and make this a subjective rather then an objective decision. The elements going into this equation range widely from the patients co-morbidities and other illnesses are in determining whether they are "fit" for surgery or "high risk", to whether the patient will follow up and be compliant with surveillance imaging, to what the patients expectations and knowledge are about the purposed intervention to outside influences such as the wishes, knowledge-base and influence family, friends and loved ones have. Putting all of these patient variables together is often a difficult and arduous task that can greatly influence the treatment modality chosen perhaps more then any other variable outlined.

3. Size

The anatomical size, in transverse diameter, has long been established as one of the main indications for treatment vs. observation. The commonly accepted size for the initiation of intervention is 5.5 cm based on several landmark publications and the accepted risk of 1% rupture below this threshold. A threshold diameter of 5.5 cm has been the point of separation commonly used based on the United Kingdom Small Aneurysm trial [5] and the US Veterans Administration Aneurysm Detection and Management [12] Study. These trials showed no benefit in overall survival to early repair over continued observation for AAAs less then 5.5 cm in diameter, and demonstrated an annual rupture risk for such small AAAs (4.0 cm to 5.4 cm) to be low approximately 1%. These studies where based on open aneurysm intervention. The natural history, despite the treatment threshold, of aneurysms is to continue to grow and then eventually to rupture. In the United Kingdom Small Aneurysm Trial [5], over 60% of those initially assigned to surveillance had AAA repair by 4 years, and most of those with greater then 5.0 cm AAAs had a repair within 1 year. As a result, many clinicians have dropped the threshold for intervention for AAAs to 5.0 cm in diameter. It is more appropriate to think of size as an indication of when to consider, not whether to consider AAA repair. However when to treat endovascularly remained an open question EVAR has been reported to achieves better outcomes in smaller AAAs [13] and the importance of size in EVAR outcomes has been recently underscored by an analysis of the European Collaborators on Stent-Graft Techniques for Abdominal Aortic Aneurysm Repair (EUROSTAR) database, which showed a statistically significant correlation between size (4.0 to 5.4 cm versus 5.5 to 6.4 cm versus >6.5 cm diameter) and all five outcomes studied (Type

1 endoleak, total mortality, aneurysm-related death, conversion to open repair, and post-EVAR rupture) [14 15] . Endovascular repair has been shown to be safer than open surgical repair in patients with large aneurysms, prompting a randomized trial of early endovascular repair vs surveillance in patients with small aneurysms[16]. In the PIVOTAL trial the researchers randomly assigned 728 patients with 4 to 5 cm AAAs to early endovascular repair (366 patients) or ultrasound surveillance (362 patients), and Concluded the early treatment with endovascular repair and rigorous surveillance with selective aneurysm treatment as indicated both appear to be safe alternatives for patients with small AAAs, protecting the patient from rupture or aneurysm-related death for at least 3 years [16]. In the Comparison of Surveillance Versus Aortic Endografting for Small Aneurysm Repair (CAESAR) Trial the researchers randomly assigned patients with AAA of 4.1-5.4 cm in a 1:1 ratio, to receive immediate EVAR or surveillance by ultrasound and computed tomography (CT) and repair only after a defined threshold (diameter ≥5.5 cm, enlargement >1 cm /year, symptoms) was achieved. Between 2004 and 2008, 360 patients (early EVAR = 182; surveillance = 178) were enrolled. They reported that mortality and rupture rates in AAA <5.5 cm are low and no clear advantage was shown between early or delayed EVAR strategy. However, within 36 months, three out of every five small aneurysms under surveillance might grow to require repair and one out of every six might lose feasibility for EVAR. Concluding that surveillance is safe for small AAA if close supervision is applied.[17] Depending on interpretation and resources this information may help determine when to treat patients with smaller AAA at an earlier stage. Further, it has been suggested that the threshold in women be even lower (e.g., 4.5 cm in diameter) based on women's relatively smaller aortic dimensions, which appear to play a role in their higher risk of rupture and its attendant mortality and in their [18] lower anatomical suitability for EVAR [14,18,19]

While in the past there was "no disagreement about appropriate treatment for large AAAs in patients with unsuitable anatomic characteristics that preclude EVAR, these patients should have conventional open repair, which has been reported to have low morbidity and mortality rates[14]. The advancement of technology has steadily whittled away at these anatomic criteria and continues to push the safe and acceptable anatomical criteria further into what was once considered to be the experimental or anatomically unacceptable range. With this push and the increasing use and availability of the EVAR technology there has been an over all shift in the general clinical practice in many institutions towards the implantation of EVAR, with less and less consideration being given to the surgically fit patient. This has led many clinicians to consider EVAR as the first line treatment for AAA regardless of the patient's characteristics, such as fitness for surgery, or ability to undergo a large abdominal procedure. In many ways this is the trend first set out by the laparoscopic revolution that swept through general surgery some 20-30 years ago. It is rare now to see an open cholecystectomy, and rarer still to see this as a planned first line intervention. The open cholecystectomy is often reserved for the failed laparoscopic approach. So to, it would appear, is the fate of open abdominal reconstruction. While EVAR Has boasted well-documented benefits[20-22] over open repair including a reduction of aneurysm-related mortality, a decrease in perioperative cardiopulmonary complications as well as of hemorrhage, graft infection and colonic ischemia, as well as reduced patient trauma, reduced hospital stays and faster recovery [20]. Even in the face of the EVAR 1 data suggesting that After 12 months there was negligible difference in Health Related Quality of Life (HRQL) between the two groups (EVAR vs Open) [23]. The obvious benefits noted clinically by the patient and surgeons alike have propelled EVAR forward despite all oppositions.

While the above benefits are well documented and the trends outlined it is more apparent that obtaining similar results with less pain and less procedure are the true drivers behind EVAR. The argument against EVAR citing the need for long follow up and the possibility for re-intervention as a downside is far out weighed by the realization of both clinicians and patients alike that a little "check-up" every year or 6 months trumps a week in the hospital and a possible ICU stay for all concerned. Cost is a driving negative force, but if the same results are obtainable with less pain, people, especially Americans will put up with nothing less. Re-interventions often sited as a complication of EVAR are viewed by many patients as simply tune-ups, and despite the extensive reports documenting reintervention as a negative or down side to EVAR these are often well tolerated and the surgical conversion and explantation of EVAR has become much like the open cholecystectomy.

The shift and trend is now towards EVAR first both in clinicians and patients minds. The drive has been both evidence based and human nature. When looking at an AAA needing repair most surgeons' in this era first check to see if the patient is an EVAR candidate. Almost all other criteria are secondary. If the patient is young and could undergo a big open operation the surgeon and the patients' response is more and more commonly becoming "why" from the sociological point of view. The argument has been posed that a young patient is generally a productive member of society and no matter how well they do with open repair, arguably given EVAR they would rejoin the work force much sooner and even in the face of continued "check-ups" and possible intermittent "tune-ups" they would still be a more productive, over a longer period of time then where they to undergo a open procedure with its associated recovery time and potential risks.

4. The high risk patient

The management of AAA in patients considered to be high-risk remains a challenge. While EVAR was initially studied in this group as an alternative to the open procedure in patients that where considered unfit for the open surgical intervention the pendulum has now swung in the opposite direction. Initially the question of feasibility was addressed using this patient population, now that feasibility is no longer a question and EVAR has been well established as an acceptable method for aneurysm treatment the consideration of appropriateness has come into question.

The EVAR-2 Trial which used the cohort of patients that where excluded for the EVAR-1 trial as mentioned earlier concluded after a mean 4 years of follow up that EVAR had a considerable 30-day operative mortality in patients already unfit for open repair of their aneurysm. EVAR did not improve survival over no intervention and was associated with a need for continued surveillance and reinterventions, at substantially increased cost. Ongoing follow-up and improved fitness of these patients is a priority[24] published in 2005.

Endovascular aneurysm repair (EVAR) is associated with superior short-term mortality rates but unclear long-term results and has not been shown to improve survival in patients unfit for open repair (OR)[25]. A group using the Swedish vascular registry conducted population-based study with the aim evaluating the outcome after elective EVAR compared with OR in a high-risk patient cohort. They reported that elective OR of aortic aneurysms seems to have a better outcome compared with EVAR in this specific, population-based, high-risk patient cohort after adjusting for covariates, and that they cannot confirm the benefit of EVAR from previous registry studies concluding that in clinical practice, OR may be at least as good as EVAR in high-risk patients fit for surgery. [25](Swedish study)

This prompted a Department of Veteran Affairs analysis citing that "recent results after endovascular abdominal aortic aneurysm repair (EVAR) have brought into question its value in patients deemed at high-risk for surgical intervention."[26] The Department of Veteran Affairs (VA) National Surgical Quality Improvement Program (NSQIP) is the largest prospectively collected and validated United States surgical database representing current clinical practice. Utilizing this database a study was designed to evaluate outcomes after elective EVAR performed in high-risk veterans. This retrospective review analyzed 2296 pts (EVAR, n = 788; open, n = 1580) who underwent elective aneurysm repair from May 2001 to December 2004 and met the high risk criteria. High-risk criteria analyzed included age > or =60 years, American Society of Anesthesiology (ASA) classification 3 or 4, and the comorbidity variables of history of cardiac, respiratory, or hepatic disease, cardiac revascularization, renal insufficiency, and low serum albumin level. The primary end points were 30-day and 1-year all-cause mortality.[26] The investigators concluded that veterans deemed high-risk for surgical therapy, outcomes after elective EVAR are excellent, and the procedure is relatively safe in this special patient population. Our retrospective data demonstrate that patients with considerable medical comorbidities and infrarenal abdominal aortic aneurysms benefit from and should be considered for primary [26] EVAR.

Another American group conducted an interesting study in response the the EVAR-2 publication to determine the outcome in the United States after endovascular repair (EVAR) of infrarenal abdominal aortic aneurysms (AAAs) in patients at high-risk for open surgery. They independently audited, high-compliance, chart-verified data sets, and compared those results with open surgery. Interestingly in an attempt for head to head comparability they defined High-risk to match the EVAR-2 trial and included age of > or =60 years with aneurysm size of > or =5.5 cm, plus at least one cardiac, pulmonary, or renal comorbidity. They then analyzed data from five multicenter investigational device exemption clinical trials leading to Food and Drug Administration (FDA) approval finding 565 EVAR patients that met the high-risk criteria, and 61 OPEN patients that met high-risk criteria. Primary outcome comparisons included AAA-related death, all-cause death, and aneurysm rupture. Secondary measures were endoleak, AAA sac enlargement, and migration.

After analysis they concluded that endovascular repair of large infrarenal AAAs in anatomically suited high-surgical-risk patients using FDA-approved devices in the United States is safe and provides lasting protection from AAA-related mortality. EVAR mortality remained comparable with OPEN up to 4 years.[27]

An Italian group animalized their data to determine the best treatment for high-risk patients with abdominal aortic aneurysms (AAA) using the ASA classification guidelines and found a total 375 patients who underwent AAA repair, 168 (45%) belonged in ASA classes III and IV (85 OPEN and 83 EVAR). After analysis they concluded that except patients with small aneurysms (< 6 cm), in whom the risk of death at 1-year due to comorbidities exceeds the risk of a ruptured aneurysm, all patients at high surgical risk (ASA class IV) benefit from AAA repair. Patients with small aneurysms must undergo strict surveillance to assess growth and aneurysmal wall changes to prevent unexpected rupture.[28]

Another American investigation looked at The 2001-2004 Nationwide Inpatient Sample in a direct response to EVAR-2 hypothesizing that The nationwide in-hospital mortality for patients with the highest risk undergoing EVAR in the United States is lower than that reported in EVAR trial 2. They found that 65 502 EVARs were performed with an in-hospital mortality of 2.2%. Risk-adjusted in-hospital mortality rates ranged from 1.2% to 3.7% compared to the substantial in-hospital mortality after EVAR (9%) reported in EVAR 2.

They concluded that The EVAR procedure is currently being performed in the United States with low in-hospital mortality, even in patients with the highest risk. Therefore, EVAR should not be denied to high-risk patients with abdominal aortic aneurysms in the United States on the basis of the level I evidence from the United Kingdom study. [29]
Another group utilizing Department of Veteran Affairs data attempted to further investigate this issue by examining the influence of age, aneurysm size, and patient fitness on suitability for endovascular aortic aneurysm repair. They examined 186 male patients referred for evaluation of nonruptured AAAs. Suitability for EVAR was determined by neck anatomy, iliac artery morphology, and total aortic aneurysm angulation and tortuosity according to the clinicians' experience and current practice. They found that aortic neck length (odds ratio [OR]=1.2, 95% confidence interval [CI] 1.1-1.2) and diameter (OR=0.78, 95% CI 0.63-0.96) were the only independent predictors for EVAR suitabilityn and concluded that Overall, EVAR suitability is not influenced by age, aneurysm size, or patient fitness.[30]

5. The elderly and ethics

5.1 The elderly

The elderly group is a cohort is not well documented in the world literature with relation to management of AAA. There are few large series in this population which may reflect a unique survivability in this population. The average life expectancy has been steadily increasing world wide. The United Nations World Population Prospective 2006 revision showed an average life expectancy from birth in the united states of 77.4 from 2000-to-2005 and predicted an increase to 78.2 from 2005-to-2010 and to 78.9 for 2010-to-2015. Due to the increasingly aging populations of the industrialized countries, the prevalence of vascular disorders is increasing, with an emerging patient subgroup of 80 years and older (octogenarians), often multi-morbid with an increased risk of anaesthesiological and surgical complications [31]. Abdominal aortic aneurysms (AAAs) occur in approximately 5% of the population older than 50 years and up to 10% within the male population over 80 years [32]. According to the United Nations World Population Prospective 2006 revision globally, the number of persons aged 60 years or over is expected nearly to triple, increasing from 673 million in 2005 to 2 billion by 2050. Over the same period, the share of older persons living in developing countries is expected to rise from 64 per cent in 2005 to nearly 80 per cent in 2050. A recent analysis of the nationwide sample of intact AAA repairs from 2001 to 2006 demonstrated a 69% increase in the total number of asymptomatic AAA repairs in patients more than 85 years of age in comparison to their younger counterparts [33]. Moreover the estimated life expectancy of a centenarian in the United States in 2004 was 2.3 years. (National Vitals Statistics System. Available at: http://www.cdc.gov/nchs/data/nvsr/nvsr56/nvsr56_09.pdf. Accessed June 10, 2010.)
The Question of age as a defining category of AAA repair becomes more difficult when analyzing the outcomes of the studies in the literature, many of which demonstrate favorable outcomes. Numerous articles have reported acceptable results for octogenarians treated with both open and endovascular techniques. [34]. Open repair of AAAs in octogenarians has been associated with increased life expectancy in comparison to untreated AAAs [35]. With respect to treatment of AAA mortality rate, while higher than in younger patients, is acceptable in carefully selected octogenarians [36]. While other investigators looking at EVAR vs. Open repair concluded that there was no difference in the long-term survival benefit between open repair

and EVAR in 150 octogenarians. [37] With attention to the population of octogenarian-to-nonagenarians (age range 80-95) Prenner et al report a series of 322 patients that underwent elective EVAR from January 1997 to November 2007. The mean age was 84 years +/- 3.4 years. They reported a perioperative 30-day mortality rate of 3.1% with a mean follow-up of 25.7 months. Freedom from aneurysm-related mortality was 95.4% at 1 year and 92.9% at 5 years. They concluded that EVAR in octogenarians is associated with high procedural success and low perioperative morbidity and mortality. [38]
In the Nonagenarian population Halpern et al report the largest retrospective review of EVAR over a 10-year period. While this remains a small cohort of only 23 patients. The mean age was 91.5 (range 90-94) and the perioperative mortality was only 4.3%. There were no aneurysm-related deaths beyond the 30-day postoperative period. They also reported that the mean survival beyond 30 days was 800 +/-459 days following EVAR. These results suggest that despite their advanced age, these patients benefit from EVAR with low morbidity, low mortality, and mean survival exceeding 2.4 years. Survival appears best in those patients with ≤5 comorbidities. With or without symptoms, patients over the age of 90 should be considered for EVAR [39]. Another relatively large study from a single institution analysis of endovascular repair (EVAR) in nonagenarians analyzed 18 nonagenarians (age range 90-95). They reported 100% technical success with a mortality rate of 5.6%, 41.2% and 58.3% at 30 days, 365 days, and 2 years, respectively. Mean survival of the 11 patients who expired beyond the first 30 days was 17.5 months. EVAR is safe in nonagenarians despite their advanced age and significant surgical risk factor profile. The procedure can be performed with excellent technical success and a low rate of perioperative complications. However, mortality rates after 30 days are significant. The substantial long-term mortality raises the question of possible treatment futility in this unique population. While age should not be a contraindication for EVAR, recommendations for the procedure should be based on individual patient selection. [40] In a recent review Demirel and colleges examined Vascular Surgery in the Elderly and made Recommendations for Clinical Practice. They state that with suitable morphology of the aneurysm, endovascular aneurysm repair (EVAR) is the therapy of choice for abdominal aortic aneurysm (AAA). In elderly patients unfit for open repair and with a life expectancy of less than 4 years, EVAR does not offer any survival benefit compared with no intervention. In such patients, conservative therapy should be taken into consideration [31]

5.2 The ethical dilemma

The ethical dilemma of age is mirrored on every level of patient treatment and the decision for any surgery. The question of age however perhaps underscores these considerations more strongly then any other patient related characteristics because the emphasis must be placed on the individual. There are patients that are in the most advanced chronological category that are much healthier from a physiological stand point then some patients that are very much younger in years. This gives rise to the concept of physiological age of the patient, which is far more important then the chronological age when considering surgery. The ethical discussion in the health care arena centers around 4 main concepts. These briefly outlined are as fallows. First are the basic ethical principals of beneficence and nonmaleficence. These state that the procedure or treatment in question should be beneficial and not do harm. While this is often not totally possible it may be extended in thought and practice to have the potential benefits out weigh the potential risks. Second is the principal of autonomy. This simply stated is the patents right to make decisions for themselves and has been expanded in modern medicine to be the basis of the informed consent. Given all of the information available and a clear understanding of the first principal the patient has the right to guide his or her own care. The third principle is that of justice. This principle brings into account the population or community as a whole. It is concerned with the allocation of limited vital healthcare recourses and whom these should be made available to. The dichotomy of this prospective, simply stated, is should valuable resources be adjudicated to the largest amount of people that could benefit from them or on the people that need them most. The final issue is the respect for human life. This brings into account religion, cultural beliefs, and moral values both of the individual and of society and may differ around the world.

Abdominal aortic aneurysms (AAAs) occur in approximately 5% of the population older than 50 years and up to 10% within the male population over 80 years. (Cosford PA, Leng GC. Screening for abdominal aortic aneurysm. Cochrane Database Syst Rev 2007;2:CD002945.)

Schwarze et al5 analyzed a nationwide sample of intact AAA repairs from 2001 to 2006 and demonstrated a 69% increase in the total number of asymptomatic AAA repairs in patients more than 85 years of age in comparison to their younger counterparts. [33]

6. Nonagenarians

Jim et al6 reported a single institution analysis of endovascular repair (EVAR) in nonagenarians. The study analyzed 18 nonagenarians (age range 90-95) and reported 100% technical success with a mortality rate of 5.6%, 41.2% and 58.3% at 30 days, 365 days, and 2 years, respectively. Mean survival of the 11 patients who expired beyond the first 30 days was 17.5 months. They concluded that EVAR is safe in nonagenarians despite their advanced age and significant surgical risk factor profile. [34]

Halpern et al reported a largest retrospective review of nonagenarians that underwent EVAR over a 10-year period. They analyzed 23 patients with mean age of 91.5 (range 90-94) and reported a perioperative mortality of 4.3%. There were no aneurysm-related deaths beyond the 30-day postoperative period. Mean survival beyond 30 days was 800 +/- 459 days following EVAR. Their results demonstrated nonagenarians' benefit from EVAR with low morbidity, low mortality, and survival exceeding 2.2 years despite their advanced age and, therefore, they should be considered for EVAR with or without symptoms. [39]

7. Octogenarians-to-nonagenarians

A series of 322 patients that underwent open and EVAR in octogenarians and nonagenarians (age range 80-95) was reported by Stuart Prenner and colleagues.8 The perioperative 30- day mortality rate was 3.1% with a mean follow-up of 25.7 months. Freedom from aneurysm-related mortality was 95.4% at 1 year and 92.9% at 5 years. Their results demonstrated EVAR in octogenarians is associated with low rates of perioperative morbidity and mortality and low long-term aneurysm-related mortality despite the high rates of comorbidities in these patients. [38]

8. The ruptured aneurysm

An interesting and natural advancement to endovascular technology has resulted in another group not previously mentioned which has benefited from EVAR with increasingly promising results in the literature. This is the rupture population. EVAR has now been used with excellent results in some centers not only for prevention rupture, but also for the treatment of ruptured abdominal aortic aneurysms, and is now growing in acceptance as a life saving procedure. Foster and collogues reviewed the literature to answer the question whether a policy for endovascular repair as the primary mode of treatment for ruptured abdominal aortic aneurysms (rAAAs) would improve outcomes. They reviewed One thousand three hundred and twenty-eight papers and concluded that conclude that, within the limitations of the published literature to date, endovascular repair as the primary treatment for rAAA is achievable and appears to be associated with favorable mortality over open repair with appropriate case selection. [41] More recently Bosch et al reviewed their results from April 2002 until March 2008 from a single center in the Netherlands comparing their open to their EVAR experience in the ruptured setting and concluded that In EVAR-suitable patients, an absolute perioperative mortality reduction of 25.5% of rEVAR over open surgery was found, which was still present at 6 months of follow-up. These data suggest that rEVAR is a superior treatment option for EVAR-suitable patients with an rAAA compared with an open surgery. [42] Setacci and the university of Siena group reported that despite this evidence, EVAR for rAAA remains prerogative of few centers worldwide. In conclusion only larger study or registry could assest the real role of EVAR in the management of rAAA. [43] In an attempt to further explore this question Davenport et al from the University of Kentucky examined the Thirty-day NSQIP database outcomes of open versus endoluminal repair of ruptured abdominal aortic aneurysms. They identified A total of 427 patients the majority of which (76.8%) underwent open repair. However in review of the data they found that composite 30-day morbidity risk is lower after EVAR vs open repair of rAAA. Open repair is associated with increased transfusion requirements. Performance of EVAR in rAAA patients with favorable anatomy could potentially result in improved outcome as compared with open repair. [44]

9. Inherent problems in study design

In the era of clinical and research based medicine otherwise known as evidence based medicine a great deal of positive information and tools to assist in clinical judgment have been generated. However along with the need for research to both explain what we do and document its positive or negative effects there has evolved an overwhelming amount of information. This information is not free of error and in even the gold standard randomized control study can be manipulated. While these statistical acrobatics are generally not malicious in intent a lot can ride on the outcome of study both with respect to surgical and to a broader extent medical decision making and to the bottom line of reimbursement which drive the hospitals and clinics. Whatever the reason it is important to recognize that in particular many of the "land mark studies" in AAA have a very serious problem associated with their general design, despite the fact that superficially these appear to represent the "gold standard." These studies are the randomized clinical trials (RCTs) offering an observation/no treatment (OBS/NoRx) arm as control and which are focused on the management of a condition with potentially life-threatening consequences, however small the risk, often experience a significant rate of crossover to treatment by those randomized to the OBS/NoRx arm. [45] this type of design was initially designed for Medication and drug testing. Intent-to-treat data analytic strategy was developed for drug trials in which some patients dropped out (after 10-12 weeks) before receiving full treatment. To determine whether the full treatment worked, you could just use the subjects who completed treatment when analyzing outcome data for these studies. Hence preserving data for the statistical analysis, however in a life threatening, or perceived life threatening condition, where there can be no "blinding" of the patient this type of design often leads to a significant degree of error in the form of the cross over effect. The frequency with which patients cross over may either confound the outcomes of these trials and/or undermine the acceptance of conclusions based on an intent-to-treat analysis, which should not be used in this situation. [45] Yet the very fabric on which a great many of our clinical decisions are based is from just such studies. Studies of abdominal aortic aneurysms with this design that exemplify this dilemma, with crossovers ranging from 27% to over 60% include EVAR II, UKSAT, ADAM, and PIVOTAL. Results of these trials are frequently used as level I medical evidence and their potential impact on clinical decision-making and reimbursement can be quite significant and long-lasting. [45]

10. Analysis of available studies

In 2005 the findings from the United Kingdom EVAR 1 Trial where released in the British journal, the Lancet titled "Endovascular aneurysm repair versus open repair in patients with abdominal aortic aneurysm (EVAR trial 1): randomized controlled trial". This randomized controlled trial prospectively randomized 1082 patients aged 60 years or older who had aneurysms of at least 5.5 cm in diameter and who had been referred to one of 34 hospitals proficient in the EVAR technique. The patients were both anatomically suitable for EVAR and fit for an open repair to EVAR or open repair cohorts. [24] The primary endpoint was all-cause mortality at 4 years and EVAR and OPEN were found to be similar in this regard, with mortality rates of approximately 28% (hazard ratio, 0.90; 95% CI, 0.69–1.18; P = 0.46). One of the secondary endpoints, AAA-related death, showed a 3% advantage to EVAR, which was maintained for 4 years (perioperative mortality: EVAR 1.7% versus OPEN 4.7%; midterm mortality: EVAR 26% versus OPEN 29%). Other secondary endpoints showed that patients undergoing EVAR had a much higher complication rate (41% versus 9%, $P < 0.0001$) and reintervention rate (20% versus 6%) than those having OPEN. Mean hospital (not total) costs were roughly estimated to be about 30% higher in the EVAR group. Additionally, at 12 months follow-up, there was no difference in healthrelated quality of life. The Authors concluded that Compared with open repair, EVAR offers no advantage with respect to all-cause mortality and HRQL, is more expensive, and leads to a greater number of complications and reinterventions. However, it does result in a 3% better aneurysm-related survival. The continuing need for interventions mandates ongoing surveillance and longer follow-up of EVAR for detailed cost-effectiveness assessment.

However a closer examination of the statistical breakdown of the EVAR 1 protocol raises several issues with regards cohort assignments. Of the 1082 patients ultimately randomized from the original 4799 persons assessed for the study, 453 were assigned to EVAR and 539 were assigned to open repair. Thus, only 23% of those assessed for eligibility were ultimately randomized. This eliminated close to two thirds of the candidates from the EVAR group. Reasons for exclusion included AAA was considered too small for repair in 9%; the AAA morphology was unsuitable for EVAR in 54%, and the patients were unfit for open repair in 1.5%. Adding further confusion is the all cause mortality. As demonstrated in the EVAR cohort where 10 patients died while waiting EVAR, in effect they where randomized to this group, but never availed the benefit of the intervention. Another 15 patients randomized to the EVAR group had OPEN repair. Three of these deaths were directly ascribed to AAA rupture. In the OPEN group, there were 13 deaths, of which 7 had ruptured AAAs and 18 patients received EVAR. This demonstrates a significant cross-over effect between the groups and further clouds the final analysis. The average delay from randomization to actual treatment was 57 days, despite a mean AAA size of 6.7 cm, which provides a likely explanation for the high pretreatment rupture rates. The increased availability of devices and the "off-the shelf" combinations in most large center stocks as well as the more expedient progression from diagnosis to treatment in the United states as well as many other countries world wide make delayed treatment extremely unlikely or even unacceptable in this day and age.

Another problem with the initial reporting in EVAR 1 is that only 24% of participants' data were included in the 4-year cutoff point for analysis, with 72% being still alive and uncensored at 4 years. Indeed, 25.3% of the open cohort and 21.6% of the EVAR cohort were ASA class 1; thus, this trial represented relatively healthy individuals [46] view of the above, these results, although contributory to the current body of knowledge, really only represent midterm outcomes.

In 2010 the United Kingdome EVAR trial investigators produced a subsequent analysis in the publication of Endovascular versus open repair of abdominal aortic aneurysm in the New England journal of medicine. Here the United Kingdome EVAR trial investigators examined their data from 1999 through 2004 at 37 hospitals in the United Kingdom. They randomly assigned 1252 patients with large abdominal aortic aneurysms (> or = 5.5 cm in diameter) to undergo either endovascular or open repair; 626 patients were assigned to each group. Patients were followed for rates of death, graft-related complications, reinterventions, and resource use until the end of 2009. In this group the initial 1082 patients included in a planned midterm analysis that was reported in 2005 and an additional 170 patients who were enrolled between January 2004 and August 2004, who were not included in the midterm analysis. There were no significant differences between the two treatment groups with respect to baseline characteristics. The patients in EVAR 1 were randomly assigned to undergo either open repair or endovascular repair. Patients were encouraged to undergo repair within 1 month after randomization, although such scheduling was not always possible for logistic or other reasons. [47] Despite this the For patients undergoing aneurysm repair, the median time from randomization to surgery was 44 days (interquartile range, 29 to 70) in the endovascularrepair group and 35 days (interquartile range, 20 to 57) in the open-repair group [47]. Representing, again, a delay that would still be considered unacceptable by many. Of the 12 patients in the endovascular-repair group who did not undergo aneurysm repair, 7 died within 6 months after randomization (3 as a result of rupture), 3 became physically ineligible, 1 declined surgery, and 1 became anatomically unsuitable because of a change in the shape of the aorta. Of the 24 patients in the open-repair group who did not undergo aneurysm repair, 7 died within 6 months after randomization (3 as a result of rupture), 7 became physically ineligible, 8 declined surgery (of whom 3 died), and 2 had an unknown reason (of whom 2 died). [47] They report that the 30-day operative mortality was 1.8% in the endovascular-repair group and 4.3% in the open-repair group (adjusted odds ratio for endovascular repair as compared with open repair, 0.39; 95% confidence interval [CI], 0.18 to 0.87; P=0.02). The endovascular-repair group had an early benefit with respect to aneurysm-related mortality, but the benefit was lost by the end of the study, at least partially, because of fatal endograft ruptures (adjusted hazard ratio, 0.92; 95% CI, 0.57 to 1.49; P=0.73). By the end of follow-up, there was no significant difference between the two groups in the rate of death from any cause (adjusted hazard ratio, 1.03; 95% CI, 0.86 to 1.23; P=0.72). The rates of graft-related complications and reinterventions were higher with endovascular repair, and new complications occurred up to 8 years after randomization, contributing to higher overall costs. [47]

In response to these findings Jetty et al in their manuscript Long-term outcomes and resource utilization of endovascular versus open repair of abdominal aortic aneurysms in Ontario. This retrospective analysis was based on hospital discharge abstracts. They examined all patients who underwent elective AAA repair between April 2002 and March 2007. Clinical outcomes included time to all-cause death and discharge to a nursing home or long-term care facility. Resource utilization outcomes included imaging utilization, hospital utilization, and reintervention rates. They identified 6461 patients underwent treatment of nonruptured AAAs, comprising 888 EVARs and 5573 open repairs. EVAR patients were older and had more comorbidities. The adjusted mortality was significantly lower in the EVAR group at 30 days (adjusted odds ratio [adj-OR], 0.34; 95% confidence interval [95% CI], 0.20-0.59), but long-term mortality was similar (adj-OR, 0.95; 95% CI, 0.81-1.05). EVAR patients were significantly less likely to be discharged to a nursing home or other chronic care facility (adj-OR, 0.55; 95% CI, 0.41-0.74). Imaging utilization as well as urgent and vascular readmissions were significantly higher in the EVAR group. However, the EVAR group had a significantly shorter length of stay and less intensive care unit use for the index hospitalization and decreased hospital length of stay during follow-up. There was a trend toward a slightly increased risk of reintervention with EVAR (adj-OR, 1.3; 95% CI, 0.98-1.75).They concluded that compared with open repair, EVAR significantly reduced short-term but not long-term mortality. The EVAR patients spent less time in health institutions, including long-term care facilities, but underwent more imaging studies. Future improvements in EVAR could result in further decreases in reinterventions and subsequent radiologic monitoring.[48] .

The Dutch DREAM trial was similar to EVAR 1 in that it was a prospective randomized study comparing EVAR to OPEN among patients with AAAs 5 cm or greater in diameter who were fit for open repair, but the number recruited was significantly smaller in this trial than in EVAR 1—only 351 patients. This study initially reported its 30-day mortality endpoint but it also performed a composite endpoint analysis of mortality and moderate or severe complications. Much like EVAR 1, there was a roughly 3% advantage to EVAR in perioperative mortality (EVAR 1.2% versus OPEN 4.6%), and interestingly, even though at 1 year the all-cause mortality was not different (EVAR 20.4% versus OPEN 20.3%), AAA-related death was higher for OPEN at 2 years (EVAR 2.1% versus OPEN 5.7%). Health-related quality-of-life measures were improved at 6 months in patients having EVAR; however, they were equivalent thereafter. Also, significantly higher costs were again documented in the EVAR cohort. The authors' conclusion was that the "Initial mortality advantage was lost at one year because of non-aneurysm related deaths."

The Dream trial was also updated in 2010 with a follow up carried out to 6 years titled Long-Term Outcome of Open or Endovascular Repair of Abdominal Aortic Aneurysm published in the New England Journal of medicine. Here they conducted a long-term, multicenter, randomized, controlled trial comparing open repair with endovascular repair in 351 patients with an abdominal aortic aneurysm of at least 5 cm in diameter who were considered suitable candidates for both techniques. They randomly assigned 178 patients to undergo open repair and 173 to undergo endovascular repair. The primary outcomes were rates of death from any cause and reintervention. Six years after randomization, the cumulative survival rates were 69.9% for open repair and 68.9% for endovascular repair (difference, 1.0 percentage point; 95% confidence interval [CI], −8.8 to 10.8; P = 0.97). The cumulative rates of freedom from secondary interventions were 81.9% for open repair and 70.4% for endovascular repair (difference, 11.5 percentage points; 95% CI, 2.0 to 21.0; P = 0.03). Further more similar to the original trial Six patients did not undergo aneurysm repair after randomization: four declined treatment (three in the open-repair group and one in the endovascular-repair group), one died from a ruptured abdominal aortic aneurysm before undergoing open repair, and one died from pneumonia before undergoing endovascular repair. There were eight in-hospital deaths after open repair and two after endovascular repair. The median follow-up was 6.4 years (range, 5.1 to 8.2). All patients were followed for 5 years, 79% for 6 years, and 53% for 7 years. The completeness of follow-up was 99.3% (11,589/11,673 months) for open repair and 99.7% (11,193/11,232 months) for endovascular repair. At the date of censoring, 106 patients had died during followup after hospital discharge (51 in the open-repair group and 55 in the endovascular-repair group). Five years after randomization, CT was performed in approximately one fourth of patients in the open-repair group and in almost all patients in the endovascular-repair group. They concluded that Six years after randomization, endovascular and open repair of abdominal aortic aneurysm resulted in similar rates of survival. The rate of secondary interventions was significantly higher for endovascular repair. [49]

Although the DREAM trial was criticized for being underpowered, and drawing this conclusion, most of its findings were in concert with EVAR 1, And subsequently validated in comparison to the EuroStar registry by Leurs el at. Here the Data of 177 patients of the DREAM trial with randomization to EVAR and 856 patients selected in the EUROSTAR-registry were compared. Baseline characteristics were comparable between the EUROSTAR-cohort and EVAR-arm of the DREAM-trial. The 36-month survival-rate was 87.6% for EVAR-arm in the DREAM-trial similar to the 86.8% found in this EUROSTAR-study population. The freedom of secondary procedures reached after 3 years 85.7%, and 86.9% in the DREAM and EUROSTAR-cohort, respectively. They concluded that comparable characteristics and outcomes between patients of comparable risk class of the EUROSTAR-registry and the EVAR-cohort of the DREAM-trial. This demonstrates the following: first, the EUROSTAR-data provide reliable information, and further comparisons of registry data with patients treated by conventional AAA surgery may be justified. Secondly, the various outcomes of the randomised DREAM trial appear generalisable, as it agrees with observations in a broad common practice derived database. [50] In summary, both EVAR 1 and DREAM showed no difference their primary endpoint of overall mortality but both demonstrated about a 3% advantage for EVAR in perioperative and AAA-related death, at 4 and 2 years, respectively, with similar results over long-term analysis. Complications, reinterventions, and costs were much higher in the studies' EVAR cohorts, with no improvements seen in health-related quality-of-life measures lasting beyond the initial period.

11. EVAR 2 trial

EVAR 2 utilized patients that where excluded fro the EVAR1 trial who were considered to be physically ineligible for open repair but who were candidates for endovascular repair were offered enrollment in the EVAR 2 trial [24,47]. Citing that Endovascular aneurysm repair (EVAR) to exclude abdominal aortic aneurysm (AAA) was introduced for patients of poor health status considered unfit for major surgery. The investigators instigated EVAR trial 2 to identify whether EVAR improves survival compared with no intervention in patients unfit for open repair of aortic aneurysm. In this randomized controlled trial of 338 patients aged 60 years or older who had aneurysms of at least 5.5 cm in diameter and who had been referred to one of 31 hospitals in the UK. They assigned patients to receive either EVAR (n=166) or no intervention (n=172). Primary endpoint was all-cause mortality, with secondary endpoints of aneurysm-related mortality, health-related quality of life (HRQL), postoperative complications, and hospital costs. Analyses were by intention to treat. The 30-day operative mortality in the EVAR group was 9% (13 of 150, 95% CI 5-15) and the no intervention group had a rupture rate of 9.0 per 100 person years (95% CI 6.0-13.5). By end of follow up 142 patients had died, 42 of aneurysm-related factors; overall mortality after 4 years was 64%. There was no significant difference between the EVAR group and the no intervention group for all-cause mortality (hazard ratio 1.21, 95% CI 0.87-1.69, p=0.25). There was no difference in aneurysm-related mortality. The mean hospital costs per patient over 4 years were UK pound sterling 13,632 in the EVAR group and pound sterling 4983 in the no intervention group (mean difference pound sterling 8649, SE 1248), with no difference in HRQL scores. This data evoked several interpretations and conclusions at variance with those proposed by the trialists, who basically concluded that there was no mortality advantage to EVAR in managing large AAAs in patients unfit for open repair and, since this treatment modality costs much more than observation alone, a policy of no treatment was endorsed. The paradox here is that it is precisely for such high-risk patients that EVAR was first proposed, as a lower risk alternative to open repair, yet the EVAR 2 trial appeared to refute this expectation, concluding it to be no better than no treatment! [14] Interestingly, the reported 30- day mortality rate of 9% for EVAR and the 4-year mortality of 64% are both much higher than previously reported in high-risk patient cohorts, and, while these observations provided a basis for much criticism, the published results of EVAR 2 have clearly complicated patient and provider decision-making, in addition to potentially influencing policymaking and reimbursement practices.

As an Update to the 2005 Lancet publication EVAR 2 was further examined in the 2010 publication tilted Endovascular repair of aortic aneurysm in patients physically ineligible for open repair. Presented in the New England Journal of Medicine. From 1999 through 2004 at 33 hospitals in the United Kingdom, 404 patients with large abdominal aortic aneurysms (> or = 5.5 cm in diameter) who were considered to be physically ineligible for open repair where randomly assigned to undergo either endovascular repair or no repair; 197 patients were assigned to undergo endovascular repair, and 207 were assigned to have no intervention. Patients were followed for rates of death, graft-related complications and reinterventions, and costs until the end of 2009. The 30-day operative mortality was 7.3% in the endovascular-repair group. The overall rate of aneurysm rupture in the no-intervention group was 12.4 (95% confidence interval [CI], 9.6 to 16.2) per 100 person-years. Aneurysm-related mortality was lower in the endovascular-repair group (adjusted hazard ratio, 0.53; 95% CI, 0.32 to 0.89; P=0.02). This advantage did not result in any benefit in terms of total mortality (adjusted hazard ratio, 0.99; 95% CI, 0.78 to 1.27; P=0.97). A total of 48% of patients who survived endovascular repair had graft-related complications, and 27% required reintervention within the first 6 years. During 8 years of follow-up, endovascular repair was considerably more expensive than no repair (cost difference, 9,826 pounds sterling [U.S. $14,867]; 95% CI, 7,638 to 12,013 [11,556 to 18,176]). The Trialists presented a similar conclusion to there first publication stating that in this randomized trial involving patients who were physically ineligible for open repair, endovascular repair of abdominal aortic aneurysm was associated with a significantly lower rate of aneurysm-related mortality than no repair. However, endovascular repair was not associated with a reduction in the rate of death from any cause. The rates of graft-related complications and reinterventions were higher with endovascular repair, and it was more costly. Suggesting that observation alone should be considered in patients unfit for open repair which redecorates many of the same arguments previously invoked by the fist publication.

In response to the initial EVAR 2 study data an American group from the University of Texas Southwestern Medical Center performed a Population-based, cross-sectional study analysis to look at The nationwide in-hospital mortality for patients with the highest risk undergoing EVAR in the United States they closely matched the time period of EVAR 2 reviewing the 2001-2004 Nationwide Inpatient Sample identifying EVAR procedures for nonruptured abdominal aortic aneurysms. Risk stratification was based on comorbidities and the Charlson comorbidity index, a validated predictor of in-hospital mortality after abdominal aortic aneurysms repairs. Weighted univariate and logistic regression analyses were used to determine the association between comorbidity measures and risk-adjusted in-hospital mortality. They found that During the 4-year period, 65502 EVARs were performed with an in-hospital mortality of 2.2%. Risk-adjusted in-hospital mortality rates ranged from 1.2% to 3.7%. Stratified analyses, including only elective EVAR procedures, revealed that in-hospital mortality was significantly higher in patients with the most severe comorbidities (1.7%) vs those with lower comorbidity (0.4%; P<.001). Patients with high risk had only a 1.6-fold increased risk of adjusted in-hospital mortality (odds ratio, 1.6; 95% confidence interval, 1.2-2.2) compared with patients with low risk. They concluded that the EVAR procedure is currently being performed in the United States with low in-hospital mortality, even in patients with the highest risk. Therefore, EVAR should not be denied to high-risk patients with abdominal aortic aneurysms in the United States on the basis of the level I evidence from the United Kingdom study. [29]

12. United States experiences with EVAR in high-risk cohorts

Randomized clinical trials had been lacking in the United States, which prompted the V.A. trilists to launch an investigation comparing endovascular to open abdominal aneurysm repair, which was recently published in JAMA. A randomized, multicenter clinical trial of 881 veterans, over the age of 49 years, from 42 Veterans Affairs Medical Centers with AAA that were at least 5 cm in size, or associated with an iliac aneurysm of 3 at least 3 cm in size, or had rapid expansion over a 6-to-12 month period who were candidates for both elective endovascular repair and open repair of AAA. This ongoing report detailed the time period between October 15, 2002, and October 15, 2008 Elective endovascular (n=444) or open (n=437) repair of AAA. Multiple variables and data points where extensively collected which included the main outcome measures, procedure failure, secondary therapeutic procedures, length of stay, quality of life, erectile dysfunction, major morbidity, and mortality. The mean follow-up was 1.8 years after which the American investigators concluded that short-term outcomes after elective AAA repair, perioperative mortality was low for both procedures and lower for endovascular than open repair. The early advantage of endovascular repair was not offset by increased morbidity or mortality in the first 2 years after repair. Longer-term outcome data are needed to fully assess the relative merits of the 2 procedures. The overall study has id still underway with the primary outcome of long-term (5-9 years) all-cause mortality (October 15, 2002-October 15, 2011) and has not yet been completed. (Outcomes Following Endovascular vs Open Repair of Abdominal Aortic Aneurysm)[51]

13. Remaining controversies

Several issues remain unresolved and to a certain extent have been touched on already in this chapter. A clear and comparable system that is widely accepted and used for AAA reporting would greatly forward the global knowledge base and increase understanding and transparency. The issues with randomized control tried and the intention to treat arm have been discussed above. While this practice may improve statistics it does not improve the real numbers that clinicians need when trying to evaluate a patient and determine a care-plan strategy. Another issue is the all cause mortality arm of many studies. This, like the intention to treat, may provide more numbers for statistical analysis and to a certain extent some comparability and useful information however it has been confused in certain situations with aneurysm related death, which would be a much more useful piece of information to know about in the clinical setting.

Aneurysm-related death can only be accurately determined by directly witnessed objective information, e.g., postmortem examination or rupture seen on an imaging study prior to death[14]. This however is difficult to obtain with decreasing numbers of autopsies being performed, deaths outside of the hospital and incomplete communication amongst healthcare systems. One possible solution would be a requirement in study designs for all participants to undergo a postmortem fine cut cat-scan however this has not yet been done. This would have the added benefit of having the patient locked into the system so to speak and could perhaps increase the autopsy rates. Another problem with AAA-related death outside of the abouve mentioned situation is that, taken alone, is a soft endpoint and one, which tends to preserve any initial/perioperative mortality advantage of one method of repair over another, with respect to aneurysm treatment [12] The data set would have likely been very different in the interpretation of the United Kingdom small aneurysm and Aneurysm Detection and Management trials if AAA-related death had been used as the primary end- point, rather than all-cause mortality. This was the goal of the Positive Impact of endoVascular Options for Treating Aneurysm early trial, or PIVOTAL trial which used as its primary endpoints aneurysm rupture and AAA-related deaths at up to 36 months after randomization[52] This trial was recently completed after enrolling 728 patients (13.3% women; mean age, 71 +/- 8 years) with 4 to 5 cm AAAs to early endovascular repair (366 patients) or ultrasound surveillance (362 patients). Rupture or aneurysm-related death and overall mortality in the two groups were compared during a mean follow-up of 20 +/- 12 months. The investigators concluded Early treatment with endovascular repair and rigorous surveillance with selective aneurysm treatment as indicated both appear to be safe alternatives for patients with small AAAs, protecting the patient from rupture or aneurysm-related death for at least 3 years[16]. Which provided useful information with regards to the size at which aneurysms should be treated with EVAR vs. surveillance. However there was still a significant cross-over rate from surveillance to the interventional arm Among patients randomized to surveillance, 31% underwent aneurysm repair during the course of the study[16] Cross over-over rates provide useful information as long as the setting is not in the intention to treat model as outlined above[45] The crossover rates in the PIVOTAL trial where about ½ that of the original UKSAT trial[53]. In the recently published mid-term results of the European-based 17-site Comparison of surveillance vs Aortic Endografting for Small

Aneurysm Repair (CAESAR) of small AAAs (4.1-5.4 cm) for surveillance or EVAR with the Zenith stent-graft with the primary endpoint of all-cause mortality at 54 months. However they included information on Aneurysm-related mortality, aneurysm rupture and major morbidity rates which where similar perhaps indicating a trend towards interpretable information[17] Inline with the information provided by the PIVOTAL trial they authors conclude that Mortality and rupture rates in AAA <5.5 cm are low and no clear advantage was shown between early or delayed EVAR strategy. However, within 36 months, three out of every five small aneurysms under surveillance might grow to require repair and one out of every six might lose feasibility for EVAR. Surveillance is safe for small AAA if close supervision is applied. [17] However a clear recommendation can not yet be made on the size for which small aneurysms should be treated, and we are left with the interpretation that aneurysms as seen above and in many other studies have the natural history to continue to increase in size and that many patients in the observation arm of trials, 27% to over 60% (EVAR II, UKSAT, ADAM, PIVOTAL), crossovers to the treatment arm[45].

Further controversy revolves around large AAA greater then 5.5 cm and the question of treatment in the healthy patient vs the infirmed or unfit for open surgery patients as discussed above. Though the question is somewhat being answered by the trends in AAA management in clinical practice. Studies using large administrative databases in the United States have documented a trend whereby the majority of patients undergoing elective abdominal aortic aneurysm (AAA) repair in the United States are being repaired using endovascular techniques[54] In a recently published single center study from the United States investigators retrospectively analyzed non-suprarenal AAA repairs between January 1, 1996, and December 31, 2008. Patients were stratified by endovascular AAA repair (EVAR) or open repair and the presence or absence of rupture. During a 13-year period, 721 patients underwent AAA repair, comprising 410 (56.9%) with EVAR and 311 (43.1%) with open repair. This study included a time period prior to the availability of EVAR 1996 through the period when EVAR became widely available 2008, and showed that between 2005 and 2008, average EVAR use increased to 84%. [55] This is exemplary of the increased use of EVAR over open AAA. Another group analyzed Medicare Part B data sets for 2001 through 2006 with respect to open vs endovascular AAA repair. A total of 31,965 OSRs for AAA were performed in Medicare beneficiaries in 2001, dropping to 15,665 by 2006 (-51%). In contrast, EVAR was carried out in 11,028 instances in 2001, increasing to 28,937 by 2006 (+162%). The utilization rate per 100,000 for OSR dropped from 90 to 42 (a rate decrease of 48) during the study period, while the rate for EVAR increased from 31 to 77 (a rate increase of 46)[56]. The investigators drew the obvious conclusion that the newer, less invasive, and less risky procedure (EVAR) is replacing the older and more invasive procedure (OSR) to a considerable degree[56]. In another study looking at large national administrative in-hospital database to compare utilization and age-specific outcomes between open repair (OAR) and endovascular (EVAR) repair for the treatment of abdominal aortic aneurysm (AAA). The estimated number of elective AAAs treated with EVAR increased from 11,171 in 2001 to 21,725 in 2006 ($P = .003$). The number of elective AAAs treated with OAR declined from 17,784 to 8451 during the same period ($P < .001$). By 2006, EVAR was more frequently used than OAR for patients of all ages. Compared with the younger age groups, patients aged >or=85 years had a significant increase in the total number of asymptomatic AAA repairs, driven almost entirely by an increase in the use of EVAR [33]. These authors noted that as short-term surgical outcomes are consistently improving for patients undergoing AAA repair, elective EVAR has replaced OAR as the more common method of repair in the

United States. The introduction of this technology has been rapidly adopted, particularly for the oldest-old surgical patients, aged >or=85 years, who previously may not have been offered surgical intervention for asymptomatic AAA. [33] This being said there are still significant unknowns with respect to long term out comes of EVAR despite the trend outlined above. The rapid improvements in EVAR design and deliverability have lead to changes in the anatomical criteria, and expanded usage. The EVAR device of today is very different then that of 10 years ago, however the outcomes data for "long-term follow up" is based on these older devices. The durability of these devices is a question that is difficult to answer, as this has been a constantly moving target as improvements to devices are made. Despite the increasing trend to treat all comers with EVAR, or at least the majority, the longitudinal data is not available or appropriate to make a solid recommendation. The durability of open grafts is proven with by the test of time there relatively low-tech nature and static design, this can however not be said about the endograft and the question of placing an endograft in a relatively young or fit patient with the concern that they may out-live the life of the endograft has not yet been answered.

Physician bias and training as well add to the difficulty in patient decision-making. As EVAR has gained in popularity open surgical repair has decreased and younger surgeons have less experience with open repair. The experience gained in many training programs has been that of difficult AAA repair in patients with unsuitable anatomy, which are relatively uncommon. To add to this dilemma as EVAR devices improve the pool of anatomically unfit patients decrease. Another issue is that AAA is no longer solely treated by surgeons and the decision to treat or observe a patient might be made on the clinicians inability to provide both the endovascular and open services.

14. Recommendations for the up-to-date patient decision-making with respect to the repair of abdominal aortic aneurysms

Based on the available literature and the global experience with larger studies and data-base analysis the general principles governing patient selection can be suggested as follows:

(1) in medically fit patients with AAAs large enough to justify consideration of intervention, current-day EVAR is preferable for those with suitable anatomy and with comorbidities likely to limit their longevity commensurate with the estimated durability of the device used. The argument for EVAR in all patients with suitable anatomy has been extended by some prominent figures in the vascular surgery community at recent meetings. The suggestion here is that even the first generation devices have been shown to be durable over time and that with current improvements in device and delivery system that the longevity of these devices has been clearly demonstrated. On the other hand, good risk patients with a projected longevity clearly beyond the known limits of device durability should receive OPEN, has been a standard approach. While this is an acceptable statement, there is no question that EVAR is less invasive, has a faster recovery time and a shorter hospitalization period. The aspect that has generally been looked over is that in a young, fit patient that is a productive member of society, despite their likely ability to heal and continue working with either approach is more likely to be able to do so in a more expeditious way following an endovascular strategy. [57]

(2) High-risk patients with large AAAs, who are unfit for OPEN, first deserve intensive treatment of their comorbidities, followed by EVAR, if they improve, and continued observation if they do not. Here a difficult decision has to be made which brings up

questions of ethical and moral responsibility. While the exact nuances of are left to the practitioner to decide the cautionary note here is not do something like EVAR, or any procedure for that matter, just because it can be done. While this was the patient population in which EVAR was initially studied and designed in we have proven feasibility and this question has been answered. One must look closely at the quality of life and life expectancy as well as comorbidities to make this decision.
(3) Patients with small AAAs deserve continued surveillance, with the threshold diameter being 5.0 cm diameter for males (based on the UKSAT trial follow-up data cited) and even lower, (4.5 cm diameter) for female patients, based on their relatively smaller anatomical dimensions, their attendant higher risk of rupture and higher rupture mortality, and a lower anatomical suitability for EVAR. This being said there appears to be some role in repair of smaller aneurysms in certain patient and closer or more frequent follow up in others. The opportunity for such early decision-making should be afforded by the recently approved national AAA screening program under Medicare, with screening having been shown to not only be cost effective for older men [58] but also for women as well [57]

15. Conclusions

Trusting as we do in the inevitable progress of newer technology, we believe that, in the future, the great majority of AAAs will be repaired via EVAR. This trend has been demonstrated and to a certain degree the pendulum has been set in motion. EVAR in many institutions world wide is the preferred mode of treatment and the first choice procedure. The de- vices will continue to improve, as will deployment techniques, and hopefully, patient selection will be driven more by evidence than a biased view of the options. EVAR is recommended for most patients with large AAAs and "suitable anatomy," specifically those who are deemed to be poor risk for open repair and/or have a limited life expectancy. Based on the data we have presented and contrary to the conclusions of EVAR 2, we also recommend EVAR for high-risk patients who respond to an intensive treatment of their comorbidities. Ultimately, patient and physician choice must take precedence when deciding between EVAR and no treatment in those with unsuitable anatomy for EVAR who are also unfit for open repair. The treatment of AAA like the treatment of many modern diseases needs to be individualized to the patient taking into account the many complex social and physiological considerations to formulate an appropriate management strategy

16. References

Bush, R.L., *et al.* Outcomes of care of abdominal aortic aneurysm in Veterans Health Administration facilities: results from the National Surgical Quality Improvement Program. *Am J Surg* 198, S41-48 (2009).

Ingraham, A.M., Richards, K.E., Hall, B.L. & Ko, C.Y. Quality improvement in surgery: the American College of Surgeons National Surgical Quality Improvement Program approach. *Adv Surg* 44, 251-267 (2010).

van Keulen, J.W., Moll, F.L., Tolenaar, J.L., Verhagen, H.J. & van Herwaarden, J.A. Validation of a new standardized method to measure proximal aneurysm neck angulation. *J Vasc Surg* 51, 821-828 (2010).

Steinmetz, E., *et al.* Analysis of outcome after using high-risk criteria selection to surgery versus endovascular repair in the modern era of abdominal aortic aneurysm treatment. *Eur J Vasc Endovasc Surg* 39, 403-409 (2010).

Mortality results for randomised controlled trial of early elective surgery or ultrasonographic surveillance for small abdominal aortic aneurysms. The UK Small Aneurysm Trial Participants. *Lancet* 352, 1649-1655 (1998).

Elkouri, S., *et al.* Most patients with abdominal aortic aneurysm are not suitable for endovascular repair using currently approved bifurcated stent-grafts. *Vasc Endovascular Surg* 38, 401-412 (2004).

Woodburn, K.R., Chant, H., Davies, J.N., Blanshard, K.S. & Travis, S.J. Suitability for endovascular aneurysm repair in an unselected population. *Br J Surg* 88, 77-81 (2001).

Abbruzzese, T.A., *et al.* Outcomes following endovascular abdominal aortic aneurysm repair (EVAR): an anatomic and device-specific analysis. *J Vasc Surg* 48, 19-28 (2008).

Sternbergh, W.C., 3rd, Carter, G., York, J.W., Yoselevitz, M. & Money, S.R. Aortic neck angulation predicts adverse outcome with endovascular abdominal aortic aneurysm repair. *J Vasc Surg* 35, 482-486 (2002).

Sternbergh, W.C., 3rd. Endo-exuberance and abdominal aortic aneurysm management: have we gone too far? *Expert Rev Cardiovasc Ther* 1, 605-609 (2003).

Ohki, T. & Veith, F.J. Patient selection for endovascular repair of abdominal aortic aneurysms: changing the threshold for intervention. *Semin Vasc Surg* 12, 226-234 (1999).

Lederle, F.A., *et al.* Immediate repair compared with surveillance of small abdominal aortic aneurysms. *N Engl J Med* 346, 1437-1444 (2002).

Zarins, C.K., *et al.* AneuRx stent graft versus open surgical repair of abdominal aortic aneurysms: multicenter prospective clinical trial. *J Vasc Surg* 29, 292-305; discussion 306-298 (1999).

Bush, R.L., Mureebe, L., Bohannon, W.T. & Rutherford, R.B. The impact of recent European trials on abdominal aortic aneurysm repair: is a paradigm shift warranted? *J Surg Res* 148, 264-271 (2008).

Peppelenbosch, N., Buth, J., Harris, P.L., van Marrewijk, C. & Fransen, G. Diameter of abdominal aortic aneurysm and outcome of endovascular aneurysm repair: does size matter? A report from EUROSTAR. *J Vasc Surg* 39, 288-297 (2004).

Ouriel, K., Clair, D.G., Kent, K.C. & Zarins, C.K. Endovascular repair compared with surveillance for patients with small abdominal aortic aneurysms. *J Vasc Surg* 51, 1081-1087 (2010).

Cao, P., *et al.* Comparison of surveillance versus aortic endografting for small aneurysm repair (CAESAR): results from a randomised trial. *Eur J Vasc Endovasc Surg* 41, 13-25 (2011).

Harthun, N.L., Cheanvechai, V., Graham, L.M., Freischlag, J.A. & Gahtan, V. Prevalence of abdominal aortic aneurysm and repair outcomes on the basis of patient sex: Should the timing of intervention be the same? *J Thorac Cardiovasc Surg* 127, 325-328 (2004).

Dillavou, E.D., Muluk, S.C. & Makaroun, M.S. A decade of change in abdominal aortic aneurysm repair in the United States: Have we improved outcomes equally between men and women? *J Vasc Surg* 43, 230-238; discussion 238 (2006).

Marty, B. & Enzler, M. The role of elective endovascular aneurysm repair today. *Vasa* 36, 3-4 (2007).

Cuypers, P.W., *et al.* Randomized study comparing cardiac response in endovascular and open abdominal aortic aneurysm repair. *Br J Surg* 88, 1059-1065 (2001).

Fulton, J.J., *et al.* Endovascular stent-graft repair of pararenal and type IV thoracoabdominal aortic aneurysms with adjunctive visceral reconstruction. *J Vasc Surg* 41, 191-198 (2005).

Endovascular aneurysm repair versus open repair in patients with abdominal aortic aneurysm (EVAR trial 1): randomised controlled trial. *Lancet* 365, 2179-2186 (2005).

Endovascular aneurysm repair and outcome in patients unfit for open repair of abdominal aortic aneurysm (EVAR trial 2): randomised controlled trial. *Lancet* 365, 2187-2192 (2005).

Wahlgren, C.M. & Malmstedt, J. Outcomes of endovascular abdominal aortic aneurysm repair compared with open surgical repair in high-risk patients: results from the Swedish Vascular Registry. *J Vasc Surg* 48, 1382-1388; discussion 1388-1389 (2008).

Bush, R.L., *et al.* Performance of endovascular aortic aneurysm repair in high-risk patients: results from the Veterans Affairs National Surgical Quality Improvement Program. *J Vasc Surg* 45, 227-233; discussion 233-225 (2007).

Sicard, G.A., Zwolak, R.M., Sidawy, A.N., White, R.A. & Siami, F.S. Endovascular abdominal aortic aneurysm repair: long-term outcome measures in patients at high-risk for open surgery. *J Vasc Surg* 44, 229-236 (2006).

Sbarigia, E., *et al.* What is the best management for abdominal aortic aneurysm in patients at high surgical risk? A single-center review. *Int Angiol* 24, 70-74 (2005).

Timaran, C.H., *et al.* Endovascular aortic aneurysm repair in patients with the highest risk and in-hospital mortality in the United States. *Arch Surg* 142, 520-524; discussion 524-525 (2007).

Timaran, C.H., *et al.* Influence of age, aneurysm size, and patient fitness on suitability for endovascular aortic aneurysm repair. *Ann Vasc Surg* 22, 730-735 (2008).

Demirel, S., *et al.* [Vascular Surgery in the Elderly - Recommendations for Clinical Practice.]. *Zentralbl Chir* (2011).

Cosford, P.A. & Leng, G.C. Screening for abdominal aortic aneurysm. *Cochrane Database Syst Rev*, CD002945 (2007).

Schwarze, M.L., Shen, Y., Hemmerich, J. & Dale, W. Age-related trends in utilization and outcome of open and endovascular repair for abdominal aortic aneurysm in the United States, 2001-2006. *J Vasc Surg* 50, 722-729 e722 (2009).

Lath, N.R., Rai, K. & Alshafie, T. Open repair of abdominal aortic aneurysm in a centenarian. *J Vasc Surg* 53, 216-218 (2011).

Van Damme, H., Sakalihasan, N., Vazquez, C., Desiron, Q. & Limet, R. Abdominal aortic aneurysms in octogenarians. *Acta Chir Belg* 98, 76-84 (1998).

Henebiens, M., Vahl, A. & Koelemay, M.J. Elective surgery of abdominal aortic aneurysms in octogenarians: a systematic review. *J Vasc Surg* 47, 676-681 (2008).

Paolini, D., *et al.* Elective endovascular and open repair of abdominal aortic aneurysms in octogenarians. *J Vasc Surg* 47, 924-927 (2008).

Prenner, S.B., *et al.* Outcome of elective endovascular abdominal aortic aneurysm repair in octogenarians and nonagenarians. *J Vasc Surg* 51, 1354-1359 (2010).

Goldstein, L.J., *et al.* Endovascular aneurysm repair in nonagenarians is safe and effective. *J Vasc Surg* 52, 1140-1146 (2010).

Jim, J., *et al.* Acceptable risk but small benefit of endovascular aneurysm repair in nonagenarians. *Ann Vasc Surg* 24, 441-446 (2010).

Foster, J., Ghosh, J. & Baguneid, M. In patients with ruptured abdominal aortic aneurysm does endovascular repair improve 30-day mortality? *Interact Cardiovasc Thorac Surg* 10, 611-619 (2010).

Ten Bosch, J.A., Teijink, J.A., Willigendael, E.M. & Prins, M.H. Endovascular aneurysm repair is superior to open surgery for ruptured abdominal aortic aneurysms in EVAR-suitable patients. *J Vasc Surg* 52, 13-18 (2010).

Setacci, F., *et al.* Endovascular approach for ruptured abdominal aortic aneursyms. *J Cardiovasc Surg (Torino)* 51, 313-317 (2010).

Davenport, D.L., *et al.* Thirty-day NSQIP database outcomes of open versus endoluminal repair of ruptured abdominal aortic aneurysms. *J Vasc Surg* 51, 305- 309 e301 (2010).

Buckley, C.J., Rutherford, R.B., Diethrich, E.B. & Buckley, S.D. Inherent problems with randomized clinical trials with observational/no treatment arms. *J Vasc Surg* 52, 237-241 (2010).

Prinssen, M., *et al.* A randomized trial comparing conventional and endovascular repair of abdominal aortic aneurysms. *N Engl J Med* 351, 1607-1618 (2004).

Greenhalgh, R.M., *et al.* Endovascular versus open repair of abdominal aortic aneurysm. *N Engl J Med* 362, 1863-1871 (2010).

Jetty, P., Hebert, P. & van Walraven, C. Long-term outcomes and resource utilization of endovascular versus open repair of abdominal aortic aneurysms in Ontario. *J Vasc Surg* 51, 577-583, 583 e571-573 (2010).

De Bruin, J.L., *et al.* Long-term outcome of open or endovascular repair of abdominal aortic aneurysm. *N Engl J Med* 362, 1881-1889 (2010).

Greenhalgh, R.M., Brown, L.C., Powell, J.T., Thompson, S.G. & Epstein, D. Endovascular repair of aortic aneurysm in patients physically ineligible for open repair. *N Engl J Med* 362, 1872-1880 (2010).

Lederle, F.A., *et al.* Outcomes following endovascular vs open repair of abdominal aortic aneurysm: a randomized trial. *JAMA* 302, 1535-1542 (2009).

Ouriel, K. Randomized clinical trials of endovascular repair versus surveillance for treatment of small abdominal aortic aneurysms. *J Endovasc Ther* 16 Suppl 1, I94-105 (2009).

Long-term outcomes of immediate repair compared with surveillance of small abdominal aortic aneurysms. *N Engl J Med* 346, 1445-1452 (2002).

Upchurch, G.R., Jr., *et al.* Endovascular abdominal aortic aneurysm repair versus open repair: why and why not? *Perspect Vasc Surg Endovasc Ther* 21, 48-53 (2009).

Albuquerque, F.C., Jr., *et al.* Paradigm shifts in the treatment of abdominal aortic aneurysm: trends in 721 patients between 1996 and 2008. *J Vasc Surg* 51, 1348-1352; discussion 1352-1343 (2010).

Levin, D.C., Rao, V.M., Parker, L., Frangos, A.J. & Sunshine, J.H. Endovascular repair vs open surgical repair of abdominal aortic aneurysms: comparative utilization trends from 2001 to 2006. *J Am Coll Radiol* 6, 506-509 (2009).

Wanhainen, A., Bylund, N. & Bjorck, M. Outcome after abdominal aortic aneurysm repair in Sweden 1994-2005. *Br J Surg* 95, 564-570 (2008).

Fleming, C., Whitlock, E.P., Beil, T.L. & Lederle, F.A. Screening for abdominal aortic aneurysm: a best-evidence systematic review for the U.S. Preventive Services Task Force. *Ann Intern Med* 142, 203-211 (2005).

2

The Evidence for Management of Abdominal Aortic Aneurysms: Lessons Learned from Randomised Controlled Trials

Reza Mofidi[1] and Stuart A. Suttie[2]
[1]James Cook University Hospital, Middlesbrough
[2]University of Dundee, Dundee,
United Kingdom

1. Introduction

Abdominal aortic aneurysm (AAA) is a common life threatening condition in the western world. In England and Wales alone, over 2500 patients present to hospital with rupture of AAA annually, of whom over two thirds die of their condition[1]. The best treatment for AAA is elective repair of pre-symptomatic abdominal aortic aneurysms. Such a therapeutic strategy depends on effective identification of patients with AAA and the subgroup of patients in whom there is a real risk of aneurysm rupture. As the vast majority of patients with AAAs are asymptomatic, timely identification of AAA may be achieved through targeted screening of the at risk populations. Over the last two decades longitudinal studies of patients with smaller AAAs have provided insights into the timing of AAA repair and the need for and frequency of ultrasound surveillance if an expectant management strategy is followed. This chapter discusses the available evidence for screening for AAA as well as all the other measures which have helped to optimise therapeutic strategies in the management of patients with AAA throughout the patients' journey from the initial diagnosis to the eventual repair of AAA.

2. Targeted screening for AAA

In the past 40 years with the advent and generalised use of abdominal ultrasonography there has been an accurate, cheap and non invasive tool for the diagnosis of abdominal aortic aneurysms. Abdominal ultrasonography has been found to be an accurate and reproducible modality in measuring the dimensions of AAA. This has led to the concept of its use for screening of at risk populations. In the last 20 years there have been four population based randomised controlled trials which have assessed the value of targeted screening in reducing mortality from abdominal aortic aneurysms in the unselected elderly male population[2-5]. These trials which have been undertaken in Chichester (England)[2], England (MASS trial) [3], Viborg County (Denmark) [4] and the city of Perth and suburbs (Western Australia)[5] have together recruited over 120,000 subjects. All of these studies have reported on long term (over 10 years) follow up. Using the predefined criteria set by the US Preventative Screening Task Force USPSTF [6] the MASS trial has been classified as good with the other three trials classified as fair i.e. not meeting all the criteria but judged to have no fatal flaws[7].

The Chichester trial was the first to assess the value of screening for AAA in the at risk population. It was also unique as it included women as well as men. It identified all men and women aged between 65 and 80 years of age from 9 general practices in the catchment area of St Richard's hospital in Chichester between 1988 and 1991[2,8,9]. The subjects were randomised to undergo a single screening ultrasound (US) or a control group who were followed up. AAA rupture rates, aneurysm related mortality, and overall mortality was compared between the two groups. Upon identification of AAA the therapeutic strategy for AAAs with maximum diameters between 30-44mm was once yearly surveillance US, AAAs between 44 and 59mm underwent 3 monthly ultrasound scans, whilst aneurysms greater than 60mm in diameter were considered for repair[2,8,9]. Overall 6040 men were randomised, the authors reported a significant reduction in aneurysm related mortality which has been maintained over 15 years. However, to date this study has demonstrated no difference in the all cause mortality between the two groups. The Chichester trial has been criticized for its relative small size, a relatively high aneurysm diameter threshold for repair and including 75-80 year old patients in whom the benefits of screening are marginal. In addition 27-percent of subjects who were invited for screening refused to participate thereby diluting the benefits of screening. Despite these criticisms the Chichester study remains a land mark as it demonstrated the feasibility of US screening for AAA and its potential value and remains a blue print for other aneurysm screening studies. This study identified a low but none the less troubling rate of AAA rupture in patients who had a non aneurysmal aorta on the first screening study[2]. A population based screening study in Gloucester demonstrated that 2.2-percent of men aged 65-73 years have a maximal aortic diameter of 2.5 to 2.9 mm and suggested that this group of patients should undergo repeat US scanning at 5 yearly intervals[10].

The second RCT to study the value of population based screening for AAA was carried out in Viborg County of Denmark. In 1994 all men aged between 65 and 74 were randomised to either undergo a single screening US or the control group. In all 12639 patients were randomised[4,11,12]. This study reported a 66-percent reduction in the aneurysm related mortality which has been maintained over 14-years. In addition they reported a 2-percent reduction in overall mortality after long term follow-up which did not reach significance[4].

The Western Australia population based screening was a study of similar design. It randomised 41000 men between the ages of 65 and 85 years to a single US screening and a control groups. They reported no difference in aneurysm outcomes in the full study population but when the analysis was restricted to 65-74 year old men they reported a significant reduction in aneurysm related mortality after 5 years of follow-up[5]. Long term follow-up results of this study have not been published as a separate publication to date, however in a reply to a correspondence by Lederle, Norman and Lindholt did report a surprisingly high, 3-percent reduction in overall mortality in the restricted (65-74 year old) patient population after 10 years of follow-up from the Western Australia trial which was statistically significant[13].

The MASS trial which was a population based screening RCT for men aged between 65 and 74 years of age included 4 screening centres in the United Kingdom. This study randomised 67770 patients again to single screening ultrasound or a control group and was designed to study cost effectiveness of screening in addition to reductions aneurysm related and overall mortality[3,14,15]. This study reported a 48-percent relative risk reduction in aneurysm related mortality as a result of screening. This benefit was present at 4 years [14] and was maintained at 10 years (Figure-1)[3]. There was a reduced AAA rupture rate in the patients who were invited for screening. Most of these ruptures occurred in patients who were excluded from the potential benefits of screening, such as patients who refused or did not attend screening, patients who were lost to follow-up and those who either refused or deemed not fit for surgery[3]. The MASS trial also reported a small rate of AAA rupture in patients who did not have an AAA on the screening scan, this rate was reported as 3 per 10,000 person years after 10 years of follow up[3].

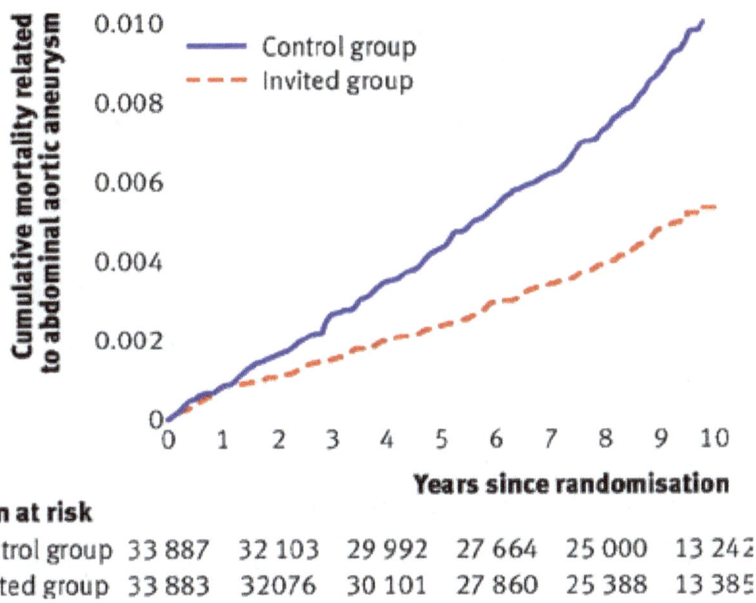

Fig. 1. Cumulative deaths related to abdominal aortic aneurysm, by time since randomisation (MASS Trial) [3]. From: Thompson SG, Ashton HA, Gao L, Scott RA and Multicentre Aneurysm Screening Study Group, Screening men for abdominal aortic aneurysm: 10 year mortality and cost effectiveness results from the randomised Multicentre Aneurysm Screening Study, BMJ 2009; 338: b2307.

In addition to the above RCTs a number of systematic reviews and meta-analyses have attempted to assess the value of population based screening in the medium and long term. Cosford and Leng in a Cochrane systematic review reported that there was significant evidence of reduction in aneurysm related mortality from AAA in men aged 65 to 80 years who undergo population based ultrasound screening, but no significant reduction in all cause mortality[16]. This review was based on the 3-5 year follow up data from the above RCTs. Subsequent to this Norman and Lindholt published a meta-analysis which showed that population based AAA screening after 7-15 years of follow up resulted in a reduction of both AAA and all cause mortality[17]. Their findings were contested as the reported 3-percent all cause mortality reduction was larger than what was expected by an approximately 50-percent reduction in aneurysm related mortality, bearing in mind that the mortality from AAA in the patient population is reported to be between 1.1 to 3-percent[18].

Takagi et al. conducted a further meta-analysis of US screening in the male population over the age of 65years using long term 10 to 15 year follow up data from the RCTs. They reported an absolute risk reduction in aneurysm related mortality of 4 per 1000 subjects screened (Figure-2). They also revealed a strong trend towards a significant reduction in all cause mortality[7]. The latter finding was surprising for the reasons mentioned already. The authors hypothesized that screening may coincide with the asymptomatic at risk population for cardiovascular disease coming in contact with health care professionals and becoming aware of smoking risk, their blood pressure etc. The resultant reduction in cardiovascular risk factors may be in part responsible for additional reduction in all cause mortality. Such a hypothesis opens the door to the possibility of risk factor alteration and institution of secondary prevention measures such as commencement of anti-platelet agents and statin therapy during screening programmes thereby increasing the value of the screening[7].

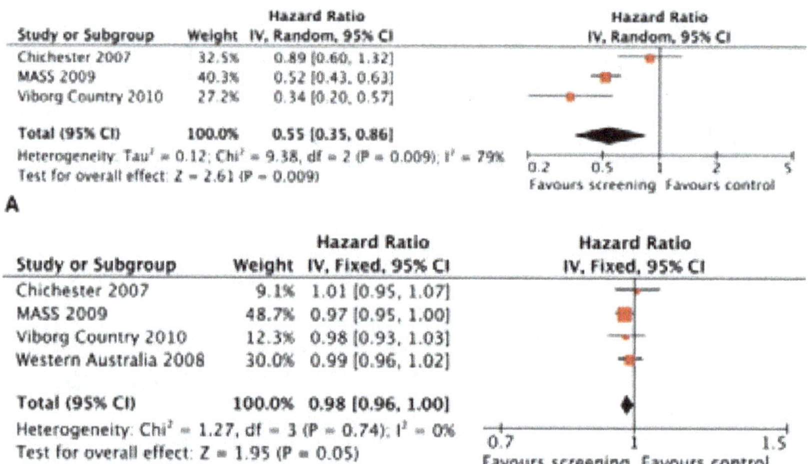

Fig. 2. Forrest Plot of illustrating the reduction in aneurysm related mortality (A) and the trend towards a reduction in overall mortality (B) as a result of population based screening of men between the ages of 65 and 80 years after 10 years of follow up[7].
From: Takagi H, Goto SN, Matsui M, Manabe H, Umemoto T. A further meta-analysis of population-based screening for abdominal aortic aneurysm. J Vasc Surg. 2010; 52(4):1103-8.

Cost effectiveness of a population based screening programme is calculated by measuring the costs of ultrasound screening as well as the extra procedures and surveillance that is required for the screen identified AAA and subtracting them from the costs of treating ruptured AAA. It is expressed in cost per life year gained. As the survival advantage in terms of life year gained continues to increase with time, the cost effectiveness of screening continues to improve. A comprehensive analysis of costs of screening was performed by the MASS trial participants. They calculated the cost per life year gained to be £41,000 after 4 years[14], £14,000 after 7 years [15]and £7600 after 10 years[3]. Using the estimated life span of men aged 65 years the cost per life year gained is estimated to be in the region of £2300, which is well below the guideline figure of £25,000 which is considered acceptable for the adaptation of new medical technologies and interventions in the National Health Service of the United Kingdom[19].
Lindholt *et al.* also performed a comprehensive cost analysis of population based AAA screening using data obtained from the Viborg trial. They reported cost per Quality

Adjusted Life Year (QALY) gained as a result of screening to be €179 albeit with relatively wide 95% confidence intervals (€-4083 to €4682) [4]. Both of these values for costs of screening are much lower than the cost analysis carried out by the USPSTF using primarily economic modelling in 2003 and suggest that population based AAA screening in men is more cost effective than the initial assessments suggested[20].

The role of screening for AAA in women remains controversial. To date there is no evidence that screening for AAA in an unselected population of women is associated with a reduction even in aneurysm-related mortality. Scott and colleagues conducted the only RCT (Chichester trial) which studied the value of screening in women over the age of 65 in an unselected population (n=9342) [21]. They reported the prevalence of AAA in women to be 1·3 percent, with other authors reporting a similar rate of 0·7–1·3 percent in unselected populations[22-24]. Scott *et al.* did not demonstrate a difference in rupture rates between the women randomized to screening and control populations of women at 5- and 10-year follow-up[21]. They concluded that screening for women was neither clinically indicated nor economically viable[21]. This study was limited by high rate of non attendance of women for AAA screening which ranged between 27 and 42-percent depending on patients age. They screened an unselected population of women without consideration of risk factors for aneurysm disease and fitness for repair; consequently a large proportion of women who were found to have an AAA did not undergo aneurysm repair[25]. The UK Small Aneurysm Trial revealed that female sex was an independent risk factor for AAA rupture; the rupture rate in women was three times higher than that in men, despite a smaller initial AP diameter. Furthermore, mean AP diameter preceding rupture was significantly lower in women than men[26]. A number of other authors have reported a higher growth and rupture rate of AAA in women [27-33]. A Finnish community-based follow-up study reported that the aortic diameter was less than 5·5 cm in 24 per cent of women with a ruptured AAA, compared with only 5 per cent of men[21]. In light of these findings the 6 cm cut off value for repair of AAA in Chichester trial may have been too large to prevent aneurysm rupture in a proportion of screened women thereby reducing the value of screening in women.

For screening to be effective in reducing aneurysm-related mortality in women, it will need to be limited to high-risk women who are fit to undergo aneurysm repair[22]. There is increasing evidence that women with atherosclerotic disease are at significantly higher risk of developing AAA. Derubertis and colleagues[22] reported that the prevalence of AAA in women with multiple (more than three) atherosclerotic risk factors was 6·4 per cent. When these findings are considered in conjunction with the increased growth rates of AAA[26] and higher aneurysm rupture rate in women, screening in women with multiple risk factors for AAA may become clinically and economically viable[34-36].

3. Optimum therapeutic strategy for small AAAs

Abdominal aortic aneurysms are treated in order to prevent rupture and the associated mortality. Aneurysm treatment has its own associated morbidity and mortality. Open surgical repair is an invasive procedure which is tolerated poorly by the subgroup of patients with multiple medical co-morbidities. Even endovascular repair cannot be accomplished without an obligatory complication rate as a result of the initial deployment of the stent graft, in addition to which a proportion of patients require secondary procedures necessary to address complications such as endoleaks, device migration and stent thrombosis requiring long term close surveillance[37]. A small proportion of patients

who have undergone endovascular repair (EVAR) succumb to rupture. Therefore the natural history of the AAA needs to be balanced against the risk associated with treatment.
Aneurysm diameter is one variable which has been consistently associated with the risk of rupture and has therefore been used to stratify patients into risk categories which decides whether US based surveillance or intervention is required to repair the aneurysm. In patients who are entered into surveillance programmes the maximum diameter of the aneurysm is used to decide on the frequency of scanning. In case of aneurysms greater than 5.5 cm there is consensus that risk of rupture mandates repair if the patient is fit to undergo the procedure. In the case of aneurysms less than 4.0 cm in diameter, most clinicians agree on a watchful waiting approach. The evidence for the optimum therapeutic strategy in the mid-sized aortic aneurysms (maximum diameter between 4.0 to 5.5 cm in diameter) has been strengthened by a number of randomised controlled trials in the last 20 years which have consolidated the modern management of AAA[26,38-41].
The UK small aneurysm trial (UKSAT) was a multicentre RCT which randomised 1090 patients, who were diagnosed as having an AAA with maximum AP diameter of 4.0 to 5.5cm and were deemed fit to undergo an open repair of AAA to either immediate open repair or 3 monthly ultrasound surveillance. They reported the rupture rate of these AAA in the surveillance group to be in the 1-percent per year. They did not find any significant difference in aneurysm related or all cause mortality between the two groups after a follow up period of 7 years (Figure-3)[26]. During the follow up period over two thirds of patients who were randomised to surveillance had undergone repair of their aneurysms based on clinical grounds. [26] Long term follow up data from the small aneurysm trial has confirmed the initial findings of the UKSAT[38].

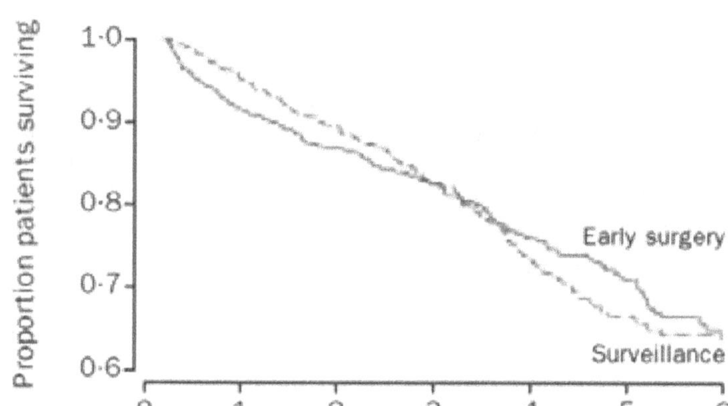

Number at risk

Surveillance	527	497	468	412	229	125	52
Early surgery	563	513	489	450	302	187	63

Fig. 3. Kaplan-Meier survival curves comparing survival of patients with small abdominal aortic aneurysms randomised to ultrasound surveillance and early surgery from UK small aneurysm trial[26]. From: United Kingdom Small Aneurysm Trial Participants. Long-term outcomes of immediate repair compared with surveillance of small abdominal aortic aneurysms. Lancet 1998;352: 1649-55.

A number of years after the publication of the UKSAT, the Veterans Affairs Cooperative Study group published the Aneurysm Detection and Management ADAM study[39]. This study involved screening of 126,196 veterans aged between 50 and 79 years of age for AAA with a single abdominal US. Those with AAA measuring 4.0 to 5.4 cm in diameter were offered entry to the trial. In all, 1136 subjects were randomly assigned to undergo early elective repair or ultrasound surveillance. Annualized rupture rate in the surveillance arm of the study was 0.6-percent, with no difference in aneurysm related and overall mortality between the two arms of the study [39]. In this study as in UKSAT the majority of patients in the surveillance arm of the study had undergone elective repair after 8 years of follow up based on clinical grounds (symptomatic aneurysm, growth to greater than 5.5cm in diameter or rapid expansion by greater than 1 cm per year) [39]. Completion of these two landmark trials which utilised open elective repair coincided with the advent and generalised use of endovascular repair as a primary modality treatment of AAA. This resulted in some authors questioning the validity of these landmark trials in the era of endovascular repair and suggested that as endovascular repair can be performed with significantly lower peri-procedural morbidity and mortality a policy of surveillance for smaller AAAs should be examined against endovascular repair.

To date two randomised controlled trials (PIVOTAL[40] and CAESAR[41]) have been conducted to compare early endovascular repair of small AAAs with ultrasound surveillance. The prerequisite for both studies was that the patients which were randomised had AAAs which were anatomically suitable for endovascular repair.

The PIVOTAL trial which was published in 2010, randomised 728 patients with AAAs measuring 40 to 50 mm in diameter to ultrasound based surveillance or early endovascular repair[40]. The mean duration of follow up was 20 months (+/-12 months) they found no difference in all cause or aneurysm related mortality between the two groups [40]. At the end of the relatively short follow up duration almost one third of patients who were in the surveillance group had undergone an aneurysm repair based on clinical grounds[40]. The other study of a similar design was the CAESAR trial which randomised 360 patients with AAAs measuring between 40 and 54 mm to early endovascular repair or a watchful waiting strategy. [41] After 54 months of follow up there was no significant difference in rupture rates, aneurysm related and overall mortality between the two groups (Figure-4). This study revealed that the probability of the patients in the surveillance arm of the study requiring delayed repair based on clinical grounds during the duration of follow up was 60-percent[41]. In addition they reported that 16.4-percent of aneurysms which upon entry into the trial were suitable for endovascular repair will be no longer suitable for EVAR after 36 months[41].

A constant finding in these trials has been that a significant proportion of AAAs under ultrasonographic surveillance come to require repair within the duration of the study[26,39]. This, taken together with the low but present annual risk of rupture has lead to differing interpretations of the results of these trials with some authors still advocating in favour of early repair of small AAA using the justification that a policy of early EVAR is as safe as a policy of US Surveillance[42]. To date there is no objective data to recommend either open or endovascular repair of smaller AAAs over a policy of watchful waiting and US surveillance. A policy of early EVAR is associated with a risk of early and delayed complications and a need for secondary procedures, thus mandating the need for close surveillance in patients who undergo early EVAR. It is therefore unlikely that there will be an economic justification for early endovascular repair.

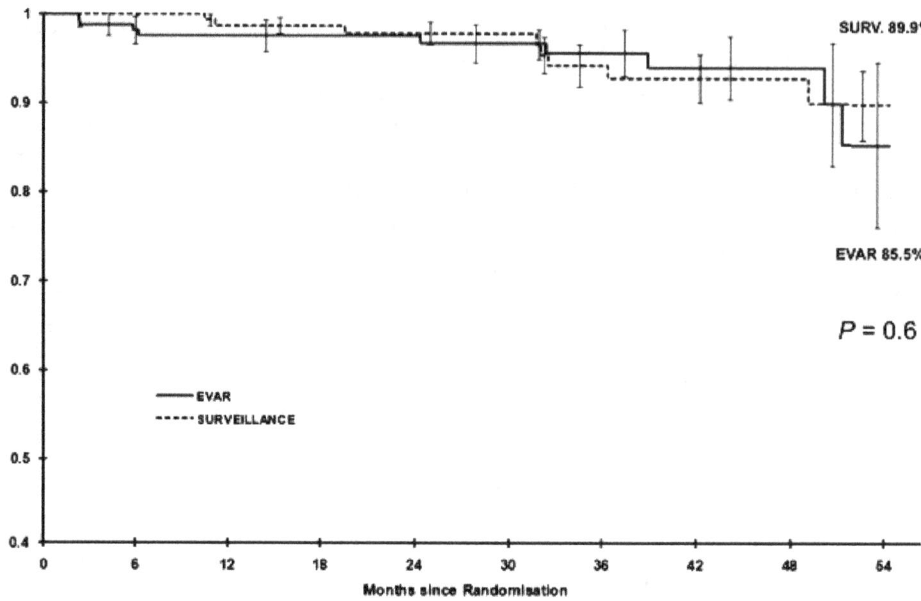

MONTHS	0	6	12	18	24	30	36	42	48	54
EVAR	182	162	157	145	128	106	83	57	37	21
SURVEILLANCE	178	162	154	139	118	98	77	60	39	29

Fig. 4: Kaplan–Meier estimates of survival at 54 months from time of randomisation in EVAR versus Surveillance groups. P = 0.6. Numbers at risk are shown. CAESAR trial[41]. From:Cao P; DeRango P, Verzini F, Parlani G et al. Comparison of surveillance vs Aortic Endografting for Small Aneurysm Repair (CAESAR) trial: results of a randomised controlled trial. Eur J Vasc Endovasc Surg. 2011; 41(1): 13-25.

4. Open versus endovascular repair of AAA

Ever since its inception, EVAR has offered the promise of reducing the perioperative morbidity and mortality which has been associated with open elective repair. By the end of last century, data from EVAR registries such as RETA [43]and EUROSTAR [44] suggested that endovascular repair, although safe was associated with an immediate complication rate in addition to events such as endoleak and device migration which mandate lifelong surveillance and in a group of patients re-intervention. As with any new or emerging technology or intervention the case for primacy of EVAR over open repair in terms of perioperative mortality rate, post operative complications and cost effectiveness needs to be made using good quality evidence. A number of trials with a similar design have been commissioned in order to compare the outcomes following EVAR and open repair of AAA in patients who are anatomically suitable to undergo endovascular repair and fit to undergo open repair. These include the Dutch Randomised Endovascular Aneurysm Management (DREAM) [45,46]trial, EVAR-1 Trial (United Kingdom) [47], ACE trial (France) [48] and Open Versus Endovascular Repair (OVER) of abdominal aortic aneurysms trial (United States)[49].
The DREAM trial which was the first to report its results enrolled 351 patients between November 2000 and December 2003 from 24 centres in the Netherlands and 4 centres in Belgium. This study focused on short term combined mortality and morbidity outcomes[45]. It

reported a significantly lower operative mortality and severe complication rates in the EVAR group compared to the patients who had been randomised to open repair. At 2 years follow up aneurysm related mortality following EVAR was still significantly lower than open repair (2.1% versus 5.7%) however after 2 years of follow up there was no significant difference in the overall survival rates or freedom from moderate to severe complications between the two groups. The conclusions drawn from this trial was that there was a significant reduction in early morbidity and mortality following EVAR compared to open aneurysm repair but this difference is not sustained past 2 years[45,46].

EVAR-1 trial was a multicentre RCT which was conducted in 37 hospitals in the UK. It randomised 1252 patients with large AAA to either open or endovascular repair. Unlike the DREAM trial, EVAR-1 was designed to perform a comparison of long term survival, graft durability, quality of life and hospital costs associated with open repair and EVAR in addition to comparing short term mortality and morbidity between the two groups[47]. They reported a significantly lower in perioperative morbidity and mortality following EVAR. Four years after randomisation, all cause mortality was similar between the two groups, although there was a persistent reduction in aneurysm related mortality in the EVAR group,(Figure-5)[47]. After 12 months there was no difference in quality of life scores between the two groups with a greater number of complications and re-interventions at 4 years in the EVAR arm of the study. The hospital costs of EVAR were 25-percent higher than open repair[47].

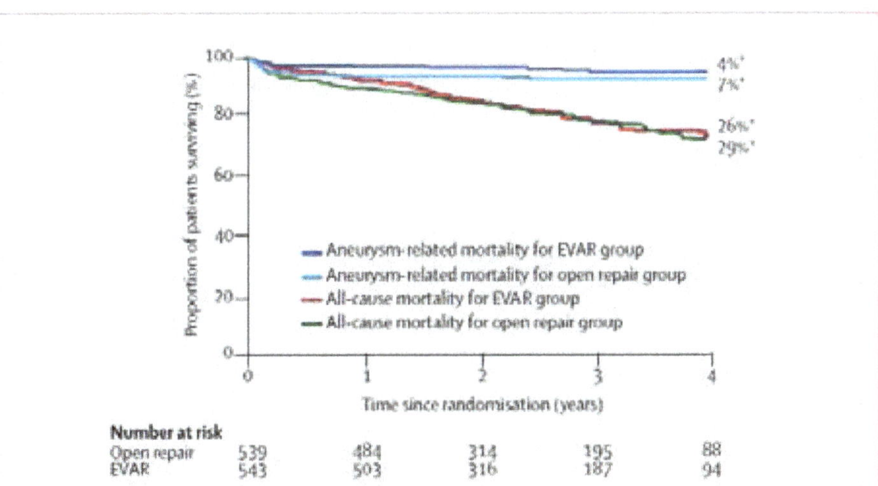

Fig. 5. EVAR-1 Kaplan-Meier survival curves comparing aneurysm related and overall mortality between patients who have been randomised to open elective and endovascular (EVAR) repair of AAA (EVAR-1 trial)[47]. From: EVAR trial participants. Endovascular aneurysm repair versus open repair in patients with abdominal aortic aneurysm (EVAR trial 1): randomised controlled trial. Lancet 2005; 365(9478): 2179-86.

The OVER trial is a RCT which included 42 Veterans Affairs medical centres in the United States. It randomised 881 patients who had AAA with a greater than 50 mm in maximal diameter, an iliac aneurysm greater than 30mm in diameter or rapid sac expansion, to elective open repair or EVAR. The preliminary results from this study indicated that the

EVAR group had significantly lower 30-day mortality as well as all cause mortality[49]. After a mean follow up of 1.8 years the complication rate was not significantly different between the two groups nor was the secondary reintervention rate. As in the DREAM trial, the reintervention following EVAR was mainly due to a device related complications whereas the commonest reason for reintervention following open repair was for incisional hernia[46,49]. Early results from the ACE trial suggest similar early mortality benefit following endovascular repair which is lost after medium term follow up[48].

Some subgroups of patients such as those who have significant co-morbidities such as cardiovascular or respiratory disease, octogenarians and women with AAA, require an individualised approach and revised criteria for the management of AAA. From its inception EVAR has provided the promise of repairing AAA in patients in whom open repair poses a high risk. Therefore armed with the knowledge that smaller AAAs are best managed by a policy of watchful waiting, EVAR appeared to be an ideal modality for the management of patients with larger AAAs which are anatomically suitable for endovascular repair, have a reasonable predicted longevity but are unfit to undergo open repair. The EVAR-2 trial was designed to answer this question. EVAR-2 trial was a randomised controlled trial of 338 patients who had an AAA with a maximum diameter of greater than 5.5cm and their aneurysm morphology was anatomically suitable for EVAR, but were medically unsuitable to undergo open repair. Primary endpoint was all-cause mortality, with secondary endpoints of aneurysm-related mortality, health-related quality of life, postoperative complications, and hospital costs[50].

The 30-day operative mortality in the EVAR group was 9.0-percent and the no intervention group had an annual rupture rate of 9·0-percent per year. Aneurysm related mortality in the patient population was 13-percent and all cause mortality after 4 years of follow up was 64-percent [50].

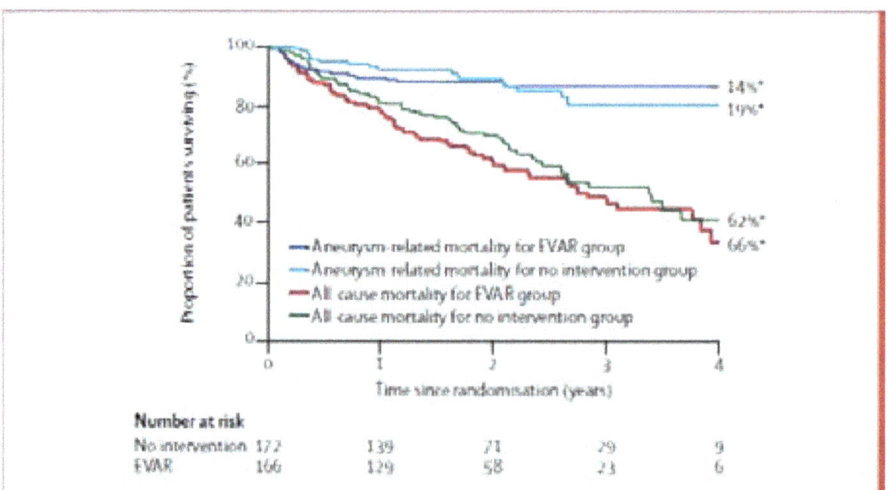

Fig. 6. Kaplan-Meier curves comparing aneurysm related and overall mortality between patients who have been randomised to EVAR and no intervention group (EVAR-2 trial)[50]. From: EVAR trial participants. Endovascular aneurysm repair and outcome in patients unfit for open repair of abdominal aortic aneurysm (EVAR trial 2): randomised controlled trial. Lancet 2005; 365(9478): 2187–92.

There was no significant difference in all-cause mortality between the EVAR group and the no intervention group (hazard ratio 1·21, 95% CI 0·87–1·69). There was no difference in aneurysm-related mortality (Figure-6) [50]. A policy of early endovascular repair was significantly more expensive than expectant management and was associated with a higher complication and reintervention rate. There was no difference in quality of life scores between the two arms of the study[50]. Therefore the conclusion drawn by the authors was that this population of patients are best served by conservative treatment. Clearly the design of such a study provides one difficulty and that is the definition of not fit for open AAA repair is subject to clinical opinion and may be related to factors that do not affect patient's longevity. The other group of patients are those with one organ morbidity such as respiratory disease or border line medical fitness, who have a large AAA and favourable anatomy for endovascular repair. Therefore clinical judgement is exercised in the application of results of EVAR-2 trial.

5. Medical treatment of patients with AAA

In addition to risk of growth and rupture, patients with AAA are at risk from other cardiovascular events by the virtue of their age, medical co-morbidities and male preponderance of AAA. Medical management of patients with known AAA follows two parallel but different aims, reducing cardiovascular event rates perioperatively and during follow up in addition to aneurysm specific therapy which is aimed at slowing aneurysm growth and reducing the risk of rupture[51-53].

Hyperlipidaemia, a known modifiable risk factor in the development of cardio-vascular disease, can be treated with the use of drugs such as the statins (3-hydroxyl-3-methylglutaryl coenzyme A reductase inhibitors). Patients with AAA are known to be at high risk of cardio-vascular disease as well as increased risk of cardio-vascular complications following AAA repair [54]. Statin therapy has been associated with improved survival due to decreased risk of cardio-vascular complications, in both open and endovascular repair [54-58]. Although the primary mechanism of statins is in reducing low density lipoproteins and total cholesterol levels along with increasing levels of high density lipoproteins, other protective non lipid mechanism may be at work. These so called pleiotropic effects describe a diversity of cellular events which have an effect on several components of the arterial wall, including: endothelial cells; smooth muscle cells; platelet function, monocytes and macrophages, which together help to modify the inflammatory process in the vessel wall. Statins have been shown to be beneficial in the secondary prevention of coronary heart disease even in those patients with normal lipid profiles[59-60].

Matrix Metallo Proteinase-9 (MMP-9) expression is closely linked to aneurysm formation in animal models. In vitro experiments have shown that addition of Cerivstatins to human organ cultures from AAA reduces tissue levels of both total and active MMP-9 in a concentration dependent manner. Evans et al reported significantly reduced MMP-9 levels in excised tissue obtained from the aneurysm sac at the time of the aneurysm repair in patients who had been started on statins 3-weeks preoperatively compared with controls[59]. Schouten et al monitored 150 patients with small AAAs for 12 months and reported a reduction in the aneurysm expansion rate in patients receiving statin therapy[60]. In an observational study of 130 patients under surveillance, Sukhija reported no aneurysm expansion in 75 patients who were on statin therapy over a 2 year follow up period[61]. Schlosser et al in an analysis of the results of a large observational cohort study which involved 5057 patients with vascular disease (Second Manifestation of ARTerial disease (SMART) study) and included 230 patients with small AAA revealed an independent association between statin therapy and reduced aneurysm growth rate. This reduced growth and rupture rates were independent of serum lipid values[62,63].

Over the years there has been some interest in β-blockers, both to slow the growth rate of AAA and to reduce perioperative morbidity form cardiovascular events. The benefit was postulated partly due to their haemodynamic properties and partly due to the effect of β-blockers on matrix proteins. In a trial reported by Lindholt and colleagues the use of Propranolol did not reduce the rate of expansion of AAA, admittedly in the treatment arm of the study the compliance was poor with only 22-percent continuing on Propranolol by 2-years[64]. Another trial which was carried out in Canada came to a similar conclusion owing to poor patient compliance in the treatment arm of the study[65].

In the last 15 years there has been significant interest in using peri-operative β-blockade as a means of increasing myocardial oxygen delivery thereby reducing the risk of perioperative myocardial infarction and death. Mangano et al randomised 200 patients who were undergoing major elective non-cardiac surgery to either receive Atenolol or placebo. This was started before the induction of anaesthesia. Patients with evidence of congestive cardiac failure, systolic blood pressure of less than 100mmHg orpulse rate of less than 55 beats /minute, 3rd degree heart block or broncho-spasm were excluded. This treatment was continued for 6 months postoperatively. They reported a significant reduction in cardiovascular event rate and death from cardiac causes[66].

Poldermans and colleagues performed a similar study in patients undergoing elective aneurysm or infrainguinal arterial reconstruction. They screened 1351 patients for cardiac disease using Dobutamine stress testing, 173 patients had a positive test of whom 59 were randomised to receive Bisoprolol and 53 placebo[67]. They also reported a significant reduction in non fatal cardiac events as well as cardiac death. In these patients β-blockade was started at least a week in advance of the operation and they were screened for bradycardia and hypotension preoperatively[67].

POISE was a large international randomised controlled trial of the use of extended release Metoprolol in patients undergoing non-cardiac surgery, the study randomised 8351 patients to either receive Metoprolol or placebo which was started 2-4 hrs before surgery and continued for 30 days. They reported a significantly reduced risk of myocardial infarction in the Metoprolol group but at the expense of higher mortality and stroke rate in the treatment arm of the study[68]. Similarly, Yang et al randomised such patients undergoing major vascular surgery, not already β-blocked, to dose adjusted Metoprolol or placebo 2 hours prior to surgery and until discharge or maximum of 5 post-operative days, and found no protective effects of β-blockade in terms of 30 day myocardial infarction and death rates[69]. β-blockade did result in significantly more episodes of bradycardia and hypotension. In light of these findings the American Heart Association guidelines regarding perioperative β-blocker therapy in patients undergoing non cardiac surgery have been altered to be more cautious and circumspective (Table-)[70].

In a large observational study, Hackham et al have shown that the use of Angiotensin Converting Enzyme Inhibitor (ACE_I) therapy taken 3-12 months prior to data analysis significantly reduced the risk of rupture from AAA, independently of blood pressure[71]. This data was obtained from a large administrative database of 3379 patients with ruptured and 11947 with non ruptured AAA. Other anti-hypertensive medications had no such effect [71]. Interestingly, patients who had stopped ACE_I therapy prior to admission were more likely to present with ruptured AAA [71]. The effect of ACE_I on expansion of AAA is still equivocal, with some studies demonstrating no protective effect of ACE_I therapy [72-73]. Thompson et al in a recent observational study of 1269 patients with small AAA who were followed up for a mean of 3.4 years, reported a significant reduction in aneurysm growth rate as a result of ACE inhibitor therapy[72]. The follow up data from UK small aneurysm trial does not support the above finding[74].

Infection with Chlamydiae pneumonia has been postulated as a risk factor for AAA expansion, as the organism has been isolated from atherosclerotic plaque and the walls of AAA [75,76]. Three small trials have aimed to elucidate the effect of the antibiotics Doxycycline and Roxithromycin in AAA growth, two of which have shown reduced aortic expansion associated with treatment [77,78], whilst another one by Baxter and colleagues showed no effect of doxycycline on aortic diameter [79]. These three trials were limited by their small numbers. In addition administration of Doxycycline has been shown to suppress MMP-9 in both human and animal studies [79-81], suggesting that the reduction in aneurysm expansion rate with administration Doxycycline may be mediated through a mechanism which is independent from treatment of Chlamydiae pneumoniae infection.

To date there is no conclusive evidence that any medical therapy is associated with a reduction in aneurysm growth or risk of rupture. However diagnosis of AAA provides a forum for instituting appropriate secondary prevention therapies, which will reduce morbidity and mortality in the peri-operative period as well reduce long term cardio-vascular risk. There is some evidence that instituting some of these treatments such as statin therapy, ACE inhibitors may well have an effect on aneurysm growth and rupture rates.

6. References

Filipovic M, Seagroatt V, Goldacre MJ. Differences between women and men in surgical treatment and case fatality rates for ruptured aortic abdominal aneurysm in England. *Br J Surg.* 2007; 94: 1096–1099.

Scott RA, Wilson NM, HA Ashton, Kay DN. Influence of screening on the incidence of ruptured abdominal aortic aneurysm: 5-year results of a randomized controlled study, *Br J Surg* 1995; 82: 1066–1070.

Thompson SG, Ashton HA, Gao L, Scott RA and Multicentre Aneurysm Screening Study Group, Screening men for abdominal aortic aneurysm: 10 year mortality and cost effectiveness results from the randomised Multicentre Aneurysm Screening Study, *BMJ* 2009; 338: b2307.

Lindholt JS, Sørensen J, Søgaard R and Henneberg EW. Long-term benefit and cost-effectiveness analysis of screening for abdominal aortic aneurysms from a randomized controlled trial, *Br J Surg* 2010; 97; 826–834.

Norman PE, Jamrozik K, Lawrence-Brown MM, Le MT *et al.* Population based randomised controlled trial on impact of screening on mortality from abdominal aortic aneurysm, *BMJ* 2004;329; 1259.

Harris RP, Helfand M, Woolf SH, Lohr KN, et al. Current methods of the US Preventive Services Task Force: a review of the process. *Am J Prev Med.* 2001;20:21-35.

Takagi H, Goto SN, Matsui M, Manabe H, Umemoto T. A further meta-analysis of population-based screening for abdominal aortic aneurysm. *J Vasc Surg.* 2010; 52:1103-8.

Scott RAP, Wilson NM, Ashton HA, Kay DN. Influence of screening on the incidence of ruptured abdominal aortic aneurysm: 5-year results of a randomised controlled study. *Br J Surg* 1995; 82: 1066–70.

Ashton HA, Gao L, Kim LG, Druce PS, et al. Fifteen-year follow-up of a randomized clinical trial of ultrasonographic screening for abdominal aortic aneurysms. *Br J Surg*. 2007;94:696–701.

Heather BP, Poskitt KR, Earnshaw JJ, Whyman M, Shaw E. Population screening reduces mortality rate from aortic aneurysm in men. *Br J Surg*. 2000;87:750-3.

Lindholt JS, Vammen S, Juul S, Henneberg EW, Fasting H. The validity of ultrasonographic scanning as screening method for abdominal aortic aneurysm. *Eur J Vasc Endovasc Surg* 1999; 17:472–475.

Lindholt JS, Juul S, Fasting H, Henneberg EW. Screening for abdominal aortic aneurysms: single centre randomised controlled trial. *BMJ* 2005; 330:750.

Lindholt JS, Norman P. Response to comment on "Screening for abdominal aortic aneurysm and overall mortality in men". *Eur J Vasc Endovasc Surg* 2008;36:621-622.

The Multicentre Aneurysm Screening Study Group. The Multicentre Aneurysm Screening Study (MASS) into the effect of abdominal aortic aneurysm screening on mortality in men: a randomised controlled trial *Lancet* 2002; 360: 1531–39

Kim LG, P Scott RA, Ashton HA, Thompson SG. et al. A sustained mortality benefit from screening for abdominal aortic aneurysm. *Ann Intern Med*. 2007;146:699–706.

Cosford PA, Leng GC. Screening for abdominal aortic aneurysm. *Cochrane Database Syst Rev*. 2007; (2):CD002945.

Lindholt JS, Norman P. Screening for abdominal aortic aneurysm reduces overall mortality in men. *Eur J Vasc Endovasc Surg*. 2008;36:167–171.

Lederle FA. Comment on "Screening for abdominal aortic aneurysm reduces overall mortality in men.". *Eur J Vasc Endovasc Surg*. 2008;36:620–621.

Rawlins MD, Culyer AJ. National Institute for Clinical Excellence and its value judgments. BMJ 2004; 329:224-7.

Fleming C, Whitlock EP, Beil TL, Lederle FA. Screening for Abdominal Aortic Aneurysm: A Best Evidence Systematic Review for the U.S. *Ann Intern Med*. 2005;142:203-211.

Scott RA, Bridgewater SG, Ashton HA.Randomized clinical trial of screening for abdominal aortic aneurysm in women. *Br J Surg*. 2002; 89:283-5.

Derubertis BG, Trocciola SM, Ryer EJ, Pieracci FM, et al. Abdominal aortic aneurysm in women: prevalence, risk factors, and implications for screening. *J Vasc Surg*. 2007; 46: 630-635.

Solberg S, Singh K, Wilsgaard T, Jacobsen BK. Increased growth rate of abdominal aortic aneurysms in women. The Tromso study. *Eur J Vasc Endovasc Surg*. 2005; 29: 145–149.

Norman PE, Castleden WM, Hockey RL. Prevalence of abdominal aortic aneurysm in Western Australia. *Br J Surg*. 1991; 78: 1118–1121.

Mofidi R, Suttie SA, Howd A, Dawson AR, Griffiths GD, Stonebridge PA. Outcome from abdominal aortic aneurysms in Scotland, 1991-2006. *Br J Surg*. 2008; 95:1475-9.

United Kingdom Small Aneurysm Trial Participants. Long-term outcomes of immediate repair compared with surveillance of small abdominal aortic aneurysms. *Lancet* 1998;352: 1649-55.

Brown LC, Powell JT. Risk factors for aneurysm rupture in patients kept under ultrasound surveillance. UK Small Aneurysm Trial Participants. *Ann Surg.* 1999; 230:289-96

Heller JA, Weinberg A, Arons R, Krishnasastry KV, et al. Two decades of abdominal aortic aneurysm repair: have we made any progress? *J Vasc Surg.* 2000; 32: 1091- 1100.

Dueck AD, Johnston KW, Alter D, Laupacis A, Kucey DS. Predictors of repair and effect of gender on treatment of ruptured abdominal aortic aneurysm. *J Vasc Surg.* 2004; 39:784-7.

Dimick JB, Stanley JC, Axelrod DA, Kazmers A, et al. Variation in death rate after abdominal aortic aneurysmectomy in the United States: impact of hospital volume, gender, and age. *Ann Surg.* 2002;235:579-85.

Semmens JB, Norman PE, Lawrence-Brown MM, Holman CD. Influence of gender on outcome from ruptured abdominal aortic aneurysm. *Br J Surg.* 2000;87:191-4.

McPhee JT, Hill JS, Eslami MH. The impact of gender on presentation, therapy, and mortality of abdominal aortic aneurysm in the United States, 2001-2004. *J Vasc Surg.* 2007; 45:891-9.

Mofidi R, Goldie VJ, Dawson ARW, Murie JA, Chalmers RTA. The influence of gender on the growth rate of abdominal aortic aneurysms. *Br J Surg.* 2007; 94: 310-314.

Norman PE, Semmens JB, Lawrence-Brown MM, Holman CD. Long term relative survival after surgery for abdominal aortic aneurysm in western Australia: population based study. *BMJ.* 1998; 317: 852-6.

Akkersdijk GJ, Prinssen M, Blankensteijn JD. The impact of endovascular treatment on in-hospital mortality following non-ruptured AAA repair over a decade: a population based study of 16,446 patients. *Eur J Vasc Endovasc Surg.* 2004; 28:41-6.

Wanhainen A, Lundkvist J, Bergqvist D, Bjorck M. Cost-effectiveness of screening women for abdominal aortic aneurysm, *J Vasc Surg.* 2006; 43:908–914.

Ouriel K. Treating Smaller Aneurysms: is there a rationale? Advanced Endovascular Therapy of Aortic Disease. Blackwell Publishing, London 2007: 171-180.

Powell JT, Brown LC, Forbes JF, Fowkes FG, et al. Final 12-year follow-up of surgery versus surveillance in the UK Small Aneurysm Trial. *Br J Surg.* 2007; 94:702-8.

Lederle FA, Wilson SE, Johnson GR, Reinke DB, et al. Immediate repair compared with surveillance of small abdominal aortic aneurysms. *New England Journal of Medicine* 2002;346:1437-44.

Ouriel K, Clair DG, Kent KC, Zarins CK; (PIVOTAL) Investigators. Endovascular repair compared with surveillance for patients with small abdominal aortic aneurysms. *J Vasc Surg.* 2010; 51:1081-7.

Cao P; DeRango P, Verzini F, Parlani G et al. Comparison of surveillance vs Aortic Endografting for Small Aneurysm Repair . *Eur J Vasc Endovasc Surg.* 2011; 41: 13-25.

Ouriel K, Srivastava SD, Sarac TP, O'hara PJ, et al. Disparate outcome after endovascular treatment of small versus large abdominal aortic aneurysm. *J Vasc Surg.* 2003;37:1206-12.

Thomas SM, Beard JD, Ireland M, Ayers S, et al. Results from the Prospective Registry of Endovascular Treatment of Abdominal Aortic Aneurysms (RETA): mid term results to five years. *Eur J Vasc Endovasc Surg* 2005; 29: 563–70.

Vallabhaneni SR, Harris PL. Lessons learnt from the EUROSTAR registry on endovascular repair of abdominal aortic aneurysm.*Eur J Radiol* 2001; 39: 34–41.

Blankensteijn JD, de Jong SECA, Prinssen M, van der Ham AC, et al. Two-Year Outcomes after Conventional or Endovascular Repair of Abdominal Aortic Aneurysms. *N Engl J Med* 2005;352:2398-405.

De Bruin JL, Baas AF, Buth J, Prinssen M, et al. Long-term outcome of open or endovascular repair of abdominal aortic aneurysm. *N Engl J Med.* 2010; 362:1881-9.

EVAR trial participants. Endovascular aneurysm repair versus open repair in patients with abdominal aortic aneurysm (EVAR trial 1).*Lancet* 2005; 365: 2179-86.

Becquemin JP, Pillet JC, Lescalie F, Sapoval M, et al; ACE trialists. A randomized controlled trial of endovascular aneurysm repair versus open surgery for abdominal aortic aneurysms in low- to moderate-risk patients. *J Vasc Surg.* 2011;53(5):1167-1173.

Lederle FA, Freischlag JA, Kyriakides TC, et. al. Outcome following endovascular vs open repair of abdominal aortic aneurysm: a randomised trial. *JAMA* 2009; 302: 1535-42.

EVAR trial participants. Endovascular aneurysm repair and outcome in patients unfit for open repair of abdominal aortic aneurysm (EVAR trial 2). *Lancet* 2005; 365: 2187–92.

Golledge J, Powell JT. Medical management of abdominal aortic aneurysm. *Eur J Vasc Endovasc Surg.* 2007; 34: 267-73.

Miyake T, Morishita R. Pharmacological treatment of abdominal aortic aneurysm. *Cardiovasc Res.* 2009; 83(3):436-43.

Baxter BT, Terrin MC, Dalman RL. Medical Management of Abdominal Aortic Aneurysm. *Circulation* 2008; 117: 1883-9.

Heart Protection Study Collaborative Group. Lancet 2002; 360: 7-22.

McNally MM, Agle SC, Parker FM, Bogey WM, et al. Preoperative statin therapy is associated with improved outcomes and resource utilization in patients undergoing aortic aneurysm repair.*J Vasc Surg* 2010:51;1390-6.

Kertai MD, Boersma E, Westerhout CM, van Domburg R, et al. Association between long-term statin use and mortality after successful abdominal aortic aneurysm surgery. *Am J Med* 2004; 116:96-103.

Leurs LJ, Visser P, Laheij RJ, Buth J, et al. Statin use is associated with reduced all-cause mortality after endovascular abdominal aortic aneurysm repair. *Vascular* 2006; 14; 1-8.

Kapoor AS, Kanji H, Buckingham J, Devereaux PJ, et al. Strength of evidence for perioperative use of statins to reduce cardiovascular risk: systematic review of controlled studies. *BMJ* 2006; 333:1149-1152.

Evans J, Powell JT, Schwalbe E, Loftus IM, Thompson MM. Simvastatin Attenuates the activity of matrix metalloprotease-9 in aneurysmal aortic tissue. *Eur J Vasc Endovasc Surg.* 2007; 34: 302–303.

Schouten O, van Laanen JH, Boersma E, Vidakovic R, et al. Statins are associated with a reduced infrarenal abdominal aortic aneurysm growth. *Eur J Vasc Endovasc Surg.* 2006; 32: 21–26.

Sukhija R, Aronow WS, Sandhu R, Kakar P, Babu S. Mortality and size of abdominal aortic aneurysm at long-term follow-up of patients not treated surgically and treated with and without statins. *Am J Cardiol.* 2006; 97: 279–280.

Schlösser FJ, Tangelder MJ, Verhagen HJ, van der Heijden GJ, et al. Growth predictors and prognosis of small abdominal aortic aneurysms. *J Vasc Surg.* 2008; 47:1127-1133.

EVAR-2 trial participants. Does aneurysm rupture risk decrease in patients who are anatomically suitable for endovascular repair. Br J Surg 2008; 95 (S1): 10

Lindholt JS, Henneberg EW, Juul S, Fasting H. Impaired results of a randomised double blinded clinical trial of propranolol versus placebo on the expansion rate of small abdominal aortic aneurysms. *Int Angiol.* 1999; 18: 52–57.

Propranolol for small abdominal aortic aneurysms: results of a randomized trial. *J Vasc Surg.* 2002; 35: 72–79.

Mangano DT, Layug EL, Wallace A, Tateo I. Effect of atenolol on mortality and cardiovascular morbidity after noncardiac surgery. Multicenter Study of Perioperative Ischemia Research Group.*N Engl J Med.* 1996; 335(23):1713-20.

Poldermans D, Boersma E, Bax JJ, Thomson IR, et al. The effect of bisoprolol on perioperative mortality and myocardial infarction in high-risk patients undergoing vascular surgery. Dutch Echocardiographic Cardiac Risk Evaluation Applying Stress Echocardiography Study Group. *N Engl J Med.* 1999; 341(24):1789-94.

POISE Study Group. Effects of extended-release metoprolol succinate in patients undergoing non-cardiac surgery (POISE trial): a randomised controlled trial. *Lancet* 2008; 371(9627):1839-47.

Yang H, Raymer K, Butler R, Parlow J, et al. The effects of perioperative beta-blockade: results of the Metoprolol after Vascular Surgery study, a randomized controlled trial. *Am Heart J.* 2006; 152:983-90.

Fleisher LA, Beckman JA, Brown KA, Calkins H, Chaikof E et al. ACC/AHA 2006 guideline update on perioperative cardiovascular evaluation for noncardiac surgery: focused update on perioperative beta-blocker therapy. *Circulation*2009;120: e169-e276.

Hackam DG, Thiruchelvam D, Redelmeier DA. Angiotensin-converting enzyme inhibitors and aortic rupture: a population-based case-control study. *Lancet.* 2006; 368: 659–665.

Thompson A, Cooper JA, Fabricius M, Humphries SE, et al. An analysis of drug modulation of abdominal aortic aneurysm growth through 25 years of surveillance. *J Vasc Surg.* 2010.52; 55-61.

Sweeting MJ, Thompson SG, Brown LC, Greenhalgh RM, et al. Use of angiotensin converting enzyme inhibitors is associated with increased growth rate of abdominal aortic aneurysms. *J Vasc Surg.* 2010; 52:1-4.

Brady AR, Thompson SG, Fowkes FG, Greenhalgh RM, Powell JT; et al Abdominal aortic aneurysm expansion: risk factors and time intervals for surveillance. *Circulation* 2004; 110:16-21.

Lindholt JS, Ashton HA, Scott RA. Indicators of infection with Chlamydia pneumoniae are associated with expansion of abdominal aortic aneurysms. *J Vasc Surg.* 2001; 34: 212–215.

Nieto FJ. Infective agents and cardiovascular disease. *Semin Vasc Med.* 2002; 2: 401–415.

Mosorin M, Juvonen J, Biancari F, Satta J, et al. Use of doxycycline to decrease the growth rate of abdominal aortic aneurysms: a randomized, double-blind, placebo- controlled pilot study. *J Vasc Surg.* 2001; 34: 606–610.

Vammen S, Lindholt JS, Ostergaard L, Fasting H, Henneberg EW. Randomized double-blind controlled trial of roxithromycin for prevention of abdominal aortic aneurysm expansion. *Br J Surg.* 2001; 88: 1066–1072.

Baxter BT, Pearce WH, Waltke EA, Littooy FN, et al. Prolonged administration of doxycycline in patients with small asymptomatic abdominal aortic aneurysms: report of a prospective multicenter study. *J Vasc Surg.* 2002; 36: 1–12.

Petrinec D, Liao S, Holmes DR, Reilly JM, et al. Doxycycline inhibition of aneurysmal degeneration in an elastase-induced rat model of abdominal aortic aneurysm: preservation of aortic elastin associated with suppressed production of 92 kD gelatinase. *J Vasc Surg.* 1996; 23: 336–346.

Curci JA, Mao D, Bohner DG, Allen BT, et al. Preoperative treatment with doxycycline reduces aortic wall expression and activation of matrix metalloproteinases in patients with abdominal aortic aneurysms. *J Vasc Surg.* 2000; 31: 325–342.

3

The Evolution of Aortic Aneurysm Repair: Past Lessons and Future Directions

Ricky Harminder Bhogal and Richard Downing
University of Birmingham & Worcestershire Royal Hospital, United Kingdom

1. Introduction

The history and evolution of aortic aneurysm repair demonstrates an important paradigm within surgery, namely the importance of surgical pioneers and innovators who have strived to achieve technical excellence and improve patient care. It also highlights the wider evolution of surgery from traditional open operative techniques to the modern minimally invasive procedures. The following chapter discusses the surgical innovators and the techniques they have described that have enabled the repair of both thoracic aortic aneurysms (TAA) and abdominal aortic aneurysms (AAA).

Aortic aneurysms represent a significant health risk particularly for the elderly population. AAA is the 14th-leading cause of death for the 60- to 85-year-old age group in the United States (10.8 deaths per 100,000 population). TAA by contrast is less frequent with an incidence of 10.4 per 100,000. Both AAA and TAA are known to increase in prevalence with advancing age and have an increased prevalence in males. The risk of aneurysm rupture increases with increasing aneurysm diameter over 5.5-6.0 cm and is the primary indication for the repair of both TAA and AAA. Therefore surgery to repair both AAA and TAA is either pre-emptive to prevent rupture or emergent to repair a rupture. Repair of TAA and AAA by either open or minimally invasive techniques significantly reduces the risk of rupture and improves patient mortality. The establishment of these techniques has required the development of procedures from embryonic thoughts in the minds of the surgeons of antiquity through to the utilisation of ever increasing modern technologies.

2. History of aortic aneurysm repair

The Ebers Papyrus of approximately 2000BC describes arterial aneurysms among diseases afflicting the Egyptians albeit the site of the aneurysms is not mentioned. Yet given Egyptian embalmers reluctance to open body cavities it is likely that the aneurysms were evident upon the external surface of the body. There is no convincing evidence to suggest that the ancient Egyptians attempted aneurysm repair, although it was advised "to treat it with a knife and burn it with a fire so that it bleeds not too much" (Thompson, 1998). Unlike atherosclerosis, no aneurysms have been found in Egyptian mummies.

The most important surgeon with respect to aortic aneurysm surgery in antiquity is the third century Greek surgeon, Antyllus, who should rightly be regarded as the 'Father of Aneurysm Surgery' if not vascular surgery as a whole. Indeed he has been described as a 'comet on the surgical horizon' for his pioneering work on aneurysm repair (Major, 1954). This innovative surgeon attempted surgical repair of abdominal aortic aneurysm which has led to the term the Antyllus method; ligation of the artery above and below an aneurysm, followed by incision into and emptying of the sac. Antyllus was also the first to recognize two forms of aneurysm. The developmental type caused by dilation, which pertains to this chapter, and those which follow arterial trauma. He also created a taxonomy related to an aneurysm's potential for rupture. Much of Antyllus's remarkable pioneering work and his surgical methods of aneurysmal repair would have been lost to history were it not for the writings of the Greek medical writer and physician Oribasius. It is clear that Antyllus also developed specific instructions for a number of operations including hydrocele repair and cataract surgery. He also listed the indications and contraindications for surgery and described the complications that could arise from the operations. In large part, Antyllus's operation for aneurysm remained the standard procedure until the 19th century thereby illustrating his surgical genius.

Antyllus's contribution toward the development of modern vascular surgery cannot be overstated. Indeed he should be held in the same regard as the dominant figure of Greek medicine, Galen who also described traumatic aneurysms and noted that rupture could be forestalled in some circumstances by external compression. Galen, the physician to the Roman gladiators, would have treated traumatic aneurysms following venesection in the cubital fossa- lesions which were easier to observe than AAA and TAA. Taken together, the work of Antyllus and Galen established the foundations for future surgeons to develop the techniques required for successful aortic aneurysm surgery and repair.

In the fifth century AD the Byzantine physician Aëtius of Amida described a now well-established principle of operative treatment of aneurysms in which proximal arterial control is followed by ligature from within the aneurysm of the orifices of inflow and outflow vessels, thus building upon Antyllus's method. In addition he described the clinical signs of aneurysms mentioning that they can occur in any part of the body including the head.

Unfortunately, there again followed a long hiatus in the history of aortic aneurysm repair. The next significant contribution was in 1452 by the French physician Jean Francois Fernel who observed that aneurysms could occur in the chest, adjacent to the spleen and within the mesentery of the bowel. It is not clear whether Fernel was referring to thoracic aneurysms at this stage. Andreas Vesalius offered the first clinical description of an aneurysm of the abdominal aorta, while his 16th century contemporary Ambroise Pare stated that arterial wall degeneration can be caused by syphilis, that aneurysms may thrombose and that injudicious incision of an inflamed pulsatile mass may cause exsanguinating haemorrhage.

The English physicians and brothers William and John Hunter portrayed a unique experimental and clinical genius rarely present in late 18th century medicine. They made significant advances in both the physiology and surgical repair of blood vessels and pioneered the treatment of peripheral aneurysms. Indeed their important contributions to vascular surgery have prevailed until today while their studies of aneurysm formation, pathology and treatment laid the foundation for modern aneurysm repair. John Hunter developed a successful operation for popliteal aneurysm based on his meticulous laboratory investigations on collateral blood flow which led to a more logical approach to these lesions with improved proximal arterial occlusion by ligature.

One of John Hunter's pupils, the English surgeon and anatomist Astley Cooper, applied Hunterian principles for ligation of aneurysms of common carotid and internal and external iliac artery aneurysms. In 1817 he was the first surgeon to ligate the abdominal aorta proximal to a leaking left iliac artery aneurysm.

The early 20th century saw an explosion in numerous novel attempts to repair and halt the inexorable growth of aneurysms in the decades before the development of modern vascular surgical techniques. Yet, despite extensive research and application of experimental techniques AAA repair remained unsuccessful until 1923 when the American surgeon Rudolph Matas renovated the approach of Antyllus and Aëtius of Amida and carried out endoaneurysmal ligature of peripheral aneurysms. The approach spared collaterals around the aneurysmal sac. Matas also first proposed the concept of endoaneurysmorrhaphy and performed the first successful aortic ligation on a human. The Canadian physician William Osler called him the 'Father of Vascular Surgery' but perhaps this would be better reserved for Antyllus. Other novel techniques for AAA repair included arterial walls that were scarified with talc, wrapped in polythene or cellophane or filled with meters of wire to which a galvanic current could be applied. Notably Albert Einstein was operated upon by Rudolf Nissen in 1949 using the polythene/cellophane technique, and survived six years after the operation when the aneurysm ruptured.

The 1950's was the decade which heralded the modern era of aortic aneurysm surgery. In 1951, Lam and Aram reported the first successful repair of a thoracic aortic aneurysm while in the same year the first successful AAA resection with allograft reconstruction was reported by Charles Dubost in Paris (Dubost C et al, 1951). In 1953 Bahnson reported a series of saccular aneurysms repaired using a technique of lateral resection with primary suture (Bahnson, 1953). The development of treatment modalities for thoracic aneurysms followed successful treatment of AAA almost akin to a domino effect. Most of the initial successful repairs involved the use of preserved aortic allografts, thus triggering the establishment of numerous aortic allograft banks. Simultaneously, Gross and colleagues successfully used allografts to treat complex thoracic aortic coarctations, including those with aneurysmal involvement (Gross et al, 1948). Ascending aortic replacement required the development of cardiopulmonary bypass and was first performed in 1956 by the American surgeons Cooley and DeBakey (Cooley & DeBakey, 1957). They successfully replaced the ascending aorta with an aortic allograft. Successful replacement of the aortic arch with its inherent risk of cerebral ischaemia was understandably more challenging and was not reported until 1957 again by DeBakey *et al* (DeBakey et al, 1957). Although the use of aortic allografts as aortic replacement was widely accepted in the early 1950s, the search for synthetic substitutes was well underway prompted by the inevitable aneurysmal degeneration of such allografts. The synthetic material Dacron was introduced by DeBakey and by 1955, Deterling and Bhonslay believed that Dacron was the best material for aortic substitution (Deterling & Bhonslay, 1955), a conclusion which pertains to the present time.

Finally, in 1966, Oscar Creech, a pupil of Rudolf Matas, emphasized the virtues of intra-saccular graft interposition now universally used for open aortic aneurysmal repair. Following in the footsteps of the ancient pioneering surgeons, later surgeons have developed the techniques of both open and minimally invasive aortic aneurysm repair.

3. Open repair of abdominal aortic aneurysm

3.1 Open AAA repair

The advances dating from Antyllus through to Oscar Creech led to the development of a standard operative procedure to repair AAA. More recently, non-invasive screening

programs and a dramatic rise in the elderly population have led to an increased incidence of asymptomatic AAA. Despite adopting an aggressive surgical posture toward elective repair of AAA the incidence of ruptured AAA has continued to increase. Annually 35 000 to 40 000 aneurysms are repaired in the United States. AAAs are conventionally defined as a ≥50% increase in aortic diameter compared with the normal proximal aorta. Indications for surgical replacement of aneurysms are determined by weighing the risk of rupture against the surgical morbidity and mortality rates. Repair is generally indicated when the diameter of the aneurysm exceeds 5.5 cm (Lederle et al 2002), the annual expansion rate exceeds 1 cm per year or when the aortic aneurysm becomes symptomatic.
Comprehensive radiological imaging forms the basis of planning open AAA repair. Figure 1 shows the typical appearance of an AAA on transverse computed tomography (CT).

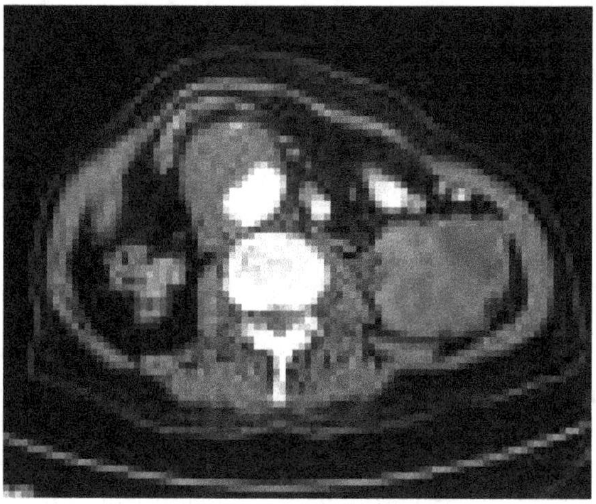

Fig. 1. Typical appearance of a fusiform AAA as seen on transverse CT. The aneurysm contains thrombus with radio-contrast seen within the lumen.

CT defines the aneurysm in terms of morphology, either fusiform or saccular, but more importantly defines the anatomy of the aneurysm neck. Ninety five per cent of AAA are infra-renal, ie. the neck of the aneurysm originates below the origin of the renal arteries and thus aneurysm replacement is associated with fewer post-operative complications when compared to supra-renal AAA replacement when the aneurysm neck originates above the renal arteries (see below). Aneurysms that involve the descending thoracic and abdominal components of the aorta can be described by the Crawford classification (Table 1). This classification is of practical use when considering intervention, for example, in choosing the extent of the incision and planning implantation. For instance a laparotomy will often suffice for repair of a type IV aneurysm whilst a thoraco-laparotomy is required for a type II aneurysm.
Open aneurysm repair using homografts and subsequently Dacron has successfully been employed to prevent rupture since the 1950s. Since Matas's original description of the surgical repair of AAA the operation has evolved to be applied in both the elective and emergency setting. The open surgical approach in the modern era is performed either via a trans-peritoneal or retroperitoneal exposure to obtain proximal and distal aortic control using vascular clamps (Figure 2).

Type	Proximal Extent	Distal Extent
I	Left subclavian artery	Visceral Aorta (usually suprarenal)
II	Left subclavian artery	Infrarenal aorta
III	Mid-thoracic aorta	Infrarenal aorta
IV	Diaphragm	Infrarenal aorta
V	Mid-thoracic aorta	Visceral aorta (usually suprarenal)

Table 1. Crawford classification of thoraco-abdominal aneurysms.

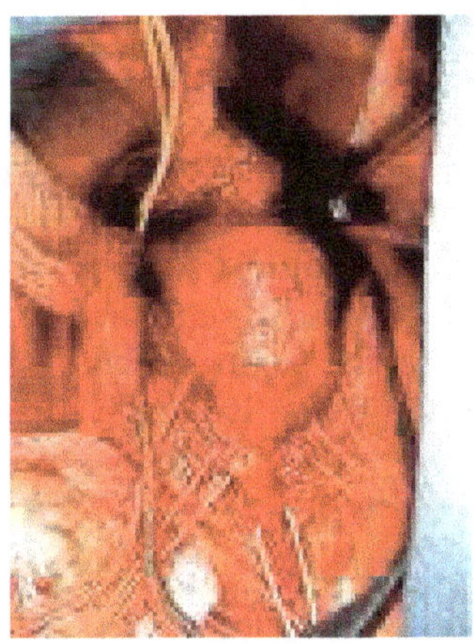

Fig. 2. An infrarenal AAA during surgical repair. A typical infra-renal AAA is seen with placement of a clamp to establish proximal aortic control. The iliac vessels have been controlled with vascular sloops to be clamped to achieve distal aortic control.

Intravenous heparin is administered, the aneurysm sac opened and back-bleeding branch arteries (lumbar and inferior mesenteric) are ligated. A prosthetic graft, usually made of Dacron, is sutured to the proximal aorta and the aorta proximal to the bifurcation (Figure 3).

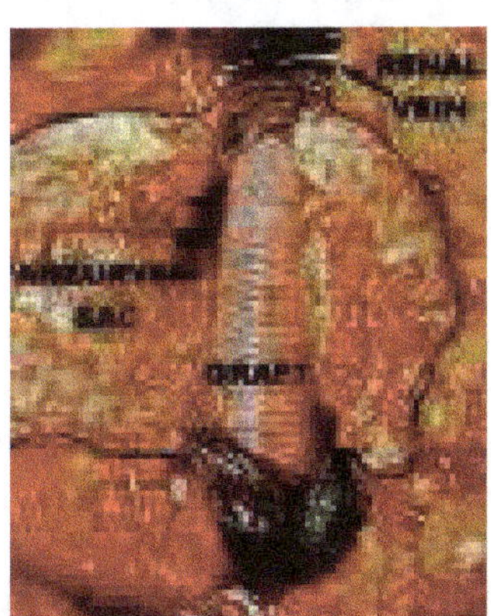

Fig. 3. An orthotopic Dacron graft has been sutured to replace the AAA.

Demonstrates the satisfactory position of a Dacron graft sutured into the original site of the AAA.

If the AAA is aorto-iliac ie. the iliac arteries are also aneurysmal a bifurcated graft or 'Y-graft' is used and sutured to the iliac segments usually at the iliac bifurcation. Flow is restored to the lower extremities and the aneurysm sac closed over the synthetic graft. Although effective and durable in treating AAA and preventing rupture the operation has been associated with mortality rates of >4% since the 1980s although in large volume units, rates of 1-2% are now reported. This has provided the impetus for the development of minimally invasive or endovascular techniques. However, traditional open aneurysm repair may still be considered superior to endovascular repair (EVAR) because it provides secure fixation at all anastomotic sites, ligation of all lumbar branches and other aortic branches with virtual elimination of the possibility of endoleaks associated with EVAR (see below). In addition, open AAA repair offers complete treatment of aneurysmal disease with obliteration of the aneurysmal sac and debridement of its clot and atheromatous debris and most importantly is of proven durability. Of all the technical advantages of open repair, secure fixation at all anastomoses is probably the most important. Many authors submit that suture fixation with continuous polypropylene is superior to metallic barbs, hooks, and struts that are part of the current generation of EVAR devices (Clagett, 2008). Also it remains to be determined whether endostaplers, used during EVAR to provide aortic fixation, will adequately penetrate the diseased aneurysmal aortic wall. Hence, open repair still has a prominent role in the surgical treatment of aortic aneurysmal disease.

3.2 Complex open AAA repairs

Five per cent of AAAs are supra-renal where the aneurysm neck originates at any point above the origin of the renal arteries. Most infra-renal AAAs can be repaired safely under infra-renal aortic cross-clamping using the technique detailed above (Figure 2). However, juxtarenal (ie. an infrarenal neck inadequate for clamp placement) and suprarenal AAA's necessitate control of the aorta using suprarenal, inter-visceral, or supra-celiac aortic clamps. The procedure for repair remains essentially the same with suturing of a Dacron graft to the proximal and distal aorta following exclusion of the aneurysm but may necessitate mesenteric and/or renal arterial implantation into the graft. Anecdotal evidence suggests that inappropriate infra-renal clamping may cause renal embolization and a higher incidence of para-anastomotic pseudoaneurysms. Supra-renal clamping induces the risk of renal and gastrointestinal complications. Clamping between the renal arteries and the superior mesenteric artery (SMA) is associated with a disturbingly high rate of complications and should be avoided (Crawford et al, 1986). However, supra-celiac clamping avoids the need for retraction and manipulation of large aneurysms and may reduce the risk of embolization during dissection. In a study by Green and colleagues, patients whose aortas were clamped immediately above the renal arteries had higher peri-operative mortality rates and a higher incidence of renal failure requiring dialysis than did patients whose aortas were clamped at the supra-celiac or infra-renal level (Green et al, 1989). However, some researchers have noted no differences in mortality rates with regard to the site of aortic clamping and comparable or even favourable cardiac morbidity rates with more proximal clamping (El-Sabrout & Reul, 2001.). Direct comparison of early mortality after supra-renal and supra-celiac clamping with infra-renal clamping appeared to reveal a strikingly higher mortality rate after supra-renal and supra-celiac clamping. However, in-depth analysis reveals that most patients in the supra-renal and supra-coelic group had considerably more risk factors and underwent more extensive procedures than did those in the infra-renal group (Green et al, 1989). Myocardial infarction or congestive heart failure in the early post-operative period developed more often after supra-renal and supra-coelic clamping than after infra-renal clamping and was associated with a higher patient mortality. In a study by Sasaki *et al*, post-operative renal dysfunction developed in 50% of patients after bilateral supra-renal clamping, in comparison with only 8.4% after infra-renal clamping (Sasaki et al, 2000). Other authors have reported that the rates of transient postoperative renal dysfunction after elective supra-renal and supra-coeliac clamping was 12.6% as opposed to 3.35% after infra-renal clamping (Barratt et al, 2000). Importantly, chronic renal failure is a rare complication of openAAA repair.

3.3 Complications of open AAA repairs

Complications which may follow open AAA repair include not only cardiac and respiratory dysfunction but also visceral ischaemia/ischaemic colitis, trash foot, aorto-enteric fistula, sexual dysfunction, persistent chronic peri-aortitis and acute renal failure.

In 1974 Willard *et al* reported in a series of 6100 patients an incidence of visceral ischaemia and/or infarction of 1.5% (Willard et al, 1974). Such early studies advocated the re-implantation of the inferior mesenteric artery (IMA). The incidence of this complication has changed little over the decades but selective IMA re-implantation is now preferred if there is evidence or suspicion of colonic ischaemia.

Acute lower limb ischaemia following aortic surgery is commonly termed 'trash foot', an unwelcome complication that is associated with a high morbidity and mortality.

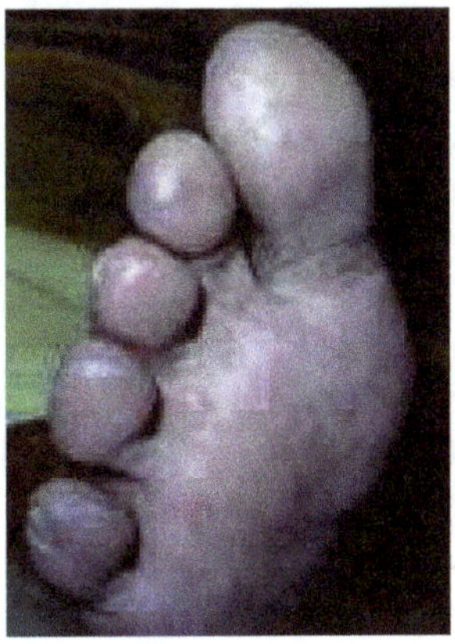

Fig. 4. The typical appearance of a trash foot following open AAA repair. The aetiology remains uncertain. Embolectomy may be required to restore limb perfusion.

The exact cause of the ischaemia remains uncertain, but it has been attributed to either athero-emboli from native arteries, thrombo-emboli from the prosthetic graft or thrombosis of small vessels in the distal arterial tree. It's reported incidence is 1.4% for open AAA repairs and may result in early or delayed amputation of digits or limb (Kuhan et al, 1997). The 30-day mortality can be as high as 25%. Attempts to reduce the incidence involve early mobilization and clamping of the iliac arteries, and irrigation of the aortic anastomosis and graft with heparin saline solution (Kuhan et al, 1997).

Aorto-enteric fistulas (AEF) are abnormal communications between the aorta and the intestine. It may occur after previous aortic aneurysm surgery with the duodenum as the most frequent site of fistulation (Saers et al, 2005). Presentation of AEFs is usually with massive gastrointestinal haemorrhage with or without associated aortic or graft sepsis. AEFs are difficult to diagnose with a high an index of suspicion needed in patients with previous aortic aneurysm surgery. If not treated promptly, AEFs are fatal (Voorhoeve et al 1996; Song Y et al 2008). Surgery offers the only definitive treatment. The favoured technique involves aortic debridement, repair of the intestinal defect and *in situ* aortic replacement which remains a high risk procedure with an operative mortality of 30-40%. Extra-anatomic bypass is performed in patients with extensive local sepsis and is associated with an even higher mortality (Song Y et al, 2008). Endovascular techniques can achieve rapid control of bleeding associated with AEFs and avoid intervention in a hostile abdomen, while eliminating the complications associated with open surgery. However, placing new prosthetic material in an infected field may be hazardous. A recent review found that 44% of such patients developed recurrent graft infection; this complication was more likely in patients who had evidence of sepsis pre-operatively and resulted in a higher 30-day and overall mortality; importantly life-long antibiotic therapy did not reduce recurrent sepsis (Antiniou et al, 2009). Hence AEFs require multi-modal and multi-disciplinary management to optimise patient outcome.

Surgical treatment of AAA's is appreciated to adversely affect sexual function, with the incumbent negative impacts upon the quality of life. The reported level of sexual dysfunction after open AAA repair is 30% (Jimenez et al, 2004). Moreover, the incidence rises during the first post-operative year. Of course, patients with aortic aneurysms have atherosclerosis in other regions of the vascular tree and often have pre-existing sexual dysfunction. After AAA repair patients undergoing open repair report a greater magnitude of sexual dysfunction when compared to those undergoing EVAR (Prissen et al, 2004). Importantly EVAR and open elective AAA repair both have an impact on sexual function in the early postoperative period but EVAR appears to offer improved sexual function over the longer term (Jimenez et al, 2004).

As with any prosthetic material, Dacron, can become infected and result in an inflamed aorta/graft termed chronic peri-aortitis. This process can result in peri-aortic fibrosis and/or ureteral obstruction. Diagnosis involves clinical and radiological findings allied to blood inflammatory markers while treatment involves surgical intervention. However fibrosis and/or ureteral obstruction may recur (van Bommel et al, 2008).

The incidence of acute renal failure following complex AAA repair is discussed in detail above. Recent studies report the incidence of acute renal failure as approximately 10% (Kim GS et al, 2011). Despite this incidence the number of patients requiring dialysis after AAA repair remains low. However the reduction in relative incidence of acute renal failure after AAA repair using EVAR is a definite advantage of the minimally invasive approach. In a large cohort study by Wald *et al* the incidence of acute renal failure was reported as 6.7% (Wald et al, 2006). However EVAR was associated with lower odds of acute renal failure and acute renal failure requiring dialysis.

A recent study has shown that patient mortality after open AAA repair is most closely correlated with surgeon rather than institutional case volume (McPhee et al, 2011).

4. Open descending thoracic aortic aneurysm repair

4.1 Introduction to open TAA repair

Diseases of the thoracic aorta remain among the most lethal of conditions and the most difficult to treat. Not surprisingly, the surgical techniques required to achieve successful TAA repair took longer to develop than those applied to open AAA repair but have evolved significantly during the past 20 years.

The procedure and outcome of ascending TAA repair are discussed within another chapter of the book and will not be considered here. The outcome from open repair of the descending TAA has steadily improved (Svennson et al, 1993). Many factors are responsible including advancements in anaesthesia, improved operative techniques, and advances in critical care. Although open surgical repair of this type of aneurysm once entailed great operative risk, experienced surgical centres now report acceptable surgical mortality and morbidity rates despite the inherent complexity of the repair.

4.2 Surgical technique of open descending TAA repair

Pre-operative assessment forms a key part of patient selection. Identification of pre-existing cardiovascular, pulmonary or renal risk factors enables development of a customised approach to open descending TAA repair. For example, the use of diaphragm-sparing techniques may be particularly helpful in patients with poor pulmonary reserve (Engle et al, 1999). The procedure is performed under general anaesthesia with the patient positioned in the right lateral decubitus position. A cerebrospinal fluid (CSF) catheter is placed in the third or fourth lumbar space to allow CSF drainage and pressure monitoring. The benefits of general hypothermia are well-established and for open descending TAA repair many centres routinely reduce the core body temperature to 32-34°C during surgery. Organ ischaemia remains a major source of morbidity. Moderate systemic heparinisation, permissive hypothermia and sequential aortic clamping are used routinely. The kidneys may be intermittently perfused with cold (4°C) crystalloid to maximise renal hypothermia which affords better protection against acute renal dysfunction. To reduce the risk of peri-operative coagulopathy and bacterial translocation after the aorta is opened adjacent to the visceral branches, separate balloon perfusion catheters may be used to selectively perfuse the coeliac axis and superior mesenteric artery by connection to a left heart bypass (LHB) circuit. Oxygenated blood flows to the abdominal viscera while the intercostal and visceral branches are reattached to the graft substantially reducing mesenteric ischaemic time. After repair of the aneurysm the operative field is rewarmed with warm saline to reverse cooling.

A modified thoraco-abdominal incision is utilised for open descending TAA repair. The incision begins in the abdomen 3 cm below the costal margin and continuing over the sixth rib before curving cephalad just posterior to the tip of the scapula. Following division of the relevant muscular layers the lung is deflated, and the sixth rib is usually excised. The incision is completed by dividing the costal cartilage. The diaphragm is partially incised circumferentially to improve exposure and to avoid traction injury to the phrenic nerve. The pericardium is opened posterior to the phrenic nerve, and the patient given intravenous heparin to reduce the risk of thrombotic complications and to preserve perfusion of the intercostal and lumbar arteries which reduces the risk of spinal cord ischaemia. The left atrium is cannulated through the left pulmonary vein or the left atrial appendage. A pump with an inline heat exchanger is attached to the cannula, and the arterial inflow established through the left femoral artery or the descending thoracic aorta. Distal aortic perfusion is commenced when the cross-clamp is applied. By maintaining distal aortic perfusion during aortic reconstruction, LHB reduces spinal and visceral ischaemic time and prevents many of the complications seen after open AAA repair. Aortic control is established using the familiar proximal and distal paradigm using appropriate vascular clamps. It is vital at this stage to allow the important lower intercostal arteries to be perfused from below during of arterial construction of the proximal anastomosis and decrease the spinal cord ischemic time. This period requires carefully maintenance of normal proximal aortic pressure.

Vascular clamps are placed on the aortic arch between the left common carotid and left subclavian arteries. A vascular clamp is also applied to the left subclavian artery. The aorta is opened longitudinally and divided circumferentially a few centimetres beyond the proximal clamp. The haemodynamic effects of clamping and unclamping the aorta have been investigated since the mid-20th century as these effects are major contributors to the development of post-operative organ dysfunction (see below). Sequential clamping of the aorta remains an effective strategy for reducing ischaemic times. As the aorta is replaced from the proximal to the distal extent of the lesion, the aortic clamp is moved sequentially to lower positions along the graft to restore perfusion to newly reattached branch vessels. After the proximal anastomosis is completed using a non-absorbable continuous suture, the aortic clamp is repositioned onto the graft, flow restored to the left subclavian artery and the remainder of the aneurysm is opened longitudinally. An open distal anastomosis completes the repair.

As an alternative to the "clamp and sew" technique described above, left heart bypass can be used selectively to provide distal aortic perfusion during the repair. In this technique the aorta is opened longitudinally and separated from the oesophagus. Stay sutures are applied to the aneurysm wall, and haemostasis obtained by oversewing any bleeding intercostal or bronchial arteries. Blood salvage is accomplished using a cell-saving device, while blood may be re-infused using a rapid infuser system. The length of aorta that is replaced is dependent upon as assessment of the aneurysm at the time of exploration. Once adequate haemostasis is obtained, an appropriately sized, woven Dacron tube graft is anastomosed to the proximal aorta with a running polypropylene suture. The graft is then cut in a bevelled fashion to accommodate the intercostal arteries. Re-implantation of patent, lower intercostal arteries (T8 through T12) is also performed. The distal anastomosis is completed and the graft flushed. The aortic clamps are slowly removed, and suture lines checked for haemostasis. The patient is weaned from left heart bypass once the rectal or bladder temperature reached 36°C. Protamine is usually administered and the atrial and femoral cannulae removed.

4.3 Complications of open descending TAA repair

Although recent advances in surgical techniques have improved the outcome of open descending TAA repair, significant mortality and morbidity is still encountered. Twenty seven percent of patients experience respiratory complications with prolonged postoperative ventilation (longer than 48 hours) and 11% require tracheostomy. Available data demonstrates that pre-operative renal insufficiency and the extent of the aneurysm are important predictors of respiratory complications (Etz et al, 2007). Paraplegia is the most devastating sequel to TAA repair. Debate still pervades the optimal approach to peri-operative spinal cord protection. Early experimental data showed that aortic clamping increased CSF pressure which is now kept less than 10 mmHg for 3 days postoperatively by appropriate drainage through a CSF catheter. After removal of the drain delayed neurologic deficit should prompt its reintroduction to reduce CSF pressure (Estrera et al, 2003). The use of atrio-femoral bypass may have a protective effect in reducing paraplegia (Svennson et al, 1993). Subsequent to this latter study, other authors have reported encouraging results in reducing paraplegia rates by using only the clamp and sew for open descending TAA repair (Coselli et al, 2004). However, in a recent study involving 347 patients who had undergone descending open TAA repair and were specifically analyzed using propensity score analysis, the authors concluded that left heart bypass did not reduce paraplegia during repair (Coselli et al 2004). Although the overall incidence of paraplegia is low at 2.6%, it can be concluded from the available literature that simple clamp and sew technique can be performed safely with acceptable results. The incidence of acute renal failure after open descending TAA repair is 3-14%. If subsequent dialysis is required, patient mortality may rise to 30-60%. The risk of renal failure also increases if shunting and bypass techniques are not utilised. Aside from the techniques outlined above mannitol may also improve post-operative renal function by increasing renal perfusion and by acting as a free radical scavenger.

A recent meta-analysis by Jonker et al conclusively showed the reduced rates of cardiac complications following minimally invasive TAA repair when compared to open repair. (Jonker et al, 2010). The incidence of myocardial infraction was 11.1% following open repair compared to 3.5% after TEVAR. The reported incidence of stroke after open TAA repair varies between 2-18% (Moon et al, 2007). Again in their systemic review Jonker *et al* showed that the TEVAR reduced the incidence of stroke (4.1% TEVAR versus 10.2% open repair). It is important note that many of these studies have assessed total complications in the particular patient groups and clinically some patients with invariably suffer more than one complication.

5. Aneurysm repair in the modern era

5.1 Minimally invasive aortic aneurysm repair

In accord with the advancements in general surgery, the late 1990's witnessed the pioneering of thorascopic and laparoscopic aortic aneurysm repair. Unfortunately the introduction and advancement of endovascular techniques have overshadowed and perhaps forestalled major development of these surgical approaches. A brief overview follows.

5.2 Thorascopic TAA repair

The premise for the development of thorascopic TAA repair was to minimize surgical trauma and aid improved patient outcome relative to open TAA (Fukada et al, 2002). The use of thoracoscopy in thoracic surgery is known to decrease post-thoracotomy pain and lead to enhanced patient recovery (Dajczman et al, 1991; Kirby et al, 1993). The literature consists of only limited case reports and case series detailing the technique of thorascopic descending TAA repair although the advent of endovascular techniques have impaired the major development of this facet of aortic aneurysm repair, thorascopy have been invaluable for the field of thoracic surgery. Historically thorascopic TAA repair was not attempted in humans over concern of prolonged aortic cross-clamp time necessitated by a minimally invasive procedure. As discussed above, during open descending TAA repair, the duration of the aortic clamp period, intercostal artery reimplantation critical to spinal cord blood flow and the completeness of spinal cord reperfusion are risk factors for paraplegia. However, shortening aortic clamp time and complete reconstruction of the intercostal artery were considered problematic if visualisation were as restricted as the original pioneers of thorascopic TAA repair envisaged. However, the thorascopic approach would certainly reduce patient morbidity, post-thoracotomy pain and ventilatory complications (Dajczman et al, 1991).

As with conventional open and endovascular repairs, preoperative radiological imaging is essential. Contrast CT and Magnetic Resonance Imaging (MRI) may help to prevent post-operative paraplegia by visualizing the spinal artery of Adamkiewicz. The patient is placed in a right lateral decubitus position, as with open repair. The initial insertion site of the thoracoscope in the middle axillary line in the 4th intercostal space. A second thorascopic port is inserted through which a fan retractor is placed at a point 5 cm anterior to the first incision. Under direct thoracoscopic visualization of the TAA a mini-thoracotomy is made in the 7th intercostal space. This incision could be extended according to the location of the aneurysm. The third port placed in the 5th intercostal in the anterior axillary line is used for additional thorascopic views. The posterior surfaces of the aortic necks are dissected by the operator's hand introduced through the mini-thoractomy to avoid injuring the hemi-azgous vein. Umbilical tapes are placed around the aortic necks. Femoro-femoral cardiopulmonary bypass may be used at this stage. Two custom-made vascular cross-clamps are introduced via the first port and a fourth puncture wound made 4 cm anterior to the edge of the mini-thoractomy (Castronuovo et al, 2000). The aortic necks are transected after the placement of a proximal cross-clamp distal to the 9th intercostal space and a distal clamp. Video-assisted graft replacement of the aorta is performed with continuous sutures by conventional instruments. Single re-implantation of the artery of Adakiewicz by use of a side-arm graft can be considered if radiological imaging has been obtained (Yamada et al, 2000). The principal benefits of the technique is that it enables the thoractomy wound to be made smaller by introduction of aortic clamps through puncture wounds, and while enabling a more accurate determination of the intercostal space to be incised by pre-observation of the thoracic cavity using a thoracoscope. However these techniques have not progressed to the establishment of total thorascopic TAA repair.

5.3 Laparoscopic AAA repair

The gold standard in the treatment of AAA remains repair with a prosthetic graft through an open approach (Creech et al, 1966). In the last 10 years EVAR has become an established alternative as a result of low failure rates and reduced mortality in the short term (Brewster et al, 2002; Brewster et al, 2003). However, over longer follow-up, complications following EVAR such as endoleaks, endograft migration, occlusion, and aneurysm rupture (see below) have been reported leading to reintervention rates in the order of 10% to 34% of cases (Verhoeven et al, 2004; Sampram et al, 2003; Becquemin et al, 2004). While EVAR has been gaining widespread popularity, the laparoscopic technique (through either a fully laparoscopic or a laparoscopy-assisted approach) for AAA repair has been under development (Dion et al, 1993; Kline et al, 1998; Cerveira et al, 1999; Edoga et al, 1998). Laparoscopic AAA repair was developed to overcome specific technical challenges during open surgery, such as bowel manipulation, bleeding control, and, mainly, the performance of vascular anastomoses, which might jeopardize the procedure success rate (Kolvenbach et al, 2004; Coggia et al, 2004). In some instances the insertion of a hand inside the insufflated abdominal cavity restores tactile feedback to the surgeon, who is able to locate the aneurysm neck and iliac arteries, thus adding to the visual evaluation of the anatomy and quality of the tissues. The internal hand also compensates for lack of the tri-dimensional vision encountered in laparoscopy.

For total laparoscopic AAA repair the patients the patient is positioned at 45-degree right decubitus position. The abdomen is hyper-extended and draped from the right mid-clavicular line to the left posterior axillary line.

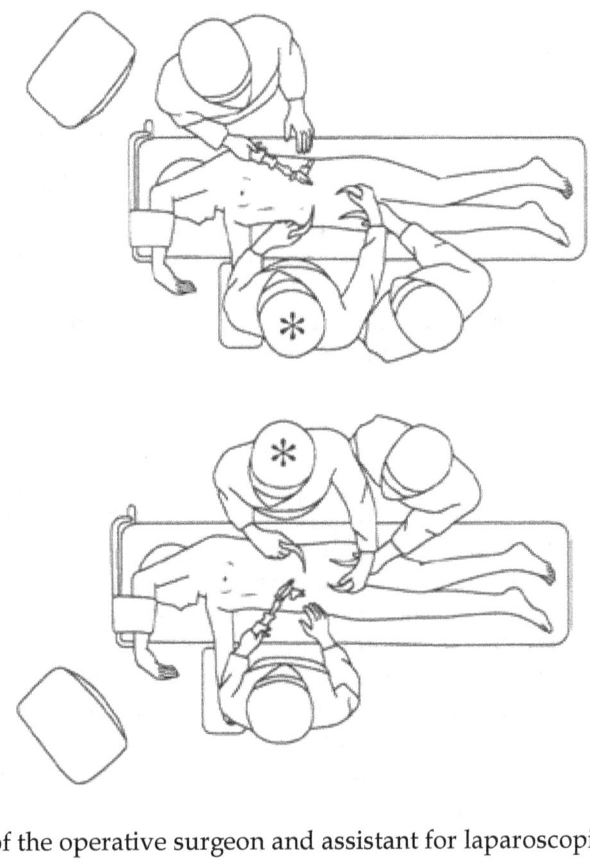

Fig. 5. The position of the operative surgeon and assistant for laparoscopic AAA repair.

Figure 5 demonstrates the position of the operating team at the commencement of the procedure. The patient lies in the semi-decubitus position on the right. The operating surgeon (*) stands on the right of the patient. After retrocolic dissection the operating surgeon (*) stands on the left of the patient (lower panel) to perform endoaneurysmorrhaphy and laparoscopic anastomosis. (Taken from Chiu et al, 2008)

Initially, a sub-umbilical incision is made and a Veress needle inserted into the abdominal cavity to create a carbon dioxide pneumoperitoneum. A laparoscopic port is then inserted. Two additional laparoscopic ports are inserted in the midline above and below the first one port. By using these three ports, the peritoneal cavity is inspected. In hand-assisted laparoscopic AAA repair a midline mini-laparotomy incision of approximately 7-8 cm is first made for insertion of a laparoscopic omni-port-site device. Through the omni-port, the non-dominant hand of the surgeon is introduced into the abdominal cavity without any loss of insufflation. After the mini-laparotomy is performed, a laparoscopic port is placed in the epigastrium. With their non-dominant hand, the surgeon gently pushes bowel loops toward the right side of the abdominal cavity aided by tilting the operating table to the right and in the Trendelenburg position (not exceeding 30°).

Whether total laparoscopic or hand assisted AAA repair is used the initial dissection and mobilisation of the descending and sigmoid colon is carried out. The paracolic gutter is incised to expose the retroperitoneum and the splenic flexure detached from the splenic hilum. The descending mesocolon is dissected medially leaving Gerota's fascia, the ureter and gonadal vein intact. Following the landmark of the gonadal vein, the dissection is performed cephalic to the renal vein. The surgeon and assistant then move to the left side of the patient (Figure 5).

Three additional laparoscopic ports are then inserted. Three sutures serve as stay sutures to hold the left hemicolon apron. The traction sutures and right decubitus position help exposure of the retroperitoneal space. A laparoscopic fan retractor is used to keep the visceral organs away from the dissection. The aneurysmal neck and bilateral common iliac arteries can be isolated to facilitate the clamping of the aorta. The lumbar arteries behind the aneurysm and the IMA can be visualised, clipped and divided. Heparin is given prior to aortic clamping. Two additional laparoscopic ports are inserted for laparoscopic vascular clamps. A stab incision over the aneurysm allows assessment of the amount of collateral flow. The aorta is transected. The entire aneurysm is dissected free using electrocautery. A segment of Dacron graft is inserted into the abdomen and the proximal anastomosis between the aorta and the prosthesis is performed under direct vision with conventional but long instruments, according to the technique described by Oscar Creech (Creech et al, 1966). The proximal anastomosis is carried out using a 15 cm suture staring from the far side and running the dorsal aspect of the anastomosis. The other suture is used to finish the remaining anastomosis. The distal anastomosis is performed in the same way. The laparoscopic clamps are then removed. Afterward, the IMA is sewn or re-implanted, depending on left colon vascularisation. The aneurysm wall and the posterior parietal peritoneum are closed to cover the prosthesis in the conventional manner. Laparoscopic AAA repair has been applied to the repair of even complex AAA such as juxta-renal repair (Coggia et al, 2008).Although there remain proponents within centres performing laparoscopic AAA repairs routinely, it is likely that the approach will remain a niche in the field of surgical options for AAA.

6. Endovascular aneurysm repair (EVAR)

In tandem with a global movement towards minimally invasive techniques in all branches of surgery, endovascular techniques have become the treatment of choice for many aneurysmal conditions of the aorta reinforced by the mortality of open aneurysm repair. The concept centres on the endoluminal deployment of a covered stent graft which effectively shields the aneurysm wall from systemic arterial pressure and thereby, prevents aneurysm rupture. Since the first published report of stent graft implantation for AAA in humans in 1991 suggested that this approach was feasible (Parodi et al, 1991), a surge in both the number of EVARS performed and technological improvements in stent graft design account for a steady upward trend in stent graft use as reflected in administrative databases. Indeed, some consider EVAR to be the procedure of choice for

AAA (Cowan et al, 2006; McPhee et al, 2007). The pace of technological evolution of EVAR has been rapid in comparison to the two millennia required for the development of successful open aneurysm repair.

Diffusion of this technology, although widespread, has been met with both enthusiasm and scepticism. Advocates of traditional open surgical techniques maintain that EVAR is costly and that long-term outcomes for patients are inferior. Rather than relying on sutures to provide fixation, as in open repair, endovascular stent grafts rely on radial forces of self-expanding stents for fixation or self expand in concert with active fixation using hooks or barbs at the proximal aorta fixation site. With longer follow-up now being achieved after EVAR, >97% 5-year and >94% 9-year rupture-free survival has been observed (Brewster et al, 2006). Pre-procedural planning using CT as its backbone is the most critical component of a technically successful EVAR. Advances in imaging have had a major role in the development of these complex endovascular procedures: CT images are reconstructed on three dimensional imaging work-stations and 'centreline of flow' reconstructions are used to design the customised endoprotheses (Figure 6).

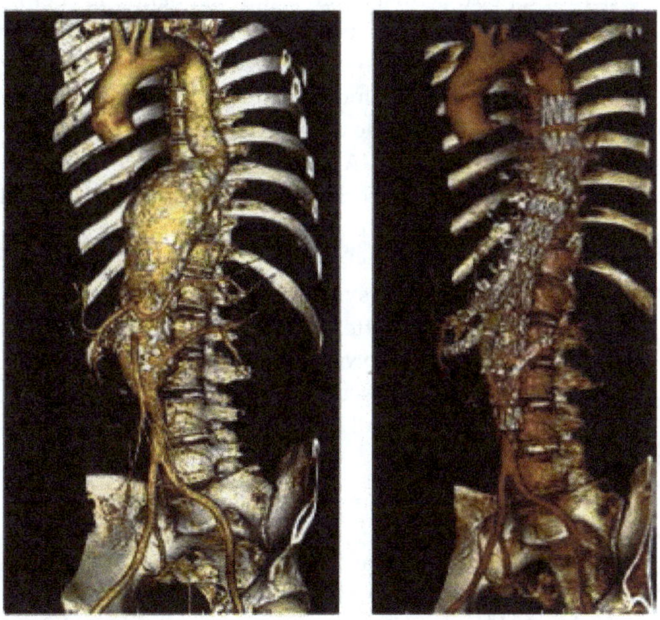

Fig. 6. Three-dimensional volume rendering reconstruction of a computed tomography angiogram performed before (left) and after (right) implantation of a four-branch endograft to treat a type III thoracoabdominal aneurysm. The bridging stents between the branches and the four target vessels are implanted from a brachial approach (Taken from Haulon et al, 2011).

Furthermore, intra-operative imaging can now incorporate on-table CT with 3-D reconstruction to improve the accuracy of graft placement and decrease fluoroscopy time and contrast media volumes. EVAR is a great advance but one must not lose sight of the fact that from a purely technical standpoint, open aneurysm repair is a superior operation. EVAR has been adapted for the treatment of AAA (herein termed EVAR) and TAA (TEVAR). Each procedure is discussed below.

6.1 Anaesthetic considerations for TEVAR & EVAR

Anaesthesia for TEVAR must accommodate the potential risk of conversion of the operation to open TAA repair. The risk of open conversion of TEVAR is decreasing with improvements in endoluminal prostheses and increased surgical expertise. Pre-operative assessment for TEVAR has tended to address the typical issues relating to general anaesthesia in a vascular patient. TEVAR should be classified as a high risk surgical procedure. The intra-operative anaesthetic goals during TEVAR are to provide haemodynamic stability while preserving cardiac, spinal and splanchnic blood flow. In addition, the maintenance of intra-vascular volume, adequate tissue oxygenation and body temperature is required. Accordingly, both general and regional anaesthetic techniques have been used successfully in the treatment of patients with descending TAA When combined with neurological monitoring and trans-oesophageal echocardiography (TOE). Care must be taken to ensure tachycardia and hypertension is avoided as this may impair spinal cord perfusion. The use of new self-deploying stents has meant that earlier manoeuvres such as ventricular asystole (Dorros et al, 1996) and ventricular fibrillation (Kahn et al, 1998) are not required for a 'still' operating field. Whilst an endoluminal balloon is being used to 'seal' the aortic wall after stent deployment (see below), a patient may experience significant haemodynamic stress, especially if baseline cardiac function is poor. Vasopressors and inotropes must be available to manage haemodynamic instability. Cardiac complications are the most common serious peri-operative adverse events of EVAR (Prissen et al, 2004) and the most common cause of late death (EVAR Trial 1, 2005). Hence patient selection must include careful risk stratification of co-morbidities. The Society for Vascular Surgery of America has recommended a medical co-morbidity grading system for EVAR that emphasizes cardiac, pulmonary, and renal status but also includes hypertension and patient age as relevant risk factors. This scoring system aids in patient selection and provides a framework for uniform data collection patterns intended to facilitate analysis of outcomes for EVAR. When a decision is made to proceed with EVAR, it can be performed under general anaesthesia, local aesthetic with sedation, epidural, or spinal block. Again for a patient undergoing EVAR the very small risk of conversion to open repair must be accommodated in operation planning.

6.2 EVAR for TAA (TEVAR)

Non-invasive repair of descending TAA has become particularly attractive but to justify its use the associated mortality and morbidity rates need to be equal to or better than those of open surgical repair. Dake *et al* reported the first endovascular TEVAR in 1994 (Dake et al, 1994) which ushered in a new era in the treatment of thoracic aortic disease. TEVAR is emerging as the preferred treatment strategy in a majority of patients, as increasing data suggests that it may be performed with lower peri-operative morbidity and mortality rates with similar mid-term survival, when compared with standard open TAA repair (Bavaria et al, 2007; Jackson et al, 2007). However, anatomic constraints, principally related to required endograft landing/seal zones and the suitability of femoral and iliac access vessels for endograft introduction excludes a significant number of patients, many of whom are not ideal candidates for open surgery (Jackson et al 2007). With regard to landing zones, both length and diameter must be considered with a required seal zone length of ≥2 to 2.5 cm for all available devices. The endografts are usually oversized by 10% to 15%, and thus, the adequate seal zone diameter ranges from 18 to 42 mm depending on the device used.

Conventional TEVAR seal zones generally extend from zone 2 to zone 4 using a landing zone map.

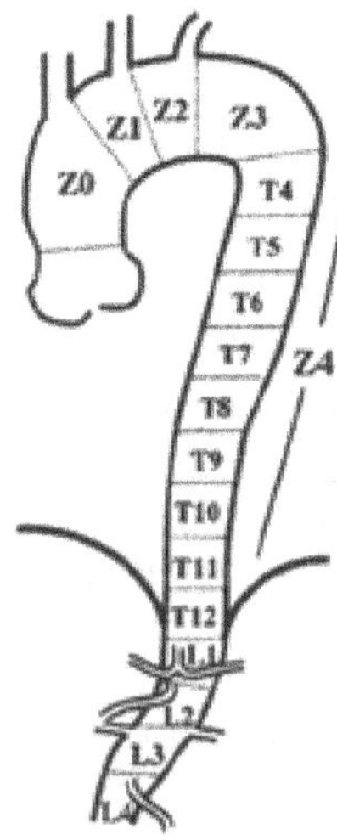

Fig. 7. The landing zones required for TEVAR.

Fig. 7 demonstrates the aortic landing zone map devised by Ishimaru. Conventional TEVAR landing zones are between zone 2 just distal to the left common carotid artery, and zone 4 to the level of the celiac axis. Distal landing zones in zone 4 may be preformed in conjunction with visceral debranching procedures (Ishimura 2004).

In this manner, endograft coverage may span regions of thoracic aorta between the left common carotid (CCA) and coeliac axis. The coeliac axis may occasionally be covered if necessary to achieve an adequate distal seal. Coeliac coverage is generally safe in situations in which the celiac artery is small in diameter and the SMA large and the gastroduodenal artery patent which will feed the coeliac distribution after coeliac coverage. Furthermore, if the right hepatic artery originates from the SMA, coeliac coverage should be well tolerated. Other seal zone considerations include the absence of excessive thrombus or calcification, which might impair endograft apposition to the aortic wall. For conventional TEVAR, the endografts are generally introduced via the femoral vessels, although introduction via the iliac arteries or even the infra-renal aorta may be necessary in some cases if the femoral vessels are unsuitable because of inadequate size or heavy calcification. The proximity of the oesophagus to the aorta in the intra-thoracic and upper abdominal regions makes TOE an attractive imaging modality for guiding placement of the endograft and detecting endoleaks after endograft deployment (see below). Precise placement of the endograft is essential to ensure exclusion of the aneurysmal sac from aortic flow. The endograft system can be clearly visualised in the aorta, from guidewire insertion, to balloon inflation and stent expansion. Aside from TOE, intra-operative CT and/or fluoroscopy can also be used to monitor the endograft system.

6.3 EVAR for AAA (EVAR)

Despite the reduction in mortality rates of open AAA repair from 20 to 5% in the past 30 years (Rickenbach et al, 2004) there are still several complications associated with this approach as illustrated above. It remains an invasive procedure with mortality rates rising sharply in those with co-morbid disease such as coronary artery disease and renal failure while recovery can be protracted resulting in reduced quality of life. Such problems combined with the high number of patients for whom open AAA was contraindicated prompted Volodos *et al* in 1991 to report their clinical experience of using self-fixing synthetic remote endoprosthetics for aorta reconstruction (Volodos et al, 1991). In the same year Parodi *et al* reported repair of AAA in five subjects using an endovascular approach with a modified stent and graft material (Parodi et al, 1991). The stent graft system reported by Parodi was initially developed and patented by Lazarus in 1987 (Lazarus et al, 1987).Although in these early studies reflux was found at the distal end of the graft which necessitated re-intervention, EVAR was established as a feasible treatment for AAA and more importantly safe for the patient.

The basic design of all endografts is similar: the aortic aneurysm is crossed by a tubular graft that has a wide diameter (~20-36 mm) and supported by stents along its length. The tube either bifurcates into two smaller diameter stent grafts that fit into the iliac arteries, or it decreases in size to locate in one iliac artery. Due to rapid commercialisation there are numerous EVAR devices available on the world wide market. The feasibility of EVAR like TEVAR depends mainly on anatomic factors that represent the important predictors of success. Aside from the indications of either an asymptomatic aneurysm of appropriate maximal diameter, or a small aneurysm with features putting it at increased risk of rupture, patients being considered for EVAR must fulfil several anatomic criteria. These include 1) ilio-femoral access vessels that will allow safe insertion and deployment of the device, adequate seal, and sufficient length to provide axial support for the graft and 2) an infra-renal aortic neck of adequate length, limited angulation, and appropriate diameter. These features, as well as the presence or absence of thrombus and calcium at each level of fixation are evaluated using CT. Anatomic selection criteria for EVAR are based principally on characteristics of the proximal infra-renal neck, aneurysm sac and iliac arteries. An unfavourable neck anatomy is the most frequent cause for exclusion from EVAR (Iezzi et al, 2001). The guidelines for EVAR are constantly being redefined, mostly as a result of increasingly operator experience and improvement in stent-graft technology. Although, with new technology the number of patient's eligible for EVAR will increase, complex aortic anatomy will be a significant limitation, at least for the foreseeable future and is likely to ensure that open AAA repair will continue to form an essential part of vascular surgery.

EVAR, as with TEVAR, begins by the surgeons gaining access to both femoral arteries typically through small groin incisions, although a totally percutaneous approach has been reported with low complication rates and high incidence of technical success (Lee et al, 2007). Therefore, both the femoral and iliac arteries must be patent, have as little tortuosity as possible, and one of them must allow a catheter, up to 24 French (Fr) (8 mm) in diameter, to be introduced to the aorta. In some patients with AAA the arteries are too small to allow access (Velazquez et al, 2001). In addition some patients have concomitant vascular disease, so the femoral and iliac arteries can be arteriosclerotic or tortuous which denies access (Wolf et al, 2001). Calcification may also compromise passage of the stent delivery sheath. After bilateral access is obtained, a marking angiogram is typical to confirm pre-operative CT measurements and identify the exact location of the lowest renal artery. Most devices follow with ipsilateral main body insertion and deployment at the infra-renal neck, wire cannulation of the contralateral "gate," contralateral limb deployment, balloon angioplasty to fully expand the device, and completion angiography. Technical success is achieved when there has been successful access to the arterial system using a remote site, successful deployment of a patent stent graft the stent graft with secure proximal and distal fixation and absence of either a type I or type III endoleak (Chaikof et al, 2002). Patients who undergo EVAR or TEVAR need regular clinical follow-up with appropriate imaging for the remainder of their lives because of the potential for stent graft migration and other causes of sac repressurization that put the patient at risk of aneurysm rupture. CT is the gold standard for follow-up imaging. Concerns with using CT for follow-up include the cumulative effects of radiation exposure and the effect of repetitive administration of intravenous contrast on renal function. MRangiography is an alternative for follow-up of most endograft devices but is costly, time consuming, and not universally available. Duplex ultrasound is preferable but bears the limitations of relatively small numbers of accredited vascular ultrasound technicians and the risk of inter-operator variability. Wireless pressure monitoring of the aneurysm sac using a small sensor implanted at the time of EVAR has been proposed as an alternative to other imaging modalities, but no long-term studies currently demonstrate its efficacy in preventing AAA rupture after EVAR (Kurosawa et al, 2007). Efforts to find the optimal method for minimizing the frequency and inconvenience for the patient of follow-up visits while maximizing freedom from aneurysm-related death are ongoing. The first generation stents were suitable only for treating infra-renal aortic aneurysms with a long narrow neck, but subsequent device evolution has led to the situation where few aortic aneurysms cannot be treated by endovascular means. Continued development of grafts is likely to lead to application of the technique to increasing numbers of complex AAA's.

6.4 Complications of TEVAR & EVAR

Many adverse events may accompany EVAR as it is a technically complex procedure typically performed on a high-risk, elderly patient population. This is particularly true of patients undergoing TEVAR. Hence, although the incidence of paraplegia is lower with TEVAR, it remains one of its most dreaded complications. The aetiology probably differs from that encountered after open surgery in that no aortic cross-clamping is required and most likely arises secondary to coverage of important intercostal or other collateral arteries supplying the spinal cord. Some institutions have introduced CSF drainage as described above for open TAA repair (Fuchs et al, 2003). However CSF catheters have their own related morbidity in the form of meningitis, CSF leak and epidural haematomas. In patients with high risk of spinal ischaemia additional intra-operative neurological monitoring with trans-cranial motor evoked potentials and/or somatosensory evoked potentials are useful.

Blood loss following EVAR can be difficult to quantify, as it is often lost around the sheaths and catheters and can be retroperitoneal in the case of EVAR if an injury to femoral or iliac vessels occurs. In addition, TEVAR involves the liberal use of radiographic contrast to assist in appropriate deployment of the graft, ensure exclusion of the aneurysmal sac and determine branch vessel patency. The administration of radio-contrast media can lead to acute kidney injury which is usually reversible albeit its development is associated with adverse outcomes (Rudnick et al, 2008). There is no specific treatment for radio-contrast induced acute renal failure other than supportive management although preventive measures such as hydration with isotonic sodium bicarbonate and administration of the antioxidant acetylcyteine may reduce the risk (Merten et al, 2004).

Myocardial responses to aortic cross-clamping are well documented. The degree of cardiovascular and systemic effects depends on the level at which the cross-clamp is applied. The higher the clamp is placed, the greater the haemodynamic disturbance. Unlike open aortic surgery, TEVAR does not involve extended periods of aortic occlusion. Although the balloon is usually deflated within 15-20 seconds during TEVAR, patients with coronary artery disease or left ventricular dysfunction may respond poorly and run a high risk of myocardial ischaemia.

The above complications of EVAR procedure relate to the peri- and post-operative period. One of the most common adverse events following EVAR is the need for a secondary intervention. Data from the EUROpean collaborators on Stent/graft Techniques for Aortic Aneurysm Repair (EUROSTAR) registry of 2846 patients treated from December 1999 until December 2004 revealed that EVAR resulted in a cumulative incidence of secondary interventions of 6.0%, 8.7%, 12%, and 14% at 1, 2, 3, and 4 years, respectively (Hobo et al, 2006). Secondary interventions are typically performed when the aneurysm has become repressurized because of incomplete exclusion of blood flow from the sac. The term "endoleak" was created in 1996 to describe this complication (White et al, 1996). An endoleak is defined as the persistence of blood flow outside the lumen of the endograft but within an aneurysm sac or adjacent vascular segment treated by the graft (White et al, 1996; Gonzalez-Fajardo et al, 2002). Endoleaks may occur because of misplacement or poor sizing of an endograft, endograft fatigue and displacement or distortion of the endograft material. These latter factors represent device failure which in the modern era has largely been overcome as a result of device development. Endoleaks have been classified into types I to IV based upon the underlying cause and anatomical site of origin. Each is discussed below.

Persistent flow around the attachment sites (proximal or distal) of the endograft due to inadequate or ineffective seal at the graft ends is classified as a type I endoleak. Type I endoleaks may occur in up to 24% of patients following TEVAR is the most frequently encountered, usually results from technical error and may eventually result in graft failure. Type I endoleaks usually require additional stent-graft deployment. .which may increase complication rates and adversely affect patient quality of life. Type I and type III endoleaks (see below) are treated immediately to halt peri-graft flow or flow between modular components.

An endoleak may also occur because of retrograde flow into the aneurysmal sac from a patent collateral branch vessel (type II endoleak) and is not of major concern. The endoleak usually resolves spontaneously after 6 months. Type II endoleaks are typically managed expectantly with intervention reserved for persistent endoleaks in the presence of aneurysm sac enlargement. The presence of a persistent type II endoleak for ≥ 6 months, however, has been associated with aneurysm enlargement, increased rate of secondary interventions, and even aneurysm rupture (Fairman et al, 2006; Jones et al, 2007). Secondary interventions can range from diagnostic angiography to endograft removal with conversion to open repair.

Flow into the aneurysmal sac because of leakage between modular segments of an endograft is classified as a type III endoleak. This is probably more common in the thoracic aorta because of greater haemodynamic stress causing early or late graft material fatigue. Management via the endovascular route using a covered stent to reline the failing endograft is usually appropriate. A related cause of endoleak and potential complication of EVAR is device failure. The integrity of stent graft materials and maintenance of proper positioning within the aneurysm are critical in preventing pressurization of the aneurysm sac and rupture. Material failure includes fracture of any of the metallic components of the stent graft, including stents, hooks, or barbs, or tears in the fabric component of the stent graft. Loss of proper stent graft position can occur for many reasons. Material failure, inadequate proximal or distal seal zone, aneurysm remodelling after EVAR, or features of the vessel, such as thrombus or calcium, that limit stent purchase, have all been implicated in the migration of stent grafts. Each of these modes of failure must be analyzed within the context of their clinical significance. A stent fracture that leaves the graft fabric intact and is not in a critical region for maintaining fixation would likely need only follow-up, whereas modular component separation resulting in a large type III endoleak will require urgent intervention to restore stent graft integrity.

Flow detected in the aneurysmal sac by completion angiography may occur due to porous graft material. This is termed a type IV endoleak and may be difficult to distinguish from other types of graft leakage. Its diagnosis is made after exclusion of any other identifiable source of endoleak. Type IV endoleaks rarely occurs with modern stent graft design.

Type V endoleaks or 'endoleak of undefined origin' (endotension), although still reported (Iyer et al, 2007), but are much less frequent after modification of the Gore Excluder device in 2004 to a low-permeability expanded polytetrafluoroethylene layer (Tanski et al, 2007). Endotension is the continued pressurisation of the sac with subsequent sac enlargement in the absence of an apparent endoleak. It is may be caused by pressure transmission through a sealed of thrombosed endoleak (Kamineni et al, 2004). Controversy surrounds the nature of this type of endoleak and its management. An increase in aneurysm size can occur with endotension, but if there is no demonstrate endoleak or the aneurysm is shrinking in size, additional intervention is usually not required. Several procedures are possible: open replacement of the graft, wrapping the endograft with a new graft at laparotomy, and endovascular relining of the stent-graft. Conversion to open repair usually treats endotension satisfactorily (Lin et al, 2003).

Stent fatigue and fracture are also a problem following endovascular procedures. Ten per cent of all stent grafts have fractured within 4 years (Jacobs et al, 2003). The fracture of a stent strut may lead to a Type III endoleak, or if the attachment barbs and hooks fracture, the stent graft may migrate to form a Type I endoleak. Many stents allow initial deployment which allows partial re-positioning, as no repositioning can be performed when the graft is fully deployed. Inaccurate deployment will also lead to the increased use of extenders, thus increasing the probability of Type III endoleak (Zairns et al, 2003). Although many of the stents grafts do allow some manoeuvrability post-implantation, this is mostly in the form of moving the stent down the aorta. Thus if barbs/anchors have been deployed, too much movement may itself cause dissection of the artery. Kinking caused by fracture of the stent or insufficient support given to the graft can result in obstructed of a bifurcated limb (Corbett et al, 2008) which often leads to the need for endovascular re-intervention being required. EVAR device migration remains a major problem. Fixation devices (endostaplers) along with new stent graft designs may be important in preventing graft migration. Such approaches appear to work in animal models with relatively thin, non-diseased aortas (Arko et al, 2005).

The primary goal of EVAR is aneurysm exclusion and depressurisation. However continued pressurisation secondary to endoleaks or endotension can be associated with late aneurysm rupture with a reported incidence of one per cent (Cho et al, 2004). Diagnosis of rupture after EVAR can be problematic. Female gender and adverse anatomy with short wide and angulated infra-renal necks may be predisposing factors (Brewster et al, 2006). The mortality for late rupture is variable and reported between 43-83%.

As discussed above, aorto-duodenal fistula (ADF) is an abnormal communication between the aorta and usually the fourth part of the duodenum which constitutes a rare but life-threatening complication of aneurysm repair. Until recently, they were primarily associated with open

AAA repair occurring at a rate 2% (Bertges et al, 2003). It is believed that local infection leads to intestinal necrosis and subsequent fistula formation. Endotension may also be a contributory factor. Treatment of ADF is graft removal, revascularisation and intestinal repair.

7. Evidence for type of aneurysm repair: In a nutshell

7.1 Open versus laparoscopic AAA repair

Reviews of published large series of open AAA repair demonstrate consistent short-term (30-day) outcomes: death, 2-5%; myocardial infarction, 2-8%; renal failure, 2-5%; pneumonia, 5%; bleeding, 2-4%; leg ischaemia 1-4%; colon ischaemia, 1-2%; and length of stay 5 to 10 days (Lerderle et al, 2000, Johnston et al, 1998, Huber et al, 2007, Richardson et al, 1991). The short term morbidity and mortality are offset by a low rate of adverse long-term (10 or more years) outcome that include anastomotic aneurysm, 4-10%; graft infection 1-2% and thrombosis, 3% (Biancari et al, 2002; Hallet et al, 1997; Schermehorn et al, 2008). These figures have been used as the benchmark against which the newer, minimal invasive repairs have been judged.

The follow-up results of laparoscopic AAA repair seem to indicate a better post-operative course when compared with standard open repair. Retrospective comparisons with open surgically treated cases are unreliable because the groups are not matched or randomized and are thus subject to the influence of uncontrolled variables. The advantages of the laparoscopic approach over the open surgical approach are likely to be real. Indeed total laparoscopic aortic surgery based on data from the reported laparoscopic AAA repair literature reports better outcomes in terms of post-operative stay when compared to hand-assisted laparoscopic surgery and open repair (Coggia et al, 2004). However with the advent of EVAR and the pace of technological development the randomized prospective trials required to assess laparoscopic and open AAA repair have not been performed. Laparoscopic AAA repair has thus largely become marginalised because of the wide adoption of EVAR.

7.2 Open versus EVAR repair

In modern aortic surgery the question has centred largely on the potential benefits of EVAR in comparison to open repair. Retrospective studies based on large administrative databases comparing open repair with EVAR document impressive superiority of EVAR in early patient outcomes (Schermehorn et al, 2008; Lee et al, 2004; Hua et al, 2005). This advantage of EVAR is all the more impressive when one considers that the EVAR was in general performed upon older and sicker patients. These results have been confirmed in the randomised trials, EVAR-1 and the Dutch Randomized Endovascular Aneurysm Management (DREAM) (Greenhalgh et al, 2004; Prissen et al, 2004). Additionally, two randomized European trials comparing EVAR to open surgery and one randomized trial comparing EVAR to no intervention were published in 2005 (Blankensteijn et al, 2005; EVAR Trial 1, 2005; EVAR Trial 2, 2005). The DREAM trial, randomised 351 patients with asymptomatic AAAs >5 cm in diameter with suitable stent graft anatomy to open surgery or EVAR. This study suggested a 30-day benefit in mortality favouring EVAR (Prissen et al, 2004). The trend toward an early mortality advantage was lost, however, 12 months into the 2-year study follow-up (Blankensteijn et al, 2005).

The second trial, from the United Kingdom, EVAR 1, was similar to DREAM in comparing EVAR to open surgery in patients with suitable stent graft anatomy and aneurysm size ≥5.5

cm (EVAR Trial 1, 2005). This study randomized 1082 patients. EVAR 1 more clearly demonstrated an early peri-operative mortality benefit for EVAR (Greenhalgh et al, 2004). Blood product use and length of hospital stay also favoured EVAR. In contrast, the primary end point of all-cause mortality did not show a lasting benefit for EVAR at the 4-year study conclusion, although aneurysm-related death was decreased (EVAR Trial 1, 2005). Complication rates and re-intervention rates were much higher for stent graft repair than for open repair. EVAR trial 2 (EVAR Trial 2, 2005) randomized 338 patients >60 years of age with aneurysms ≥5.5 cm who were deemed unfit for open surgical repair to EVAR or no intervention (EVAR Trial 2, 2005). Between the two arms of the study, 142 patients died during follow-up, which correlated to a 64% overall mortality by Kaplan–Meier estimates at 4 years. This study was complicated by long delays in EVAR after randomization and a 27% patient crossover rate from the no intervention group. In the final analysis, no benefit to EVAR over medical management was detected in either overall mortality or aneurysm-related mortality for patients unfit for open surgery.

Ongoing in the United States is the Open Versus Endovascular Repair (OVER) trial, a 9-year study that began in 2002 comparing endovascular aneurysm repair with standard open surgery using a multi-centre randomized trial through the Department of Veteran Affairs Cooperative Study Group (Lederle et al, 2006). In comparison with EVAR, open AAA repair has a highly significant 2- to 3-fold increase in mortality, a 1.5- to 2-fold increase in major morbidity, a 12-fold increase in blood transfusion requirement and a 2-fold increase in length of stay and discharge to a long-term care facility.

In conclusion, although early outcome data provided a compelling case for EVAR the outlook became clouded when long term outcomes were considered. This finding is even more pertinent when it is considered that both EVAR 1 and DREAM showed that EVAR was associated with a 4-fold increase in long-term (2-4 years) complications and a 3-fold increase in the need for re-intervention (Greenhalgh et al, 2005; Blankensteijn et al, 2005). Quality of life is heavily in favour of EVAR especially in the weeks and months immediately following the procedure. However after 6 months and longer quality of life is documented to be better in patients with open repair (Greenhalgh et al, 2005; Prissen et al, 2004a; Prissen et al, 2004b). This is likely related to the greater need for radiological surveillance with EVAR. However although earlier studies suggested that EVAR was not cost-effective (Jonk et al, 2007; Prissen et al, 2007) more recent data from the National Institute for Clinical Excellence (NICE) in the United Kingdom suggests EVAR is cost effective (Hay et al, 2009). In addition, the long-term outcomes of EVAR are not fully understood. Indeed a 7- to 8-fold increase in aneurysm-related death after 5 years of follow-up has been observed in good-risk patients treated with EVAR in comparison with open repair (Eliason et al, 2009).

7.3 EVAR for small aneurysms

Whereas randomized clinical trials have focused on establishing the proper use of EVAR for larger aneurysms, its application for the treatment of small aneurysms is still an area of controversy. Early open aneurysm repair for aneurysms <5.5 cm in diameter does not confer a long-term survival advantage (Lederle et al, 2002; UK small aneurysm trial, 2002). However, retrospective analysis of the large EUROSTAR database revealed that EVAR for aneurysms with diameters between 4.0 cm and 5.4 cm had lower incidence of type I endoleak and improved cumulative freedom from aneurysm-related death relative to two comparison groups with aneurysm diameters of 5.5 to 6.4 cm and ≥6.5 cm (Peppelenbosch et al, 2004). Level 1 evidence is lacking at this time, but the Positive Impact of EndoVascular

Options for Treating Aneurysms EarLy (PIVOTAL) and Comparison of Surveillance versus Aortic Endografting for Small Aneurysm Repair (CAESAR) trials were initiated in an attempt to provide such evidence (Cao et al, 2005). Both are device specific, randomize patients with smaller aneurysms to EVAR or surveillance, and use an FDA-approved Medtronic device or the Cook Zenith device, respectively. Until the results of these trials are published, the optimal management of small aneurysms remains ambiguous and a patient-specific approach that takes into account aneurysm morphology, biology, and patient co-morbidities should be used.

7.4 Open versus TEVAR for TAA

TEVAR benefit to risk ratio is even greater than that encountered with EVAR although TEVAR is more expensive than EVAR. In comparison to open surgery it is associated with significant reduction in blood transfusion requirements, major complications, ITU and hospital length of stay (Murphy et al, 2009). However the total hospital costs are 2-fold higher and the cost margin minus 34% in comparison with plus 6.2% for open repair (Ramagnoli et al, 2009). The extra costs for TEVAR were usually a result of the use of multiple devices to treat extensive aneurysms. Clearly, in elderly patients and in those at high risk for open repair, TEVAR is an excellent surgical option for repair. With continuing evaluation of endovascular techniques, comparisons with open repair will be made. Recently, the results from the combined experience of EUROSTAR and the United Kingdom Thoracic Endograft registries have been published (Leurs et al, 2004). From this report, overall 30-day mortality was 5.4% for elective cases, and paraplegia was 4% after aneurysm stenting; 1-year follow-up was obtained for 45% of patients of the entire cohort with an 80% survival for aneurysmal disease. Others have reported similar early results (Mitchell et al, 1999; Greenberg et al, 2000; White et al, 2004; Najibi et al, 2002, Hansen et al, 2004; Lambrechts et al, 2003). It remains striking that even with no aortic occlusion during endovascular stenting, neurologic deficit was still significant, ranging as high as 12% (with stroke as high as 7%). The overall long-term survival was 79%, 76%, 64%, and 35% at 1, 2, 5, and 10 years, respectively after open TAA repair (Svensson et al, 1993). In addition, freedom from reoperation for distal aortic related condition was 96% at 13 years. Early (1 to 2 years) survival with endovascular stenting has been reported from 73% to 81% with freedom from reintervention at 54% at almost 4 years (Mitchell et al, 1999). This report confirms that open repair for descending thoracic aortic repair remains durable for the long term and does not require multiple reinterventions. Two clinical trials have compared TEVAR with open surgery. The first published in 2002 compared 19 patients with 10 historical controls. The mean length of ITU stay and hospital stay were better in the TEVAR group. This study however was not randomised and follow up was limited (Najibi et al, 2002). The second (non-randomized) study also reported that 30 day mortality was better in the TEVAR group with fewer complications (Bavaria et al, 2007). However the two year survival was similar in both groups. A recent Cochrane review concluded that although such evidence may suggest that endovascular repair can be appropriate in selected patients, high quality studies are needed to produce generalisable conclusions (Abraha et al, 2009).

8. The future of aortic aneurysm repair

Aortic surgery has evolved at an exponential rate in the last five decades. The future lies in how we further develop these technologies to improve patient outcome. With the advent of screening programmes it is likely in the immediate future that the need for surgery will increase. How to apply these technologies for maximal patient benefit will be the future challenge to the vascular surgeon. In the next decade we can expect continuing improvements in endovascular device design to include the treatment of supra-renal and thoraco-abdominal aneurysms. The role of open repair is likely to diminish raising questions on whether centralization of complex open aortic surgery will be required.. Surgeons will need to have efficient follow-up protocols and evaluate the new stent-grafts in order to continue the advance of aortic aneurysm surgery.

9. References

Abraha, I,; Romagnoli, C, Montedori, A, Cirocchi, R (2009) Thoracic stent graft versus surgery for thoracic aneurysm. Cochrane Database Systematic Review, Vol 21, No. 1, pp. CD006796

Antoniou, GA.; Koutsias, S, Antoniou, SA, Georgiakakis, A, Lazarides, MK, Giannoukas, AD (2009) Outcome after endovascular stent graft repair of aortoenteric fistula: A systematic review. *Journal of Vascular Surgery,* Vol 49, pp. 782-789

Arko, FR,; Heikkinen M, Lee, ES, Bass, A, Alsac, JM, Zairns, CK (2005) Illiac fixation length and resistance to in-vivo stent-graft displacement. *Journal of Vascular Surgery,* Vol 41, No. 4, pp. 664-671

Bavaria, JE,; Appoo, JJ, Makaroun, MS, Verter, J, Yu, ZF, Mitchell, RS (2007) Endovascular stent grafting versus open surgical repair of descending thoracic aortic aneurysms in low-risk patients: a multicenter comparative trial. *Thoracic and Cardiovascular Surgery,* Vol 133, No 2, 369-377

Bahnson, HT (1953) Definitive treatment of saccular aneurysms of the aorta with excision of sac and aortic suture. *Surgery, Gynecology & Obstetrics,* Vol 96, No 4, pp. 383-402

Barratt, J,; Parajasingam, R, Sayers, RD, Feehally, J (2000) Outcome of acute renal failure following surgical repair of ruptured abdominal aortic aneurysms. *European Journal of Vascular and Endovascular Surgery,* Vol 20, No. 2, pp. 163-168

Becquemin, JP,; Kelley, L, Zubilewicz T (2004) Outcomes of secondary interventions after aortic aneurysm endovascular repair. *Journal of Vascular Surgery,* Vol 39, No. 2, pp.298–305

Bertges, DJ,; Villella, ER, Makaroun, MS (2003) Aortoenteric fistula due to endoleak coil embolization after endovascular AAA repair. *Journal of Endovascular Therapy,* Vol. 10, No. 1, pp. 130-135

Biancari, F,; Ylonen, K, Anttila, V, Juvonen, J, Romsi, P, Satta, J, Juvonen, T (2002) Durability of open repair of infrarenal abdominal aortic aneurysm: a 15-year follow-up study. *Journal of Vascular Surgery,* Vol 35, No. 1, pp. 87-93

Blankensteijn, JD,; de Jong, SE, Prinssen, M, van der Ham, AC, Buth J, van Sterkenburg, SM, Verhagen, HJ, Buskens, E, Grobbee, DE (2005) Dutch Randomized Endovascular Aneurysm Management (DREAM) Trial Group. Two-year outcomes after conventional or endovascular repair of abdominal aortic aneurysms. *New England Journal of Medicine,* Vol 352, No. 23, pp. 2398–2405.

Brewster, DC (2002) Do current results of endovascular abdominal aortic aneurysm repair justify more widespread use? *Surgery,* Vol 131, No. 4, pp. 363–367

Brewster, DC,; Cronenwett, JL, Hallet Jr, JW, Johnston, KW, Krupski, WC, Matsumura, JS (2003) Guidelines for the treatment of abdominal aortic aneurysms. Report of a subcommittee of the Joint Council of the American Association for Vascular Surgery and Society for Vascular Surgery. *Journal of Vascular Surgery,* Vol 37, No. 5, pp. 1106–1117

Brewster, DC,; Jones, JE, Chung, TK, Lamuraglia, GM, Kwolek, CJ, Watkins, MT, Hodgman, TM, Cambria, RP (2006) Long-term outcomes after endovascular abdominal aortic aneurysm repair: the first decade. *Annals of Surgery,* Vol 244, No. 3, pp. 426–438

Cao P, CAESAR Trial Collaborators. Comparison of surveillance vs Aortic Endografting for Small Aneurysm Repair (CAESAR) trial: study design and progress. *European Journal of Vascular and Endovascular Surgery,* Vol 30, No. 3, pp. 245–251.

Castronuovo, JJ,; James, KV, Resnikoff, M, McLean, ER, Edoga, JK (2000) Laparoscopic-assisted abdominal aortic aneuysmectomy. *Journal of Vascular Surgery,* Vol 32, No. 2, pp. 224-233

Cerveira, JJ,; Halpern, VJ , Faust, G, Cohen, JR (1999) Minimal incision abdominal aortic aneurysm repair . *Journal of Vascular Surgery,* Vol 30, No. 6, pp. 977–979

Chaikof, EL,; Blankensteijn, JD, Harris, PL, White, GH, Zarins, CK, Bernhard, VM, Matsumura, JS, May, J, Veith, FJ, Fillinger, MF, Rutherford, RB, Kent, KC (2002) Ad Hoc Committee for Standardized Reporting Practices in Vascular Surgery of The Society for Vascular Surgery/American Association for Vascular Surgery. Reporting standards for endovascular aortic aneurysm repair. *Journal of Vascular Surgery.* Vol 35, pp. 1048–1060

Chiu, KM,; Lin, TY, Chu, SH, Chen JR (2008) Total laparoscopic repair for abdominal aortic aneurysm. *J Formos Med Assoc,* Vol 107, No. 8, pp. 667-672

Cho, JS,; Dillavou, ED, Rhee, RY, Makaroun, MS (2004) Late abdominal aneurysm enlargement after endovascular repair with the Excluder device. *Journal of Vascular Surgery,* Vol 39, No. 6, pp. 1236-1242

Clagett GP, (2008) EVAR, TEVAR, FEVAR, too far? *Perspectives in Vascular and Endovascular Therapy,* Vol 20, No. 2, pp 115-119

Coggia, M,; Javerliat, I, Di Centa, I, Colacchi, G, Cerceau, P, Kitzis, M, Goeau-Brissonniere, OA (2004) Total laparoscopic infrarenal aortic aneurysm repair: preliminary results *Journal of Vascular Surgery,* Vol 40, No. 3, pp. 448–454

Coggia, M,; Cerceau, P, Di Centa, I, Javerliat, I, Colacchio, G, Goeau-Brissonniere, OA (2008) Total laparoscopic juxtarenal abdominal aortic aneurysm repair. *Journal of Vascular Surgery,* Vol 48, No. 1, pp. 37-42

Cooley, DA & De Bakey, ME (1956) Resection of entire ascending aorta in fusiform aneurysm using cardiac bypass. *Journal of American Medical Association,* Vol 162, No.12, pp. 1158-1159

Corbett; TJ,; Callanan, A, Morris, LG, Doyle, BJ, Grace, PA, Kavanagh, EG, McGloughlin, TM (2008) A review of the in vivo and in vitro biomechanical behaviour and performace of post-operative abdominal aortic aneurysm and implanted stent-grafts. *Journal of Endovascular Therapy,* Vol 15, No. 4, pp. 468-484

Coselli, JS.; LeMaire, SA, Conklin, LD, Adams, GJ (2004) Left heart bypass during descending thoracic aortic aneurysm repair does not reduce the incidence of paraplegia. *Annals of Thoracic Surgery,* Vol 77, pp. 1298-1303

Cowan Jr, JA,; Dimick, JB, Henke, PK, Rectenwald, J, Stanley, JC, Upchurch Jr, GR (2006) Epidemiology of aortic aneurysm repair in the United States from 1993 to 2003. *Annals of New York Academy of Science,* Vol 1085: 1–10

Crawford, ES,; Crawford, JL, Safi, HJ, Coselli, JS, Hess, KR, Brooks, B, Norton, HJ, Glaeser, DH (1986) Thoracoabdominal aortic aneurysms: preoperative and intraopertaive factors determining immediate and long-term results of operations in 605 patients. *Journal of Vascular Surgery,* Vol 3, No. 3, pp. 389-404

Creech, O (1966) Endoaneurysmorrhaphy and treatment of aortic aneurysm. *Annals of Surgery,* Vol 164, pp. 935–946

Dajczman, E,; Gordon, A, Kreisman, H, Wolkove, N (1991) Long-term postthoracotomy pain. *Chest,* Vol 99, No. 2, pp.270-274

Dake, MD,; Miller, DC, Semba, CP, Mitchell, RS, Walker, PJ, Liddell, RP (1994) Transluminal placement of endovascular stent-grafts for the treatment of descending thoracic aortic aneurysms. *New England Journal of Medicine,* Vol 331, No. 26, pp. 1729-34

De Bakey, ME.; Crawford, ES, Cooley, DA, Morris Jr, GC (1957). Successful resection of fusiform aneurysm of aortic arch with replacement by homograft. *Surgery, Gynecology & Obstetrics,* Vol 105, No.6, pp. 657-664

Deterling, RA & Bhonslay, SB (1955) An evaluation of synthetic materials and fabrics suitable for blood vessel replacement. *Surgery,* Vol 38, No.1, pp. 71-91

Dion, YM,; Katkhouda, N, Roleau, C, Aucoin, A (1993) Laparoscopic-assisted aortobifemoral bypass . *Surgical Laparoscopy Endoscopy,* Vol 3, No. 5, pp. 425–429

Dorros, G & Cohn, JM (1996) Adenosine-induced transient cardiac asystole enhances precise deployment of stent-grafts in the thoracic or abdominal aorta. *Journal of Endovascular Surgery,* Vol 3, No. 3, pp. 270-272

Dubost, C,; Allary, M, Oeconomos, N (1951) Aneurysm of the abdominal aorta treated by resection and graft. *Sem Hop,* Vol 27, No. 69, pp. 2678-2785

Edoga, JK,; Asgarian; K, Singh; D, James; KV, Romanelli; J, Merchant, S, Romano, D, Joostema, B, Street, J. Laparoscopic surgery for abdominal aortic aneurysm: technical elements of the procedure and a preliminary report of the first 22 patients. *Surgical Endoscopy,* Vol 12, No. 8, pp. 1064–1072

Engle, J,; Safi, HJ, Miller 3rd, CC, Campbell, MP, Harlin, SA, Letsou, GV, Lloyd MD, Root DB (1999) The impact of diaphragm management on prolonged ventilator support after thoracoabdominal aortic repair. *Journal of Vascular Surgery,* Vol 29, No. 1, pp. 150-156

Eliason, JL, & Upchurch Jr, GR (2009) Endovascular treatment of aortic aneurysms: state of the art. *Current Treatment Options in Cardiovascular Medicine,* Vol 11, No. 2, pp. 136-145

El-Sabrout, RA., & Reul, GJ (2001) Suprarenal or supraceliac aortic clamping during repair of infrarenal abdominal aortic aneurysms. *Texas Heart Institute Journal,* Vol 28, No.4, pp. 254-264

Estrera, AL.; Miller 3rd, CC, Huynh, TT (2003) Preoperative and operative predictors of delayed neurologic deficit following repair of thoracoabdominal aortic aneurysm. *Journal of Thoracic Cardiovascular Surgery,* Vol 126, pp.1288-1294

Etz, CD,; Di Luozzo, G, Bello, R, Luehr, M, Khan, MZ, Bodian, CA, Griepp, RB, Plestis, KA (2007) Pulmonary complications after descending thoracic and thoracoabdominal aortic aneurysm repair: predictors, prevention and treatment. *Annals of Thoracic Surgery,* Vol 83, No. 2, pp. S870-S876

EVAR Trial Participants (2005) Endovascular aneurysm repair versus open repair in patients with abdominal aortic aneurysm (EVAR trial 1): randomised controlled trial. *Lancet,* Vol 365, pp. 2179–2186

EVAR Trial Participants (2005) Endovascular aneurysm repair and outcome in patients unfit for open repair of abdominal aortic aneurysm (EVAR trial 2): randomised controlled trial. *Lancet,* Vol 365, pp. 2187–2192.

Fairman, RM,; Nolte, L, Snyder, SA, Chuter, TA, Greenberg, RK, Zenith Investigators (2006) Factors predictive of early or late aneurysm sac size change following endovascular repair. *Journal of Vascular Surgery,* Vol 43, No. 4, pp. 649–656

Fuchs, RJ,; Lee, WA, Seubert, CN, Gelman, S (2003) Transient paraplegia after grafting of a descending thoracic aortic aneurysm treated with cerebrospinal fluid drainage. *Journal of Clinical Anesthesiology,* Vol 15, No. 1, pp. 59-63

Fukada, J,; Morishita, K, Kawaharada, N, Yamada, A, Harada, N, Abe, T (2002) Less-invasive thoracic aneurysm repair. *Annals Thoracic Surgery,* Vol 74, No. 4, pp. 1244-1246

Gonzalez-Fajardo JA, Gutierrez V, San Roman, JA, Serrador, A, Arreba E, Del Rio, L, Martin, M, Carrera, S, Vaquero, C (2002) Utility of intraopertaive transesophgeal echocardiography during endovascular stent-graft repair of acute thoracic aoric dissection. *Annals of Vascular Surgery,* Vol 16, No. 3, pp. 297-303

Green, RM.; Ricotta, JJ, Ouriel, K, DeWeese, JA (1989) Results of supraceliac aortic clamping in the difficult elective resection of infrarenal abdominal aortic aneurysm. *Journal of Vascular Surgery,* Vol 9, pp. 124-134

Greenberg, R,; Resch, T, Nyman, U, Lindh, M, Brunkwall, J, Brunkwall P, Malina, M, Koul, B, Lindblad, B, Ivancev K (2000). Endovascular repair of descending thoracic aortic aneurysmsal early experience with intermediate-term follow-up. *Journal of Vascular Surgery,* Vol 31, pp. 147-156

Greenhalgh RM, Brown LC, Kwong GP, Powell JT, Thompson SG, EVAR Trial Participants (2004) Comparison of endovascular aneurysm repair with open repair in patients with abdominal aortic aneurysm (EVAR trial 1), 30-day operative mortality results: randomised controlled trial. *Lancet,* Vol 364, No. 9437, pp. 843–848

Gross, RE.; Hurwitt, ES. & Bill, AH Jr (1948) Preliminary observations on the use of human arterial grafts in the treatment of certain cardiovascular defects. *New England Journal of Medicine,* Vol 239, No.16, pp. 578

Hallett Jr, JW,; Marshall, DM, Petterson, TM, Gary, DT, Bower, TC, Cherry Jr, KJ, Gloviczki, P, Pairolero, PC (1997) Graft-related complications after abdominal aortic aneurysm repair: reassurance from a 36-year population-based experience. *Journal of Vascular Surgery,* Vol 25, No. 2, pp. 277-284

Hansen, CJ,; Bui, H, Donayre, CE, Aziz, I, Kim, B, Kopchok, G, Walot, I, Lee, J, Lippmann, M, White, RA (2004). Complications of endovascular repair of high-risk and emergent descending thoracic aortic aneurysms and dissections *Journal of Vascular Surgery,* Vol 40, No. 2, pp. 228-234

Haulon, S & O'Brien N (2011) Advances in endovascular repair for complex aneurysms. *British Journal of Surgery,* Vol 98, No.2, pp 163-165

Hay, N,; McCraken, F, Richardson, J, Barnett, D (2009) Endovascular stent-grafts for the treatment of abdominal aortic aneurysms: NICE technology appraisal guidance. *Heart,* Vol 95, pp. 1798-1800

Hobo, R, & Buth J (2006) Secondary interventions following endovascular abdominal aortic aneurysm repair using current endografts: a EUROSTAR report. *Journal of Vascular Surgery,* Vol 43, No. 5, pp. 896–902.

Hua, HT,; Cambria, RP, Chuang, SK, Stoner, MC, Kwolek, CJ, Rowell, KS, Khuri, SF, Henderson, WG, Brewster, DC, Abbott, WM (2005) Early outcomes of endovascular versus open abdominal aortic aneurysm repair in the National Surgical Quality Improvement Program-Private Sector (NSQIP-PS). *Journal of Vascular Surgery,* Vol 41, No. 3, pp. 382–389

Huber, TS,; Wang, JG, Derrow, AE, Dame, DA, Ozaki, CK, Zelenock, GB, Flynn, TC, Seeger, JM (2001) Experience in the United States with intact abdominal aortic aneurysm repair. *Journal of Vascular Surgery,* Vol 33, No. 2, pp. 304–310

Iezzi, R & Cotroneo AR (2001) Endovascular repair of abdominal aneurysms: CTA evaluation of contraindications. *Abdominal Imaging,* Vol 31, No. 6, pp. 722-731

Ishimaru, S (2004) Endografting of the aortic arch. *Journal of Endovascular Therapy,* Vol 11: pp. I162-I171

Iyer, VS,; Mackenzie, KS, Corriveau, MM, Steinmetz, OK (2007) Reversible endotension associated with excessive warfarin anticoagulation. *Journal of Vascular Surgery,* Vol 45, No. 3, pp. 600-602

Jackson, BM,; Carpenter JP, Fairman, RM, Moser, GW, Pochettino, A, Woo EY, Bavaria, JE (2007) Anatomic exclusion from endovascular repair of thoracic aortic aneurysm. *Journal of Vascular Surgery,* Vol 45, No. 4, pp. 662-666

Jacobs, TS,; Won, J, Gravereaux, EC, Faries, PL, Morrissey, N, Teodorescu, VJ, Hollier, LH, Marin, ML (2003) Mechincal failure of prosthetic human implants: a 10-year experience with aortic stent graft devices. *Journal of Vascular Surgery,* Vol 37, No. 1, pp. 16-26

Jimenez, JC,; Smith, MM, Wilson, SE (2004) Sexual dysfunction in men after open or endovascular repair of abdominal aortic aneurysms. *Vascular,* Vol 12, No. 3, pp. 186-191

Johnston, KW & Scobie TK (1988) Multicenter prospective study of non-ruptured abdominal aortic aneurysms. Population and operative management. *Journal of Vascular Surgery,* Vol 7, No. 1, pp. 69-81

Jones, JE,; Atkins; MD, Brewster; DC, Chung; TK, Kwolek; CJ, LaMuraglia; GM, Hodgman; TM, Cambria, RP (2007) Persistent type 2 endoleak after endovascular repair of abdominal aortic aneurysm is associated with adverse late outcomes. *Journal of Vascular Surgery,* Vol 46, No. 1, pp. 1-8

Jonker, FH,; Trimarchi, S, Verhagen, HJ, Moll, FL, Sumpio, BE, Muhs, BE (2010) Meta-analysis of open versus endovascular repair for ruptured descending thoracic aortic aneurysm. *Journal of Vascular Surgery,* Vol 51, No. 4, pp. 1032.e1-1032.e2.

Kahn ,RA,; Marin, ML, Hollier, L, Parsons, R, Griepp, R (1998) Induction of ventricular fibrillation to facilitate endovascular stent grat repair of thoracic aortic aneurysm. *Anesthesiology,* Vol 88, No. 2, pp. 534-536

Kamineni, R & Heuser, RR (2004) Abdominal aortic aneurysm: a review of endoluminal treatment. *Journal of Interventional Cardiology,* Vol 17, No. 6, pp. 437-445

Kim, GS,; Ahn, HJ, Kim, WH, Kim, MJ, Lee, SH (2011) Risk factors for post-operative complications after open infrarenal abdominal aortic aneurysm repair in Koreans. *Yonsei Medical Journal,* Vol 52, No. 2, pp. 339-346

Kirby, TJ & Rice, TW (1993) Thorascopic lobectomy. *Annals of Thoracic Surgery,* Vol 56, No. 3, pp. 784-786

Kline, RG,; D'Angelo, AJ, Chen, MHM, Halpern, VJ, Cohen, JR. Laparoscopically assisted abdominal aortic aneurysm repair: first 20 cases . *Journal of Vascular Surgery,* Vol 27, No. 1, pp. 81-87

Kolvenbach, R,; Schwierz, E, Wasilljew, S, Miloud, A, Peurschel, A, Pinter, L. Total laparoscopically and robotically assisted aneurysm surgery: a critical evaluation . *Journal of Vascular Surgery,* Vol 39, No. 4, pp. 771-776

Kuhan, G & Raptis, S (1997) 'Trash foot' following operations involving the abdominal aorta. *Australian and New Zealand Journal of Surgery,* Vol 67, No. 1, pp. 21-24

Kurosawa, K,; Ohta, H, Sumi, M, Ohki, T (2007) Physiologic monitoring data: will it change our follow-up paradigms? *Seminars in Vascular Surgery,* Vol 20, No. 2, pp. 115–120

Lam, CR, & Aram, HH (1951) Resection of the descending thoracic aorta for aneurysm: a report of the use of a homograft in a case and experimental study. *Annals of Surgery,* Vol 134, No. 4, pp. 743-752

Lambrechts, D,; Casselman, F, Schroeyers, P, De Geest, R, D'Haenens, P, Degrieck, I (2003) Endovascular treatment of the descending thoracic aorta. *European Journal of Vascular and Endovascular Surgery,* Vol 26, No. 4, pp. 437-444

Lazarus, HM (1988) Intraluminal graft device, system and method. US patent number 4,787,899

Lee, WA,; Carter, JW, Upchurch, G, Seeger, JM, Huber TS (2004) Perioperative outcomes after open and endovascular repair of intact abdominal aortic aneurysms in the United States during 2001. *Journal of Vascular Surgery,* Vol 39, No. 3, pp. 491-496

Lee, WA,; Brown, MP, Nelson, PR, Huber, TS. Total percutaneous access for endovascular aortic aneurysm repair ("Preclose" technique). *Journal of Vascular Surgery,* Vol 45, No. 6, pp. 1095–1101.

Lederle, FA,; Johnson, GR, Wilson, SE, Cute, EP, Hye, RJ, Makaroun, MS, Barone, GW, Bandyk, D, Moneta, GL, Makhoul, RG (2000) The aneurysm detection and management study screening program: validation cohort and final results. Aneurysm Detection and Management Veterans Affairs Cooperative Study Investigators. *Archives of Internal Medicine,* Vol 160, No. 19, pp 1425-1430

Lederle, FA,; Wilson, SE, Johnson, GR, Reinke, DB, Littooy, FN, Acher, CW, Ballard, DJ, Messina, LM, Gordon, IL, Chute, EP, Krupski, WC, Busuttil, SJ, Barone, GW,

Sparks, S, Graham, LM, Rapp, JH, Makaroun, MS, Moneta, GL, Cambria, RA, Makhoul, RG, Eton, D, Ansel, HJ, Freischlag, JA, Bandyk, D (2002) Aneurysm Detection and Management Veterans Affairs Cooperative Study Group. Immediate repair compared with surveillance of small abdominal aortic aneurysms. *New England Journal of Medicine,* Vol 346, No 19, pp. 1437–1444.

Lederle, FA (2006) A summary of the contributions of the VA cooperative studies on abdominal aortic aneurysms. *Annals of New York Academy of Sciences,* Vol 1085, pp. 29–38

Leurs, L,; Bell, R, Degrieck, Y, Thomas, S, Hobo, R, Lundbom, J; EUROSTAR; UK Thoracic Endograft Registry (2004) Endovascular treatment of thoracic aortic diseasescombined experience from the EUROSTAR and United Kingdom Thoracic Endograft registries. *Journal of Vascular Surgery,* Vol 40, No. 4, pp.670-679

Lin, P,; Bush, RL, Katzman, JB, Zemel, G, Puente, OA, Katzen, BT, Lumsden, AB (2003) Delayed aortic aneurysm enlargement due to endothension after endovascular abdominal aortic aneurysm repair. *Journal of Vascular Surgery,* Vol 38, No. 4, pp. 840-842

Major, RH (1954) A History of Medicine, Illinois, Charles C. Thomas, Chapter I, pp. 51-204

McPhee, JT,; Hill,JS, Eslami, MH (2007) The impact of gender on presentation, therapy, and mortality of abdominal aortic aneurysm in the United States, 2001–2004. *Journal of Vascular Surgery,* Vol 45, No. 5, pp. 891–899

McPhee, JT; Robinson 3rd, WP, Eslami, MH, Arous EJ, Messina, LM, Schanzer, A (2011) Surgeon case volume, not institution case volume, is the primary determinant of in-hospital mortality after elective open abdominal aortic aneurysm repair. *Journal of Vascular Surgery,* Vol 53, No. 3, pp. 591–599

Merten, GJ,; Burgess, WP, Gray, LV, Holleman, JH, Roush, TS, Kowalchuk, GJ, Bersin, RM, Van Moore, A, Simonton 3rd, CA, Rittase, RA, Norton, HJ, Kennedy, TP (2004) Prevention of contrast-induced nephropathy with sodium bicarbonate: a randomised controlled trial. *Journal of American Medical Association,* Vol 291, No. 19, pp. 2328-2334

Mitchell, RS,; Miller, DC, Dake, MD, Semba, CP, Moore, KA, Sakai, T (1999) Thoracic aortic aneurysm repair with an endovascular stent graft the "first generation.". *Annals of Thoracic Surgery,* Vol 67, No. 6, 1971-1974

Moon, MC,; Morales, JP, Greenberg, RK (2007) The aortic arch and ascending aorta: are they within the endovascular realm? *Seminars in Vascular Surgery,* Vol 20, No. 2, pp. 97-107

Murphy, EH,; Beck, AW, Clagett, GP, DiMaio, JM, Jessen, ME, Arko, FR (2009) Combined aortic debranching and thoracic endovascular aneurysm repair (TEVAR) effective but at a cost. *Annals of Surgery,* Vol 144, No. 3, pp. 222-227

Najibi, S,; Terramani, TT, Weiss, VJ, MacDonald, MJ, Lin, PH, Redd, DC, Martin, LG, Chaikof, EL, Lumsden, AB (2002) Endoluminal versus open treatment of descending thoracic aortic aneurysms. *Journal of Vascular Surgery,* Vol 36, No. 4, pp. 732-737

Parodi, JC,; Palmaz, JC, Barone, HD (1991) Transfemoral intraluminal graft implantation for abdominal aortic aneurysms. *Annals of Vascular Surgery,* Vol 5, No. 6, pp. 491–499

Peppelenbosch, N,; Buth, J, Harris, PL, van Marrewijk, C, Fransen, G, EUROSTAR Collaborators (2004) Diameter of abdominal aortic aneurysm and outcome of endovascular aneurysm repair: does size matter? A report from EUROSTAR. *Journal of Vascular Surgery,* Vol 39, No. 2, pp. 288–297.

Prinssen, M,; Verhoeven, EL, Buth, J, Cuypers, PW, van Sambeek, MR, Balm, R, Buskens, E, Grobbee, DE, Blankensteijn, JD (2004) Dutch Randomized Endovascular Aneurysm Management (DREAM) Trial Group. A randomized trial comparing conventional and endovascular repair of abdominal aortic aneurysms. *New England Journal of Medicine,* Vol 351, No. 16, pp. 1607–1618

Prissen, M,; Buskens, E, Nolthenius, RP, van Sterkenburg, SM, Teijink, JA, Blankensteijn, JD (2004) Sexual dysfunction after conventional and endovascular AAA repair: results of the DREAM Trial. *Journal of Endovascular Therapy,* Vol 11, No. 6, pp. 613-620

Prissen, M,; Buskens, E, de Jond, SE, Buth, J, Mackaay, AJ, van Sambeek, MR, Blankensteijn, JD, DREAM Trial participants (2007) Cost-effectiveness of conventional and endovascular repair of abdominal aortic aneurysms: results of a randomised trial. *Journal of Vascular Surgery,* Vol 46, No. 5, pp. 883-890

Richardson, JD & Main, KA (1991) Repair of abdominal aortic aneurysms. A statewide experience. *Archives of Surgery,* Vol 126, No. 5, pp. 614-616

Rickenbach, S,; Hassani, O, Thaveau, F, Bensimon, Y, Jacquot, X, Tally, SE, Geny, B, Eisenmann, B, Charpentier, A, Chakfe, N, Kretz, JG (2004) Current outcome of elective open repair for infrarenal abdominal aortic aneurysm. *Annals of Vascular Surgery,* Vol 18, No. 6, pp. 704-709

Rudnick, M & Feldman H (2008) Contrast-induced nephropathy: what are the true clinical consequences? *Clinics of Journal of American Society of Nephrology,* Vol 3, No. 1, pp. 263-272

Saers, SJ & Scheltinga, MR (2005) Primary aortoenteric fistula. *British Journal of Surgery,* Vol 92, No. 2, pp. 143-52

Sampram, ESK.; Karafa, MT, Mascha, EJ (2003). Nature, frequency and predictors of secondary procedures after endovascular repair of abdominal aortic aneurysm . *Journal of Vascular Surgery.* Vol 37, pp. 930–937

Sasaki, T,; Ohsawa, S, Ogawa, M, Mukaida, M, Nakajima, T, Komodo, K, Tachieda, R, Niinuma, H, Kawazoe, K (2000) Postoperative renal function after an abdominal aortic aneurysm repair requiring a suprarenal aortic cross-clamp. *Surgery Today,* Vol 30, No.1, pp. 33-36

Schermerhorn, ML,; O'Malley, AJ, Jhaveri, A, Cotterill, P, Pomposelli, F, Landon, BE (2008) Endovascular vs. open repair of abdominal aortic aneurysms in the Medicare population. *New England Journal of Medicine,* Vol 358, No. 5, pp. 464-474

Song ,Y.; Liu, Q, Shen, H, Jia, X, Zhang, H, Qiao, L (2008) Diagnosis and management of primary aortoenteric fistulas-experience learned from eighteen patients. *Surgery,* Vol 143, pp. 43-50

Svensson, LG,; Crawford, ES, Hess, KR, Coselli, JS, Safi, HJ (1993) Variables predictive of outcome in 832 patients undergoing repairs of the descending thoracic aorta. *Chest,* Vol 104, No. 4, pp.1248-1253.

Tanski III W & Fillinger M (2007) Outcomes of original and low-permeability Gore Excluder endoprosthesis for endovascular abdominal aortic aneurysm repair. *Journal of Vascular Surgery,* Vol 45, No. 2, pp. 243–249

Thompson JE (1998) History of vascular surgery. Chapter 6 In: Surgery: basic science and clinical evidence, pp. 1299-1312

United Kingdom Small Aneurysm Trial Participants (2002) Long-term outcomes of immediate repair compared with surveillance of small abdominal aortic aneurysms. *New England Journal of Medicine,* Vol 346, No. 19, pp. 1445–1452.

Wald, R,; Waikar, SS, Liangos, O, Pereira, BJ, Chertow, GM, Jaber, BL (2006) Acute renal failure after endovascular vs open repair of abdominal aortic aneurysm. *Journal of Vascular Surgery,* Vol 43, No.3, pp. 460-466

White, GH,; Yu, W, May, J (1996) Endoleak–a proposed new terminology to describe incomplete aneurysm exclusion by an endoluminal graft. *Journal of Endovascular Surgery,* Vol 3, No. 1, pp. 124–125.

White, RA,; Donayre, CE, Walot, I, Lippmann, M, Woody, J, Lee, J, Kim, N, Kopchok, GE, Fogarty, TJ (2001) Endovascular exclusion of descending thoracic aortic aneurysms and chronic dissections initial clinical results with the AneuRx device. *Journal of Vascular Surgery,* Vol 33, No. 5, pp. 927-934

Willard, JC.; & Nasbeth, DC (1974) Visceral infarction following aortic surgery. *Annals of Surgery,* Vol 180, pp. 312-318

Wolf, YG,; Tillich, M, Lee, WA, Rubin, GD, Fogarty, TJ, Zairns, CK (2001) Impact of aortoiliac tortuosity on endovascular repair of abdominal aortic aneurysms: evaluation of 3D computer-based assessment. Journal of Vascular Surgery, Vol 34, No. 4, pp. 594-599

van Bommel, EF,; van der Veer, SJ, Hendriksz, TR, Bleumink, GS (2008) Persistent chronic peri-aortitis ('inflammatory aneurysm') after abdominal aortic aneurysm repair: systematic review of literature. *Vascular Medicine,* Vol 13, No. 4, pp. 293-303

Velazquez, OC,; Larson, RA, Baum, RA, Carpenter, JP, Golden, MA, Mitchell, ME, Pyeron, A, Barker, CF, Fairman, RM (2001) Gender-related differences in infrarenal aortic aneurysm morphologic features: issues relevant to Ancure and Talent endografts. *Journal of Vascular Surgery,* Vol 33, pp. S77-S84

Verhoeven, ELG,; Tiellin; JFS, Prins, TR (2004) Frequency and outcome of re-interventions after endovascular repair for abdominal aortic aneurysm: a prospective cohort study. *European Journal of Vascular and Endovascular Surgery.* Vol 28, No. 4, pp. 357–364

Volodos, NL,; Karpovich, IP, Troyan, VI, Kalashnikova, YuV, Chekhanin, VE, Ternyuk, NE, Neoneta, AS, Ustinov, NI, Yakovenko, LF (1991) Clinical experiences of the use of self-fixing synthetic prostheses for remote endoprosthetics of the thoracic and the abdominal aorta and iliac arteries through the femoral artery and as intraoperative endoproshesis for aorta reconstruction. *Vasa Suppl,* Vol 33, pp. 95-99

Voorhoeve, R.; Moll, FL, de Letter, JA, Bast, TJ, Wester, JP, Slee, PH (1996) Primary aortoenteric fistula: Report of eight new cases and review of the literature. *Annals of Vascular Surgery,* Vol 10, No. 1, pp. 40-48

Yamada, N,; Okita, Y, Minatoya, K, Tagusari, O, Ando, M, Takamiya, M, Kitamura, S (2000) Preoperative demonstration of the Adamkiewicz artery by magnetic resonance angiography in patients with descending or thoracoabdominal aortic aneurysms. *European Journal of Cardiovascular Surgery,* Vol 18, No. 1, pp. 104-11

Jonk, YC,; Kane, RL, Lederle, FA, MacDonald, R, Cutting, AH, Wilt, TJ (2007) Cost-effectiveness of abdominal aortic aneurysm repair: a systematic review. *International Journal of Technology Assessment in Health Care,* Vol 23, No. 2, pp. 205-215

Zarins, CK,; Bloch, DA, Crabtree, T, Matsumoto, AH, White, RA, Fogarty, TJ (2003) Stent graft migration after endovascular aneurysm repair: importance of proximal fixation. *Journal of Vascular Surgery,* Vol 38, No. 6, 1264-1272

Part 2

Improvements in the Endovascular and Surgical Management of Aortic Disease

Endovascular Repair of Ruptured Abdominal Aortic Aneurysms

Cheong J. Lee[1], Andrew Gonzalez[2] and Mark D. Morasch[1]
[1]*Northwestern University,*
[2]*University of Illinois at Chicago, Chicago, Illinois, United States of America*

1. Introduction

Ruptured abdominal aortic aneurysms (AAAs) are catastrophic events with dismal outcomes. Even in the modern era, the overall mortality rate reaches 90%. Most ruptured aneurysms worldwide are repaired by conventional open surgery with a high operative mortality despite major medical advancements in diagnostic imaging and intensive care delivery. Over the past two decades, the in-hospital mortality rate for open repair of ruptured AAAs has remained steady at around 40%-50% (Noel et al., 2001).

Since its development in 1991 by Juan Parodi, endovascular aortic repair (EVAR) has been widely accepted as an excellent method to treat aortic aneurysms with suitable anatomy. Large prospective randomized studies have already demonstrated substantial improvements in perioperative morbidity and mortality for elective EVAR compared to elective open repair of AAA. Given the encouraging results and minimally invasive nature of EVAR coupled with yet observed dismal outcomes of open repair of ruptured AAAs, the use of EVAR in the emergent setting has been proposed. The first series of patients that successfully underwent endovascular repair of ruptured AAAs (rEVAR) with homemade grafts described by Ohki and Veith in 1999, demonstrated an operative mortality rate of only 16%, suggesting that rEVAR may potentially improve outcomes seen with open repair. In 2001, only 6% of patients with rupture AAA were treated using EVAR techniques in the United States, by 2006 that number increased dramatically to 19% (Greco et al., 2006). To put that number in some context, another recent study suggested that, as many as 33% of men, and 60% of women who present to the hospital in the United Kingdom receive no intervention at all for ruptured AAA (Filipovic et al., 2007). There are several reasons for centers to be slow to adopt the endovascular approach. These reasons include limited availability of the off-the-shelf devices on an urgent basis, lack of experienced endovascular surgical expertise, and unavailability of dedicated operating room facilities and ancillary staff who are adequately equipped to perform these procedures. As such, many patients who would qualify for EVAR still undergo the traditional open repair.

Regardless, EVAR continues to gain momentum as the preferred mode of repair for ruptured abdominal aortic aneurysms. The decision to proceed with EVAR is generally dependent upon the patient's hemodynamic stability, suitable anatomy, and an experienced center that can perform the procedure. Although no randomized controlled trials currently exist, evidence from both prospective and retrospective reviews demonstrate the feasibility and potential benefit of rEVAR. There is mounting evidence showing EVAR to be a safer, less invasive alternative to open surgery with the potential to significantly reduce in-hospital mortality and morbidity in EVAR suitable candidates despite the inherent biases that accompany the comparison.

2. A Standardized approach to endovascular repair of ruptured abdominal aortic aneurysms

To successfully treat patients with ruptured AAA using endovascular means, the practicing institution must have resources to support a multidisciplinary team approach to managing patients with ruptured AAA. Strict protocols from the emergency room to discharge planning need to be put in place to streamline patient throughput. A comprehensive protocol should address the following issues - appropriate triage and expedient imaging in the emergency department; equipment needs and necessities of the operating suite; a systematic approach to post-operative care and the management of the most common post-operative complications; a method for ensuring that the protocol includes the most up-to-date evidence-based measures; and finally, a delineation of required ancillary resources. Figure 1 below illustrates a proposed protocol for the management of patients with a suspected ruptured AAA.

A well organized team of vascular specialists should be able to address any ruptured AAA that is admitted to the hospital at any time of day or night. In order to accomplish this goal, the team must be multidisciplinary, familiar with working with each other in the context of AAAs, and have enough trained members to include 24 hour per day, 365 days per year coverage. While not an exhaustive list, the specialties required of the vascular team are vascular surgeons, vascular anesthesiologists familiar with both open and endovascular ruptured AAAs, vascular scrub nurses or technicians who have experience in both open operations and endovascular interventions, critical care nurses, surgical intensivists who are familiar with endovascular interventions, radiology technicians well versed in rapid CT protocols for delineating AAA anatomy, emergency medicine physicians familiar with ruptured AAA pre-operative requirements, a liaison in the blood bank familiar with massive resuscitation (should the case need to convert to open), and bed control managers with authority to free up appropriate ICU resources.

Ideally there should be an up-to-date inventory management system so that missing or damaged equipment are known of with enough lead time to permit transfer of the patient to a hospital with appropriate and working resources. As with the often acknowledged "door-to-balloon" time with myocardial infarction, hospitals must seek to minimize the time from diagnosis to aortic control. This includes a standardized approach to activating a dedicated team, including experienced surgeons facile with both endovascular and open techniques, anesthesiologists, nursing staff, and radiology technicians. These individuals must be experienced in performing both EVAR and open aortic repair. In a recent international, collective report of rEVAR performed by 49 centers worldwide, it was noted that staff availability and skills were a major determinant of whether a rupture AAA patient would be treated by EVAR or open repair (Veith et al., 2009). Additionally, it is advisable to have a method for the emergency room physician to put the team on notice, at the time a ruptured AAA is first suspected.

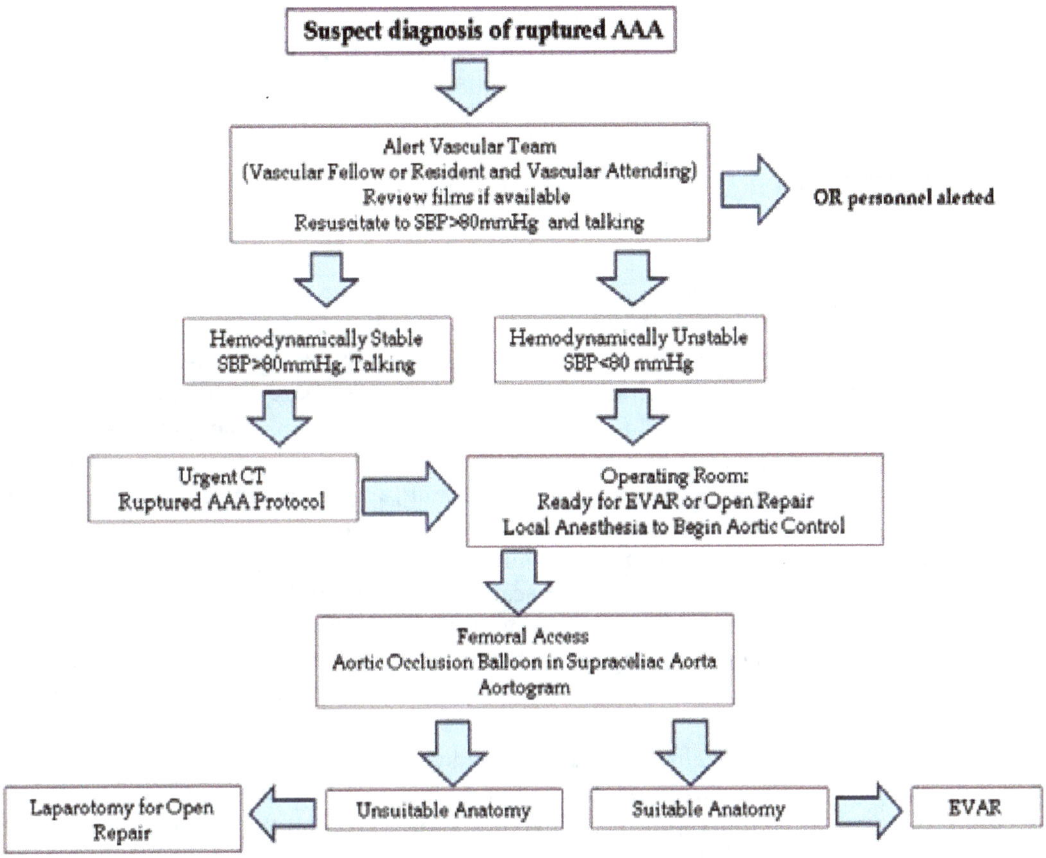

Fig. 1. Proposed protocol for rEVAR.

2.1 In the emergency room - Diagnosis and triage

When a ruptured AAA is suspected in the emergency room, the "aneurysm reflex" must be avoided where, historically, patients are aggressively resuscitated and then taken urgently to the operating room. There is evidence to suggest that a more controlled, thoughtful but expeditious approach is feasible and likely beneficial. For one, allowing "permissive hypotension" by limiting the resuscitation to maintain a detectable blood pressure (SBP >80mmHg) and maintaining mental status can help minimize ongoing hemorrhage and allow for expeditious imaging via computed tomography (CT).

The need for preoperative CT imaging prior to EVAR for ruptured AAA continues to be debated. Most centers consider such screening to be mandatory both for purposes of confirming the diagnosis as well as for morphological assessment. A few centers have developed protocols that provide for intraoperative assessment without CT delay using angiography or intravascular ultrasound. Realistically, time is usually available to send patients for CT evaluation without undue risk. Current data suggests that the majority of patients with ruptured AAA have time to undergo a CT scan. The majority of patients who are admitted to the hospital with ruptured AAA survive for a number of hours. In 2004 Lloyd et al., examined the time to death in patients with ruptured AAA who did not undergo treatment. Their findings indicated that 88% (49 of 56) of patients died >2 hours after admission with diagnosis of ruptured AAA. The median time from the onset of symptoms to admission to the hospital was 2.5 hours, and the interval between hospital admission and death was 10 hours.

2.1.1 Diagnosis and determination of anatomic suitability

Although the diagnosis of rupture AAA is generally made by CT, it is important to consider that a history along with abdominal palpation has a sensitivity of between 90-97% for patients who eventually have an operation. Once the diagnosis is suspected and the vascular team activated, the next step is to triage hemodynamically unstable patients (SBP < 80mmHg) to the operating room, and hemodynamically stable (SBP > 80mmHg) patients to the CT scanner. Given the potential for rapid and significant deterioration, it is paramount for ruptured AAA patients to have priority for the CT scanner. CT is vital in confirming the diagnosis and properly delineating the aortoiliac anatomy for EVAR suitability. At most centers, 2 hours is ample time to obtain a CT scan to assess suitability for EVAR. In the case of patients who present with true hemodynamic instability, the decision must be made to either attempt to assess the morphology, and hence the candidacy for EVAR, without axial imaging using modalities available in the procedural suite or to commit to open reconstruction.

Investigators have begun to evaluate the use of fixed C-arm imaging systems and advanced rendering softwares in the hybrid operating room to generate three-dimensional roadmaps and perform computed tomographic (CT) imaging. Eide et al used the Siemens DynaCT to generate a CT immediately following EVAR and compared those images to a standard CT angiogram performed on a standard 16 slice multidetector CT (MDCT) scanner. The authors noted no statistical differences between the intra-operative C-arm generated completion DynaCT and the postoperative MDCT. When evaluating the preoperative anatomic assessment capability in EVARs however, Nordon et al found that DynaCT provided inferior visualization of mural thrombus and calcification and underestimates vessel size. Further studies assessing CT capability of fixed C-arms in the operating room are currently underway; and as imaging technology and software continue to evolve, it will not be long before accurate three-demensional roadmaps can be rendered "on-table" to expedite assessment of anatomic suitability for EVAR.

Anatomic suitability has been reported in between 60% to 80% of patients presenting with a rupture AAA (Mehta, 2009). The range is accounted depending on strict versus liberal adherence to the generally acknowledged criteria - aortic neck length greater than or equal to 15 mm, infrarenal neck diameter less than or equal to 32 mm, aortic neck angulation less than 60 degrees, and need for both iliac arteries to be greater than 5 mm in diameter to achieve an optimal infrarenal fixation (Chaikof et al., 2009). Advancements in endograft technology continue to push the indications for use (IFU) and determination of anatomic suitability is generally dependent upon the judgment and comfort of the vascular surgeon. Accepting normally unsuitable anatomy has led a number of investigators to develop the concept of endovascular damage control, which accepts a suboptimal radiographic result in exchange for temporizing the emergency. In short, some patients will still require laparotomy for failed EVAR or for the treatment of abdominal compartment syndrome. The damage control approach can only be adopted provided patients consent to undergo vigilant late follow-up examination and understand the potential need for "preventative maintenance".

2.1.2 Triage

In the hemodynamically unstable patient taken directly to the operating suite, each respective institution should determine whether or not to proceed directly to an open operation, or alternatively attempt to determine anatomic suitability fluoroscopically or via intravascular ultrasound. The determination of whether a patient is hemodynamically unstable should not be made on an ad hoc basis, but should be explicit within the protocol beforehand. The determination of instability is based upon the level of physiologic compromise that the surgeons, anesthesiologists, emergency medicine physicians, and intensivists are comfortable and experienced with handling. In the recent 2009 survey by Veith et al., centers providing rEVAR reported a wide range of hemodynamic criteria for when a patient was too unstable to be offered EVAR:

1. All comers, regardless of hemodynamics, receive attempt at EVAR
2. Systolic blood pressure (SBP) <90 mm Hg
3. SBP <80 mm Hg
4. SBP <70 mm Hg
5. Similar SBP lower limits as above but with requirement that the level is sustained
6. SBP <50 mm Hg
7. Any SBP measurement <90 mm Hg and/or who had contained ruptures

While not stated in the Veith et al. survey, it has previously been reported that cardiac arrest is an automatic indication to proceed directly to open repair (Alsac et al., 2005).

2.1.3 Resuscitation

Clear endpoints of resuscitation should be determined when designing a standardized approach to rEVAR. Currently, limited resuscitation also called hypotensive or damage control resuscitation (DCR) has fallen back into vogue. The concept was first documented during World War I when poor outcomes were reported in battlefield patients with intravenous fluid administration (Cannon, 1818). With the recent conflicts in Iraq and Afghanistan, DCR has been extensively studied by both military and civilian trauma surgeons. In one study of civilian trauma patients it was found that limited resuscitation with a goal of maintaining systolic BP at 90 mmHg, use of isotonic intravenous fluids were limited and fresh frozen plasma (FFP) and packed red blood cells (PRBC) were transfused in a 1:1 ratio. This retrospective study found a nearly 20% decrease in 30 day mortality as well as a 50% decrease in ICU length of stay and overall hospital length of stay utilizing DCR.

Considering the age demographic of most patients presenting with rupture AAA, a study of more than 3,000 trauma patients at the Cedars-Sinai Medical Center concluded that "judicious fluid resuscitation is especially important in the elderly [age >70 years]" because the use of crystalloid volumes greater than 3 liters is associated with an 8.6 fold decrease in survival (Ley et al., 2011). Although no studies directly address the issue of survival and limited resuscitation in rupture AAA, one Dutch feasibility study found that hypotensive resuscitation with a goal SBP of 50-100 mm Hg was achievable in the majority (54%) of cases (van der Vliet et al., 2007).

2.1.4 Additional preoperative considerations

The goal of standardizing a preoperative management scheme for patients with ruptured AAA should be to make the diagnosis and get the patient safely to the operating room in 20-30 minutes. Some considerations to allow for expediency are (1) if at all possible, avoid central lines, namely femoral lines, and arterial lines (2) EKG, Chest X-rays, and Ultrasound should be avoided unless the diagnosis is in question (3) an agreed upon goals for permissive hypotension or limited resuscitation, (4) the ability to start advanced-level real time hemodynamic monitoring to minimize delays once the patient arrives at the operating suite.

2.2 In the operating room - Equipment and technical considerations

It is the authors' belief that a hybrid operating suite, which incorporates both the ability to do advanced endovascular interventions as well as traditional open operations, is essential to successfully treating ruptured AAAs. Furthermore, logistics require that the operative suite be stocked with wide range of graft sizes and types, balloons, sheaths, wires, and catheters. While the imaging quality of the cardiac catheterization lab is equal to that of a hybrid operating room, the primary advantage of hybrid operating rooms is that they permit the surgeon to emergently convert to an open procedure without the need to bring in additional equipment. Routine utilization of hybrid operating rooms should provide for a more liberal policy "EVAR first", while maintaining the option to institute an open repair should circumstances require.

2.2.1 Inventory

Concerning inventory management, there are two important considerations. First, there should be stocks of sheaths, wires, and catheters to fit various sizes of patients. There should also be a variety of sizes of aortic occlusion balloons, a power-injector, redundant back-ups for fluoroscopic equipment. A stock of endografts to match the largest aortic neck diameter and the shortest aneurysm length with a variety of iliac extensions for most AAA anatomic variations as well as a stock of Palmaz stents should be readily available. The second, and perhaps more important consideration, is that the inventory and functional status of all required equipment is must be known at all times. Because ruptured AAA are unpredictable, it must be known as soon as possible whether vital equipment (e.g. the power injector) is in disrepair so that the patient may be transferred to a hospital with the ability to carry out the intervention.

2.2.2 Anesthesia and aortic control

In rEVAR, aortic control can be performed under local anesthesia via percutaneous approach in experienced hands or general anesthesia and femoral artery cut-down. Use of local anesthesia helps to avoid the hemodynamic changes associated with muscle relaxation and general anesthesia. The significant inflammatory response related to cytokine release may be blunted with EVAR. Large doses of heparin can be avoided as well. While less invasive, the percutaneous approach suffers several physiologic, mechanical, and logistic limitations. Physiologically, it may be difficult to quickly and accurately palpate a femoral pulse in a patient who is hemodynamically unstable or undergoing permissive hypotension. This maybe obviated by the use of ultrasound guided access. From a device standpoint, the most common stents require at least an 18F sheath and may pose problems depending on patient anatomy. Logistically, cut-downs are almost invariably faster. As such, it is the recommendation of the authors to forego attempts at totally percutaneous access in any patient who is not hemodynamically stable, awake, and unable to cooperate with the operating room personnel.

2.2.3 Aortic occlusion balloons

After gaining access, an aortic occlusion balloon (AOB) is advanced via a 12-14Fr (45 cm) sheath placed into the juxtarenal aorta and advanced to the level of the supraceliac aorta. The aortic occlusion balloon is inflated as needed to maintain hemodynamic stability. A liberal usage policy with regard to AOB is recommended because of the difficulty associated with insertion at later points in the intervention. In one case series, the use of AOB was reported at 27% (Riesenman et al., 2008). It is important to remember to deflate the balloon just prior to stent deployment to prevent entrapment of the balloon between the graft and the aorta. This short period without aortic occlusion is usually insignificant to the patient's hemodynamics (Mehta et al., 2010).

2.2.4 Adjunctive procedures

The operating surgeon must be able to handle the need for unexpected adjunctive procedures as in the emergent setting, preoperative planning can be less than ideal. One such procedure that should be in the surgeon's armamentarium is knowledge and comfort in utilizing Palmaz stents to repair type I endoleaks (one of the most common operative complications of rEVAR). Further the surgeon should be comfortable with hybrid cases. For instance, if the decision is made to use an aortouni-iliac (AUI) graft or to convert a bifurcated stent graft to an AUI (as has been reported in 16% of patients), the surgeon should be comfortable performing both the primary EVAR and the femorofemoral bypass (Mehta et al., 2010).

3. Post-operative care considerations

The immediate post-operative considerations include the ability to monitor patients for the most common complications e.g. abdominal compartment syndrome. This necessitates a protocol re-activation of the operative team in the event of an emergent requirement to take the patient back to the OR.

3.1 Abdominal compartment syndrome

Abdominal compartment syndrome (ACS) is a significant complication resulting from a ruptured AAA. The pathophysiology is multifactorial resulting from existing retroperitoneal hematoma, ongoing, coagulopathic bleeding from aortic collaterals (lumbar and inferior mesenteric arteries from the disrupted aneurysm sac), and profound shock associated with ruptured AAA, which induce a systemic inflammatory response (SIRS) with increased capillary permeability and hemodynamic compromise (Mehta M., 2005). The incidence of ACS after rupture AAA is as high as 18% and carries with it a 7 fold increased risk of death (Mehta et al, 2010). Additionally, ACS is a major contributor to post operative acute renal failure and intestinal ischemia. However, both acute renal failure and intestinal ischemia can occur outside of the setting of ACS. Risk factors include massive blood transfusions, intraoperative coagulopathy and use of aortic occlusion balloons. The debate is still ongoing as to the best method for diagnosing ACS. The various options center around some combination of clinical exam findings and bladder pressure measurements. By whatever criteria, the treatment has remained decompressed laparotomy.

4. Current data on endovascular repair of ruptured aortic aneurysms

The evidence to support EVAR for ruptured AAAs is largely drawn from results of single-center case series, systematic reviews, and more recently, population-based studies arising from the United States. Although encouraging mortality rates are published, significant biases exist. First, a direct comparison between EVAR and open surgery for ruptured AAA is difficult as not all patients are anatomically suitable for EVAR. Secondly, unstable patients are by in large, directed toward traditional open repair. In a recent retrospective institutional review, Lee et al. identified this selection bias in that hemodynamically unstable patients tended to undergo open repair even when potentially anatomically suitable for rEVAR (Lee et al., 2008). Such observations may be alluding to the fact that patients stable enough to undergo CT are already a self-selecting cohort compared to those that are in extremis and cannot proceed to preoperative imaging. As experience increases with EVAR, however, hemodynamic stability may not factor as much into repair selection or else may push the choice toward rEVAR for unstable patients as access and balloon occlusion can be rapidly attained to stop hemorrhage. Despite the inherent biases that exist in studying the outcomes of rEVAR, evidence to support an EVAR first approach to managing ruptured AAAs continues to mount.

Select studies in the literature representing current data on rEVAR are summarized in Table 1 below. Many institutions that have adopted the rEVAR first approach have seen significant benefits. Of the single-center experience observational studies, the most recent report by Starnes et al. comparing outcomes before and after implementation of a rEVAR-first protocol, showed that their overall 30-day mortality fell from 54.2% to 18.5% (Starnes et al., 2009). On a larger scale, outcomes of implementing a rEVAR first protocol was reviewed in a large co-operative multicenter cohort study by Veith et al. in 2009 spanning 49 institutions in 13 countries. The study showed superiority of EVAR over open repair in terms of 30-day mortality (rEVAR 21.2% vs. Open repair 35.8%) when collectively analyzed not accounting for differences in practice variability; most centers limited the use of rEVAR to "stable" patients or those with "contained" ruptures (Veith et al., 2009). The study re-examined the results of 13 centers that were committed to performing rEVAR for all ruptured cases despite hemodynamic instability. These centers were usually those with larger volume experiences. The report showed a median 30 day mortality of 19.7% with EVAR and 36.3% with open surgery (*P*<0.0001). The power of the study is significant (1037 cases) to support rEVAR as a better treatment to managing ruptured AAAs, however, with no defined standard of practice in any participating centers and with this being a purely an observational study, the evidence is till at best level 2b.

Author, Date and Country	Study Type	Key Results
Starnes et al., (2009), J Vasc Surg, USA	Retrospective cohort study (level 2b)	Mortality reduction from 57.8% to 35.3% [absolute risk reduction 22.5%; odds ratio (OR) of 0.40]
Veith et al., (2009), Ann Surg, USA	Retrospective multi-center cohort study (level 2b)	30-day mortality amongst EVAR repair=21.2% 30-day mortality amongst open- repairs=35.8% In centers treating 24-62 rAAA overall mortality=21.0% (range 7-39%). 30-day mortality amongst centers using EVAR for 11-18 rAAA per annum=22.5% (range 6-43%). 30-day mortality for centers performing EVAR on 5-10 rAAA per annum=30%. 30-day mortality for centers performing EVAR on 1-4 rAAA per annum=35%
Karkos et al., (2009), Arch Surg, Greece	Systematic review of non-randomized observational studies (level 2a)	Meta-analysis of 19 studies reporting results of concurrent open-repair, pooled mortality after open-repair = 44.4% (95% CI, 40.0-48.8%), and pooled overall mortality for endovascular or open repair= 35% (95% CI, 30-41%)
Vogel et al., (2009), Vasc Endovascular Surg, USA	Retrospective national cohort study (level 2b)	Mortality=45.1% EVAR vs. 52.4% open-repair (P=0.21) Length of stay not significantly different between EVAR and open-repair groups
Giles et al., (2009), J Endovasc Ther, USA	Multicenter cohort study (level 2b)	Mortality=24% EVAR vs. 36% open-repair (P<0.05)
Visser et al., (2009), J Vasc Surg, Netherlands	Multi-center prospectively-recruited cohort study (level 2b)	Thirty-day mortality=26% EVAR vs. 40% open-repair (P=0.06)
Sadat et al., (2009), Eur J Vasc Endovasc Surg, UK	Prospective cohort study (level 2b)	Group 1=17 eEVAR, 29 open repairs, 4 palliated (after the introduction of rEVAR), Group 2=54 underwent open repair and 17 were palliated Significant differences in 30-day operative mortalities between the two groups 13% in Group 1 vs. 39% in Group 2 (P=0.0003)
Verhoeven et al., (2008), J Vasc Surg, Netherlands	Prospective cohort study (level 2b)	Mortality after EVAR=13.9% vs. 28.1% open-repair (P=0.092) No significant difference in mortality over 25 months follow- up between EVAR and open- repair
Ockert et al., (2007), J Endovasc Ther, Germany	Retrospective cohort study (level 2b)	30-day mortality=31% in both groups (P=1.0). Morbidity rate=55.2% EVAR vs. 62% open-repair (P=0.9)
Hinchliffe et al., (2006), Eur J Vasc Endovasc Surg, UK	Single center RCT (level 1b)	30-day intention-to-treat mortality=53% rEVAR vs. 53% open-repair Moderate or severe operative complications=77% EVAR vs. 80% amongst open-repair. Renal complications=55% EVAR vs. 8% open-repair (P=0.02) 4 patients died prior to surgery

Table 1. List of current data on endovascular repair of ruptured AAA.

Large national databases have also been used to examine the differences between open and endovascular repair for ruptured AAA. Egorova et al. examined the databases of 4 large states from 2000 to 2003 and found, even in those earlier years, that mortality in 290 rEVAR patients was lower than in 5508 open repair patients (39% versus 48%, $p<0.005$) (Egorova et al., 2008). Analysis of another large nationwide inpatient sample from 2001 to 2006 showed the increase in the use of EVAR for ruptured AAAs increased over time (5.9% in 2001 to 18.9% in 2006, $P < .0001$) while overall ruptured AAA rates remained constant (Mcphee et al., 2009). In reviewing the database, the investigators showed that rEVAR had lower overall in-hospital mortality than open repair (31.7% vs 40.7%, $P < .0001$). The benefit of rEVAR, when stratified by institutional volume, was found to be augmented in that study. Investigators also found that rEVAR patients had a shorter length of stay (11.1 vs 13.8 days, $P < .0001$), higher discharges to home (65.1% vs 53.9%, $P < .0001$), and lower cost of care ($108,672 vs $114,784, $P < .0001$) (Mcphee et al., 2009). Although these large datasets give convincing arguments to support rEVAR, reports from population-based studies are misleading because they are not able to control for significant confounders of patient physiology and morphology. In addition, it is not known whether these studies are applicable outside the United States. The study, however, noted that because of the technical requirements of the procedure, the impact of annual volume on outcomes of ruptured AAA repairs is an important factor that cannot be assessed by single institutional series.

It has been shown that there is a significant relationship between higher surgeon and hospital volume and improved patient outcomes after open surgical repair for ruptured AAA (Dimick et al., 2002). Mcphee et al found a clear mortality advantage directly related to all volume measures analyzed: annual elective open repair volume, annual elective EVAR volume, and annual RAAA volume. For each of these metrics, mortality decreased significantly as annual surgical volume increased. The absolute mortality benefit was most pronounced when analyzed according to elective EVAR volume; institutions in the high elective EVAR volume (> 40 per year) had an absolute mortality decrease of >15%(Mcphee et al., 2009). In the multicenter study by Veith et al, rEVAR related mortality is seen to be dependent upon the institutional volume of rEVARs performed. In centers treating 24–62 ruptured AAAs per year, the collective mortality rate reported is 21.0% (range 7–39%); 30-day mortality amongst centers performing 11-18 rEVARs per year is 22.5% (range 6–43%); 30-day mortality for centers performing 5–10 rEVARs per year is 30% (range 21-30%); 30-day mortality for centers performing 1–4 rEVARs per year is 35. In fact, a study by Giles et al. in 2009 showed lower mortality rates in higher volume hospitals for both open repairs and rEVAR, and a very large difference in endovascular outcomes. As such, the authors concluded that regionalization of referrals of ruptured AAA patients to high-volume centers preferentially may improve overall national outcomes.

The study by Hinchliffe et al from 2006 is the only paper published to date reporting level 1 evidence comparing rEVAR to open repair. This single-center a randomized control trial (RCT) study showed a higher EVAR related mortality compared to those reported in observational studies and did not find any overall survival advantage in the mid- to long-term with EVAR compared to open repair (Hinchliffe et al., 2006). Of those patients enrolled, 53% were deemed suitable for EVAR. The prerequisite for CT-scanning, interestingly, did not delay definitive surgery. As only 32 patients were enrolled, the study lacked sufficient power to provide definitive recommendations but did show that it is possible to recruit patients to a randomized trial of open repair and EVAR in patients with ruptured AAA.

More randomized studies have since commenced. The Amsterdam (Acute Endovascular Treatment to Improve Outcome of Ruptured Aortoiliac Aneurysms [Ajax]) trial (ISRCTN66212637) recruited 80 patients, and being underpowered, showed no significant difference in primary combined end point of 30-day mortality and serious morbidity. Recruitment for the trial has therefore been extended. The Ruptured Aorta-Iliac Aneurysms: Endo vs Surgery (ECAR) trial (NCT00577616) is currently underway and both AJAX and ECAR have been designed to recruit only the most stable patients, all of whom will be anatomically suitable for EVAR. One can argue that randomization of patients after CT scanning will not delineate the role of an rEVAR first strategy compared to open repair on an intention-to-treat basis. In consideration, the UK study Immediate Management of the Patient with Rupture: Open Versus Endovascular repair (IMPROVE) aneurysm trial (ISRCTN 48334791) will randomize patients at the time of diagnosis of ruptured AAA, either to immediate CT scan and endovascular repair whenever anatomically suitable (endovascular first), or to open repair, with CT scan being optional (normal care). The trial is set on a background of guidelines for emergency care, CT scanning and anesthesia, which incorporate the protocol of permissive hypotension. Recruitment started in October 2009 and 600 patients are required to show a 14% survival benefit at 30 days (primary outcome) for the endovascular first policy.

With the given evidence to date, the only reasonable conclusion that can be drawn is that the role of rEVAR in the management of patients with ruptured AAA remains to be proven. Due to the lack of quality data, determining the subgroup of patients that will truly gain benefit from rEVAR remains to be elucidated and we will have to await the results of level 1 evidence to answer this question.

5. Conclusion

Despite the inherent biases, information is emerging to suggest that there is a clear role for EVAR for ruptured AAA in select patients. There are a number of clear advantages to the endovascular approach given patient suitability. Patients undergoing EVAR can be treated using local anesthesia, which helps avoid the hemodynamic changes associated with muscle relaxation and general anesthesia. In addition, the morbidity associated with dissecting the aortic neck, damage to peri-aortic structures, and bleeding, can be avoided. The current literature has demonstrated decreased procedure times, reduced blood loss, and improved overall and intensive care unit lengths of stay following EVAR for ruptured AAA when compared to open surgery, but also suggests that these results are seen in select centers with adequate EVAR and open experience; supporting a direction towards regionalization of care and the management of all ruptured AAAs in large vascular centers. The routine use of EVAR for ruptured AAAs, however, remains to be proven with forthcoming level 1 evidence.

The technology behind stentgrafts continues to evolve and will further the potential for improved patient survival. If rEVAR can significantly reduce the mortality rate of patients presenting to hospital with ruptured AAA, the management of ruptured AAA would have to change as well as the organization and delivery of emergency and vascular services. The capability of performing rEVARs requires significant investment in institutional infrastructure. If feasible, however, the implementation of rEVAR capability and protocols could potentially benefit all types of repairs as the awareness and response to the arrival of a ruptured aneurysm patient is streamlined.

6. References

Alsac JM., Desgranges P., Kobeiter H., et al. *Emergency endovascular repair for ruptured abdominal aortic aneurysms: feasibility and comparison of early results with conventional open repair.* Eur J Vasc Endovasc Surg 30 (2005), pp. 632–639

Cannon W., Fraser J., Cowell E. *The Preventative Treatment of Wound Shock.* JAMA 1918:618-621.

Chaikof EL., Brewster DC., Dalman RL., et al. *The care of patients with an abdominal aortic aneurysm: The Society for Vascular Surgery practice guidelines.* J Vasc Surg. 2009:50(8S);1S - 49S.

Duchesne JC., Barbeau JM., Islam TM., et al. *Damage control resuscitation: from emergency department to the operating room.* Am Surg. 2011 Feb;77(2):201-6.

Egorova N., Giacovelli J., Greco G., et al., *National outcomes for the treatment of ruptured abdominal aortic aneurysm: comparison of open versus endovascular repairs,* J Vasc Surg 48 (2008), pp. 1092–1100.

Eide KR, Ødegård A, Myhre HO, et al. *DynaCT during EVAR - A Comparison with Multidetector CT.* Eur J Vasc Endovasc Surg. 2009;37:23-30.

Filipovic M, Seagroatt V, Goldacre MJ. *Differences between women and men in surgical treatment and case fatality rates for ruptured aortic abdominal aneurysm in England.* Br J Surg. 2007 Sep;94(9):1096-9.

Giles KA, Pomposelli F, Hamdan A, et al. *Decrease in total aneurysm-related deaths in the era of endovascular aneurysm repair.* J Vasc Surg 2009

Greco G, Egorova N, Anderson PL., et al., *Outcomes of endovascular treatment of ruptured abdominal aortic aneurysms,* J Vasc Surg 43 (2006), pp. 453–459.

Hinchliffe RJ., Bruijstens L., MacSweeney STR., et al. *A randomised trial of endovascular and open surgery for ruptured abdominal aortic aneurysm: results of a pilot study and lessons learned for future studies.* Eur J Vasc Endovasc Surg 2006;32:506–513.

Hinchliffe RJ and Braithwaite BD. *Ruptured abdominal aortic aneurysm: endovascular repair does not confer any long-term survival advantage over open repair.* Vascular 15 (2007), pp. 191–196.

Hoornweg LL., Wisselink W., Vahl A., et al. *The Amsterdam Acute Aneurysm Trial: suitability and application rate for endovascular repair of ruptured abdominal aortic aneurysms,* Eur J Vasc Endovasc Surg 33 (2007), pp. 679–683.

Kim SH, Stezoski SW, Safar P, et al: *Hypothermia and minimal fluid resuscitation increase survival after uncontrolled hemorrhagic shock in rats.* J Trauma 1997; 42:213-222.

Lederle FA and Simel DL. *Does this Patient Have Abdominal Aortic Aneurysm?.* JAMA. 1999;281:77-82.

Lee RW., Rhodes JM., Singh MJ., et al. *Is there a selection bias in applying endovascular aneurysm repair for rupture?,*.Ann Vasc Surg 22 (2008), pp. 215–220.

Lee WA., Hirneise CM., Tayyarah M., et al. *Impact of endovascular repair on early outcomes of ruptured abdominal aortic aneurysms,* J Vasc Surg 40 (2004), pp. 211–215.

Ley, EJ., Clond MA., Srour MK., et al. *Emergency Department Crystalloid Resuscitation of 1.5 L or More is Associated With Increased Mortality in Elderly and Nonelderly Trauma Patients.* Journal of Trauma-Injury Infection & Critical Care: February 2011 - Volume 70 - Issue 2 - pp 398-400

Lloyd GM, Bown MJ., Norwood MG., et al., *Feasibility of preoperative computed tomography in patients with ruptured AAA: A time to death study in patients without operation,* J Vasc Surg 39 (2004), pp. 788–791.

McPhee J, Eslami MH, Arous EJ, Messina LM, Schanzer A. *Endovascular treatment of ruptured abdominal aortic aneurysms in the United States (2001-2006): a significant survival benefit over open repair is independently associated with increased institutional volume.* J Vasc Surg 2009

Mehta M, Darling RC 3rd, Roddy SP., et al., *Factors associated with abdominal compartment syndrome complicating endovascular repair of ruptured abdominal aortic aneurysms,* J Vasc Surg 42 (2005), pp. 1047–1051.

Mehta M. *Endovascular aneurysm repair for ruptured abdominal aortic aneurysm: the Albany Vascular Group approach.* J Vasc Surg. 2010 Dec;52(6):1706-12.

Najjar SF, Mueller KH, Ujiki MB et al., *Percutaneous endovascular repair of ruptured abdominal aortic aneurysms,* Arch Surg 142 (2007), pp. 1049–1052.

Noel AA., Gloviczki P., Cherry KJ. et al. *Ruptured abdominal aortic aneurysms: the excessive mortality rate of conventional repair.* J Vasc Surg 34 (2001), pp. 41–46.

Nordon IM, Hinchliffe RJ, Malkawi AH, et al. *Validation of DynaCT in the Morphologic Assessment of Abdominal Aortic Aneurysm for Endovascular Repair.* J Endovasc Ther. 2010;17:183-189.

Parodi JC., Palmaz JC., Barone HD., et al. *Transfemoral intraluminal graft implantation for abdominal aortic aneurysms.* Ann Vasc Surg 5 (1991), pp. 491–499.

Riesenman PJ and Farber MA. *Endovascular Repair of Ruptured Abdominal Aortic Aneurysm.* Cardiovasc Intervent Radiol. 2008:31(3);496-503.

Starnes BW, Quiroga E, Hutter C, et al. *Management of ruptured abdominal aortic aneurysm in the endovascular era.* J Vasc Surg. 2010 Jan;51(1):9-17; discussion 17-8. Epub 2009 Nov 1. Erratum in: J Vasc Surg. 2010 Apr;51(4):1079.

van der Vliet JA, van Aalst DL, Schultze Kool LJ, et al. *Hypotensive hemostatis (sic) (permissive hypotension) for ruptured abdominal aortic aneurysm: are we really in control?* Vascular. 2007 Jul-Aug;15(4):197-200.

Veith FJ and Ohki T. *Endovascular approaches to ruptured infrarenal aorto-iliac aneurysms.* J Cardiovasc Surg 43 (2002), pp. 369–378.

Veith FJ, Lachat M, Mayer D, et al. *Collected world and single center experience with endovascular treatment of ruptured abdominal aortic aneurysms.* Ann Surg. 2009 Nov;250(5):818-24.

Verhoeven EL, Kapma MR, Groen H., et al., *Mortality of ruptured abdominal aortic aneurysm treated with open or endovascular repair,* J Vasc Surg 48 (2008), pp. 1396–1400.

Visser JJ, van Sambeek MR., Hamza TH et al., *Ruptured abdominal aortic aneurysms: endovascular repair versus open surgery – systematic review,* Radiology 245 (2007), pp. 122–129.

Vogel TR, Dombrovskiy V, Haser P, Graham A. *Has the implementation of EVAR for ruptured AAA improved outcomes?* Vasc Endovasc Surg 2009

5

Alternative Surgical Management of Ascending Aorta Aneurysm

Sossio Perrotta[1] and Salvatore Lentini[2]
[1]*Department of Cardiothoracic Surgery, Sahlgrenska University Hospital, Gothenburg*
[2]*Department of Cardiothoracic Surgery, University Hospital "G Martino", University of Messina, Messina*
[1]*Sweden*
[2]*Italy*

1. Introduction

The standard treatment for an ascending aorta aneurysm is radical resection and interposition of a tubular prosthesis.

Involvement of other adjacent structures has dictated the employment of more complex surgical techniques. The surgical treatment of concomitant disease of the aortic valve, aortic root and ascending aorta started in 1968 with Bentall and De Bono (Bentall & De Bono, 1968), who applied a new surgical technique bearing their names and that represents the standard surgical technique for this pathology. With this technique, the valve, aortic root and ascending aorta are resected, replaced with a prosthetic valvular conduit, and the coronary vessels are anastomised to the tubular prosthesis. Nowadays, this represents a widely accepted surgical strategy to treat concomitant disease at the three mentioned structures. Minimally invasive procedures have been reported in the treatment of these patients as well (Perrotta et al., 2008; Perrotta & Lentini, 2009).

In contrast, treatment of moderate ascending aorta dilatation associated with aortic valvular disease and with or without mild involvement of the aortic root is still controversial, especially in high risk patients (Bahnson, 1982; Prenger et al., 1994; Svensson et al., 1992).

While it is usually accepted that ascending aorta dilatation beyond 5 cm should be surgically replaced, opinions on the treatment below this limit are divided (Ergin et al., 1999). In older and high surgical risk patients, several conservative surgical techniques on the ascending aorta have been proposed, such as the "waistcoat" aortoplasty, the simple aortoplasty, the "S" shape aortoplasty and the "wrap" aortoplasty (Robicsek & Thubrikar, 1994; Mueller et al., 1997).

Radical resection of the ascending aortic aneurysm is needed in order to eliminate all the pathologic tissue of the aorta damaged by degenerative processes, such as cystic medionecrosis, aterosclerosis, and inflammatory processes. Lack of resecting part of the degenerative tissue may predispose to new aneurysmatic dilatation.

2. Histology and pathophisiology in aortic aneurysms

In the presence of mild to moderate dilatation of the ascending aorta associated with aortic valve disease, it may be difficult to ascertain if the dilatation is secondary to the hemodynamic alterations produced by the valvulopathy or by a disease of the aortic wall.

Preoperative and intraoperative studies may help to evaluate the structure of the aortic wall in relation to its thickness, elasticity and endothelium continuity. This can be done through a macroscopic analysis or through an intraoperative histopathologic evaluation on a cryostatic section of the aortic wall (Roman et al., 1989; Imaizumi et al., 1982).

The most frequent histological finding in patients with dilatation of the ascending aorta is cystic medionecrosis. However, results from histology may be very different and it is often difficult to distinguish the primary cause of dilatation (Mueller et al., 1997; Schlatmann & Becker, 1997a, 1997b; Hirst & Gore, 1976). In cystic medionecrosis it is possible to observe necrosis of the smooth muscular cells and a mucoid degeneration of the media, with accumulation of amorphic mucopolysaccaridic material in the vessel wall. Several authors (Schlatmann & Becker, 1997a; Klima et al., 1983) have observed that this is not a specific finding in patients with aortic ectasia and that positive-alcian basophile material is also present in the media of normal aortas. Furthermore, they noticed that the aortic alterations and their entities are mostly related to the patient's age and that there are more quantitative than qualitative differences between the analysed sections of normal aortas and the aneurysmatic or dissected ones. With aging, in normal aortas it is possible to observe fragmentation of the elastine, fibrosis, reduction of muscular cells and mucopolysaccarides. This may suggest that histological alterations in the aortic wall are not the expression of a degenerative disease, but the consequence of the metabolic activity of the media as a response to hemodynamic stress. With time, the hemodynamic stress prevails on the metabolic reparative processes. This process happens faster in patients with hereditary connective diseases (i.e. Marfan syndrome), in which the metabolic reparative mechanism is genetically malfunctioning.

Giving strength to the theory of hemodynamic stress, is the observation that the dilatation is more frequently localized on the lateral segment of the ascending aorta and on the aortic arch. The hemodynamic stress can be associated with an aortic valve disease. In these patients, a dilatation of the ascending aorta of various entities has been observed regardless of the presence of degenerative disease (Carrel et al., 1991).

Patients with a mild or moderate dilatation of the ascending aorta in association with an aortic valve disease often undergo only aortic valve replacement (Prenger et al., 1994; Natsuaki et al., 1998), believing it is not necessary to replace the ascending aorta. In patients with aortic valve stenosis, the replacement of the aortic valve, reducing systolic blood flow produced by the valve stenosis, eliminates the hemodynamic turbulence in the ascending aorta (Yearwood et al., 1989; Jarchow & Kincaid, 1961; Stein & Sabbah, 1976). Similarly, the surgical correction of an aortic valve insufficiency reduces the systolic hypertension and the diastolic ventricular turbulences, restoring the normal blood pressure and blood flow (Stein & Sabbah, 1976; Laske et al., 1996). In both situations the hemodynamic stress on the aortic wall is reduced (Schlatmann & Becker, 1997b; Crawford et al., 1988).

However, the removal of hemodynamic factors may not be sufficient to prevent further dilatation of the ascending aorta, and further dilatation may slowly progress according to the Laplace law (Natsuaki et al., 1998; Milano et al., 1998). For this reason, several surgical techniques of aortoplasty have been proposed in order to prevent this occurrence; some techniques modify only the aortic diameter without reinforcing (McCready & Pluth, 1979) the vessel, others instead reinforce (Robicsek, 1982) the vessel to prevent redilatation.

The efficacy of this technique is still under question since complications and redilatation may occur at follow up. These controversial results may be related to the extreme heterogeneity of the enrolled patients in the literature reports; some had aneurysms of the ascending aorta without aortic valve disease, others ascending aorta dissection or Marfan disease (Robicsek & Thubrikar, 1994; Carrel et al., 1991; Natsuaki et al., 1998; Barnett et al., 1995). These last clinical conditions are usually associated with a high frequency of redilatation (Kouchoukos et al., 1986; Carrel et al., 1993; Lawrie et al., 1993). For this reason, an accurate selection of patients and a correct surgical indication is mandatory in patients who are candidates for aortoplasty surgery.

3. Conservative treatment of an ascending aorta aneurysm

The conservative surgical treatment for an ascending aorta aneurysm takes its origin not as an elective treatment of mild or moderate dilatation of the ascending aorta, but as a surgical alternative to the traditional radical technique of resection with a tubular (Wheat et al., 1964; Ggoves et al., 1964) or a tubular valvular graft (Bentall & De Bono, 1968; Cabrol et al., 1986) (Figure 1).

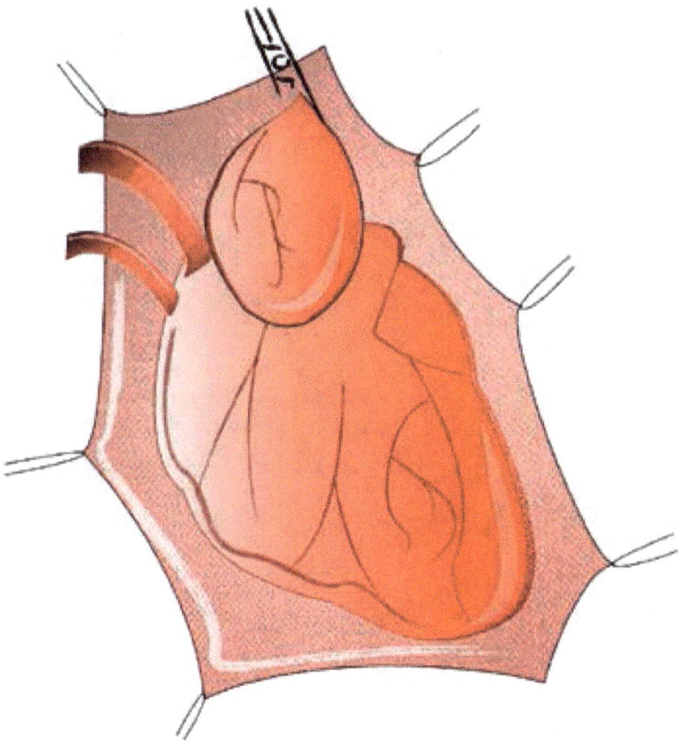

Fig. 1. Dilatation of the ascending aorta. The patient is cannulated according to standard technique; the arterial cannula is placed into the ascending aorta or aortic arch, while the venous cannula is in the right atrium. The ascending aorta is clamped before the brachiocephalic truncus. The aortic vent can be positioned according to the surgeon's preference.

It was McCready and Pluth (McCready & Pluth, 1979), who in 1979 reported the first conservative surgical technique for the treatment of an aneurysm of the ascending aorta, the so-called "simple aortoplasty"(Figure 2). They proposed an oval and longitudinal resection of the anterior wall of the ascending aorta. The aortotomy was sutured with a continuous double layer suture and in some cases reinforced by Teflon strips. In 1982, Robicsek (Robicsek, 1982) suggested his technique of aortoplasty, the so-called "external grafting" or "aortic wrap" (Figure 3), for the treatment of small aneurysms of the abdominal and thoracic aorta, and fusifom dilatation of the ascending aorta with associated valvular disease. The surgical procedure is similar to the one proposed by McCready, with an oval and longitudinal resection of the ascending aorta. The aorta is then reinforced by the application of a tubular prosthesis around the ascending aorta. The prosthesis is incised longitudinally and shaped around the vessel. The prosthesis is then stabilized by placing three sutures.

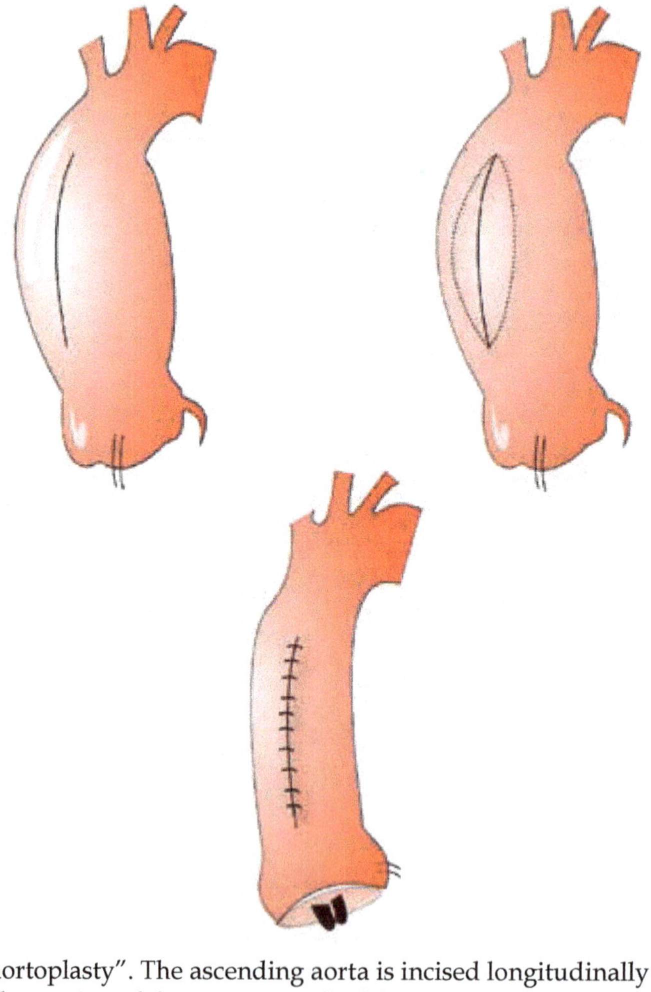

Fig. 2. "Simple aortoplasty". The ascending aorta is incised longitudinally and then an oval and longitudinal resection of the anterior wall of the ascending aorta is performed. The aortotomy can be sutured with a continuous double layer suture, or can be reinforced with Teflon felts.

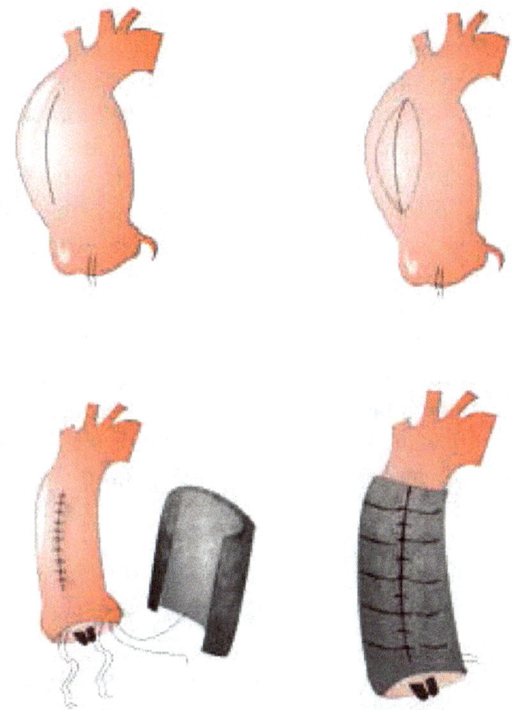

Fig. 3. "Aortic wrap aortoplasty". The surgical procedure is similar to the "simple aortoplasty". The aorta is then reinforced by the application of a tubular prosthesis around the ascending aorta. The prosthesis is incised longitudinally and shaped around the vessel. The prosthesis is then stabilized by placing three sutures at the level of the three commissures.

The results reported in the literature, both for the simple aortoplasty and for the aortic wrapping, are heterogeneous. However, most report advantages in using a conservative approach rather than radical surgery in selected cases (Carrel et al., 1991; Barnett et al., 1995).
The aortic cross clamp time and the extracorporeal circulation time are usually shorter, and this may represent an important factor in older patients requiring additional cardiac surgical procedures (Robicsek & Thubrikar, 1994; Mueller et al., 1997; Baumgartner et al., 1998).
Results from studies reporting on conservative treatment of the ascending aorta are summarized in the next paragraph.

4. Results from previous published studies

Egloff (Egloff et al., 1982), in his study, compared the results of aortoplasty surgery (both simple aortoplasty and wrapping technique) with radical surgery. He found that the incidence of cerebrovascular thromboembolic events is higher in patients undergoing radical surgery that in those undergoing conservative surgery. However, it should be mentioned that in his report, Egloff included a heterogeneous study population. Half of the patients had an acute or chronic ascending aorta dissection, while the other half had a dilatation of the ascending aorta of various entities and not always associated with an aortic valve disease. In 15% of the patients the aneurysm was related to Marfan syndrome, while in 4% of the population the aneurysm was related to syphilitic disease. There was not a specific indication for the type of surgery performed in relation to the specific pathology. This lack of specific indication may partly explain the higher incidence of redilatation of the ascending aorta after aortoplasty than after radical surgery.

Carrel (Carrel et al., 1991) reported the results of 291 patients who underwent cardiac surgery and concomitant surgery on the ascending aorta. The surgical procedures employed were aortic remodeling and external wall support in 164 patients, composite graft replacement in 81 patients and supracoronary graft in 46 patients. Elective, urgent and emergent operations were included in the study. The overall mortality was 4.8%, and he showed good results, at both medium and long term. Compared to the graft replacement and supracoronary graft, the aortoplasty group had the lowest early mortality rates (1.8% vs 9.8% vs 6.4%). The 5 and 10 year survival in the groups of patients undergoing aortic remodelling and external wall support, supracoronary graft and composite graft were, respectively, 93.5%, 82% and 80% and 83.8%, 73% and 67%. The incidence of reoperation at 10 years was 3.6% versus 2.4 %, respectively, in the group of patients that underwent conservative surgery and in the group with composite graft. The incidence of postoperative bleeding was higher in patients undergoing radical surgery rather than conservative surgery.

Barnett (Barnett et al., 1995) in 1995 evaluated the effectiveness of tailoring aortoplasty used to treat fusiform aneurysms of the ascending aorta. He reviewed results on 17 patients, of which nine had tailoring aortoplasty alone, and eight patients had aortoplasty and Dacron wrapping. In his study the author included patients with aortic valve disease associated with an aneurysm of the ascending aorta, with sizes ranging from 5 to 8 cm, confined to the tubular portion of the ascending aorta that narrowed to a normal diameter in the distal ascending aorta and with a normal diameter of the sinuses of Valsalva. All the patients underwent concomitant cardiac surgery procedures. The actuarial survival at 1 and 10 years was 81% and 63%, respectively. He concluded that in selected cases, tailoring aortoplasty can achieve long-term results comparable to those of resection and graft replacement of fusiform ascending aortic aneurysms. At the follow up (mean 4.4 years), the ascending aorta was studied with chest radiography alone without reporting any redilatation of the ascending aorta. This represents a limiting factor of the study, since the diagnosis of redilatation is important for defining the technique efficacy.

Mueller (Mueller et al., 1997), in 1997, reported on 17 consecutive patients treated by unsupported aortoplasty for an aneurysm of the ascending aorta associated with aortic valve disease. Twelve patients had predominantly regurgitation of the aortic valve, and 5 patients had stenosis. The ascending aorta diameter ranged from 5 to 5.5 cm. In 6 elderly and high-risk patients, the aorta was between 5.5 and 6 cm in diameter. He reported a hospital mortality of 12%. Survival at 7 years was 86.7%. Recurring aortic aneurysms, requiring reoperation, developed in 4 patients after a mean time of 63 months, with an event-free survival at 7 years of 41%. All of these 4 patients had aortic valve regurgitation and cystic medial necrosis. The author concludes that the high recurrence of aorta ascending aneurysm after aortoplasty in patients with aortic valve regurgitation is due to an intrinsic deficiency of the aortic wall.

In 1998 Baumgartner (Baumgartner et al., 1998) developed a modification of the reduction aortoplasty procedure as a modified "Z-plasty" (Figure 4) without the use of additional external prosthetic wrapping material. The aortoplasty was performed when moderately sized ascending aortic aneurysms were encountered during concomitant cardiac operations. The incision was S-shaped and on the lateral aspect of the ascending aorta, with biased excision of tissue predominantly in the bends of the "S". The aorta was then sutured using a double running suture. The procedure was performed in 23 patients with moderate ascending aorta aneurysms, the mean diameter being 5.0±0.7 cm, and not involving the sinuses of Valsalva; none had Marfan syndrome. Sixteen patients were studied with echocardiography at a mean follow-up of 9.9±12.6 months. Their mean intraoperative postreduction diameter was 2.9±0.65 cm, at the follow-up the aorta was 3.1±0.45 cm (p = NS). Of these, seven had a mean follow-up of 22.1±9.2 months. Their mean postreduction diameter of 2.9±0.5 cm increased to 3.1±0.35 cm (NS). The author says that this simple technique places stress on the suture line in a favorable orientation, it appears to have good mid-term results and it is best suited to moderately sized aneurysms.

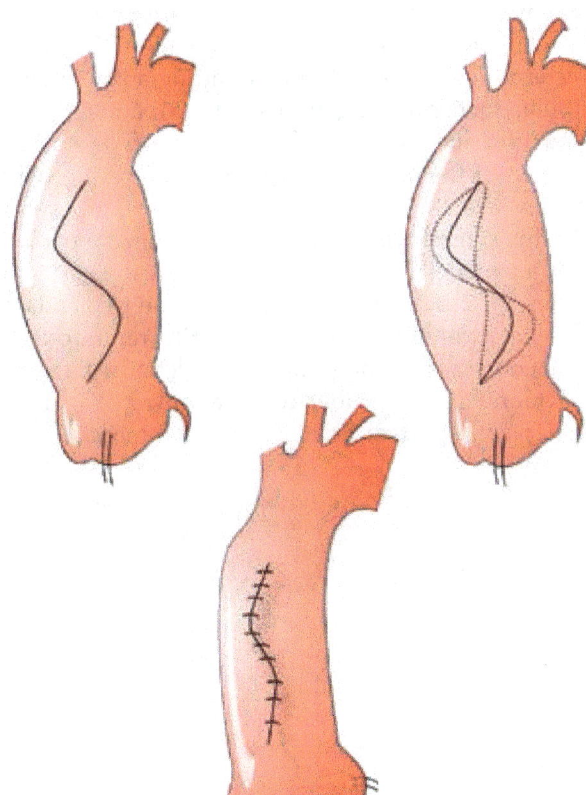

Fig. 4. "Z-plasty" aortoplasty. The incision of the ascending aorta is based on an "S-shape incision" and on the lateral aspect of the ascending aorta, with biased excision of tissue predominantly in the bends of the "S". The aorta is then sutured using a double running suture.

In 2002 Bauer (Bauer et al., 2002) reported of a total of 115 patients (36 female, 79 male) with bicuspid aortic valve and dilatation of the ascending aorta who underwent reduction aortoplasty alone or in combination with another cardiac procedure. In 106 patients (group I), reduction aortoplasty, "simple aortoplasty", was performed without additional external prosthetic support of the aortic wall. In the remaining 9 patients (group II), the aorta was externally supported by wrapping the ascending aorta with a prosthetic graft. None of the patients had characteristics of Marfan syndrome, as this surgical technique should be considered contraindicated in patients with this syndrome. The patients were postoperatively studied with CT and echocardiography during a mean follow-up time of 40 months (range 12 to 144 months). No reoperations on the ascending aorta or aortic valve during the follow-up period were reported. The 5-year survival rate was 94%±3.1%. During the late follow-up, a significant increase (> 4 mm) of the ascending aortic diameter was found in 9 patients (8.9%) from group I and in none from group II. The author observed that a factor that influenced the redilatation was the early postreduction diameter. He suggested that to avoid redilatation, the diameter of the ascending aorta should be reduced to 35 mm or less or the aorta should be supported externally by a tubular graft.

Viganó (Viganó et al., 2002), in 2002, reported the description of a different conservative surgery on the ascending aorta, named "end-to-end anastomosis" (Figure 5), designed for patients undergoing a ministernotomy approach for ascending aortic aneurysm with minor involvement of the sinotubular junction. He reported on 45 patients with a diagnosis of chronic ascending aorta aneurysm, including also patients with type A aortic dissection. To reduce the aneurysmatic section of the aorta he suggested performing two circumferential aortotomies: the first at the level of the sinotubular junction and the second at the distal border of the aneurysm. At this stage aortic valve surgery could be performed, if needed. The resulting resected wall is a cuneiform segment of the ascending aorta, that if opened on its anterior aspect, assumes a typical butterfly shape. Finally the two ends of the ascending aorta are sutured together with a running suture, eventually reinforced by Teflon strips. Patients were studied with computed tomography and echocardiography. During the follow-up period (23.7±12.3 months) a very low redilatation rate (1 of 43; 2.3%) and no incidence of pseudoaneurysm were reported; 1 patient required reoperation.

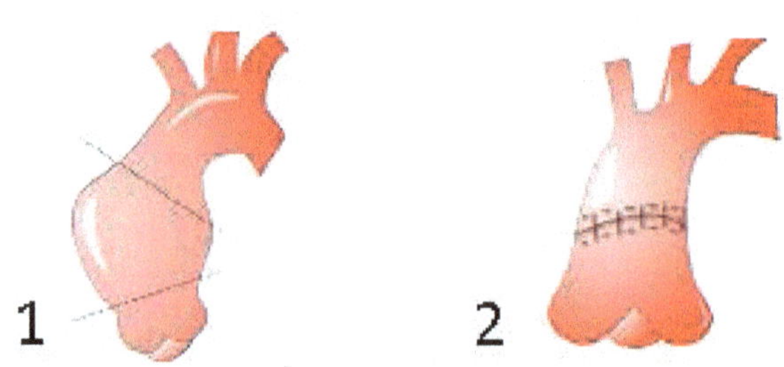

Fig. 5. After clamping the ascending aorta, distally to the aneurysm, the aorta is opened and then resected between two circumferential aortotomies: first at level of sinotubular junction and second at distal edge of aneurysm (1). Two ends of aorta, without tension, are finally sutured with a continuous (2).

Later, Masetti (Masetti et al., 2004), in a smaller series of patients undergoing "end-to-end anastomosis" suggested a modification of the previously described technique with the aim to facilitate the surgical approach. The horizontal aorta is largely mobilized, mainly by dissecting the first portion of supra-aortic trunks and by dissecting pericardial reflections adjacent to the inferior vena cava and left atrium. Then, after clamping the ascending aorta and resecting the aneurysm by two circumferential aortotomies, the two aortic ends may be sutured together with a reduced tension. The patients were postoperatively studied with CT scan during a median follow-up time of 72 months per patient (10.5±102.7 months). At the follow-up, the mean aortic diameters showed no statistically significant enlargement when compared with the findings of aortic contrast CT scan at discharge. The author concludes that cuneiform resection of the aorta ascendens and end-to-end ansastomosis provides effective long-term outcomes. This technique should be used only in patients with ascending aorta aneurysm associated with structural aortic valve disease. Patients with Marfan syndrome or other inherited connective tissue disorders should be not considered for this treatment.

Gaeta (Gaeta et al., 2009), in a recent report focused on some surgical details of the "end to end technique", reported on specific anatomic indications for this type of surgery. He recommended a preoperative CT scan spatial reconstruction of the thoracic aorta. The ideal candidate for this technique has "an elongated aorta in the antero-lateral wall; the postero-medial wall is usually restrained by the pulmonary artery and it maintains the original length".

Cotrufo (Della Corte et al., 2003; Cotrufo et al., 2003), in 2003, reported the results of 73 patients with a non-complicated dilatation of the ascending aorta associated with aortic valve structural disease, who underwent aortic valve replacement and "waistcoat aortoplasty"; some of these patients underwent plication of the sinuses of Valsalva as well. The surgical indication for associated aortoplasty was an aortic ratio >1.5 at either sinusal, tubular, or both levels. The aorta was incised longitudinally, starting from the aortic clamp towards the commissure between the right coronary sinus and the non-coronary sinus. At above 2 cm before reaching the commissure, the incision was deflected at an angle of 90° and continued towards the commissure between the left coronary and the non-coronary sinus. A triangular resection of the dilated aortic wall was then obtained by extending the incision from above the commissure to the distal end of the incision. At this point, surgery on the aortic valve was performed according the surgeon's preference. In patients with associated dilatation of the aortic sinuses, in order to treat the dilatation of the aortic sinuses and to remodel the aortic root geometry, each stitch bite placed on the aortic annulus, included the redundant subcoronary portion of the aortic wall. When implanting the prosthesis, and drawing the stitches tight, a bidimensional, longitudinal and radial plication of the three sinuses was achieved, thereby reducing the distance between the coronary ostia and the aortic annulus. The aorta was reconstructed using a double layer technique termed a "waistcoat aortoplasty". A first suture line fixed the right posterolateral free edge of the resection to the inner surface of the anterior wall, leaving a 1 to 2 cm wide anterior lap. The anterior lap was then used to cover and reinforce the neo-aortic wall, and its free margin was sutured on the right posterior wall (Figure 6 to 8). At follow-up, the ascending aorta was studied with echocardiography. The author reports that a significant postoperative reduction of Valsalva sinuses, sinustubular and ascending aorta diameters were found compared to the preoperative values. In 53 patients at a mean follow-up of 33.8±10.2 months, there was no significant enlargement of the aorta compared to 48 h postoperatively (P=0.32, P=0.15, P=0.38 respectively). Furthermore, no cases of postoperative aneurysm or aortic valve complications were recorded and the sinus plication did not interfere with the prosthesis leaflet movements. The author assesses that the "waistcoat aortoplasty", reducing the diameter of the ascending aorta and reinforcing the aortic wall, is indicated only in asymmetric dilatation of the ascending aorta associated with primary structural aortic valve disease; while in symmetrical dilatation a radical surgery is recommended.

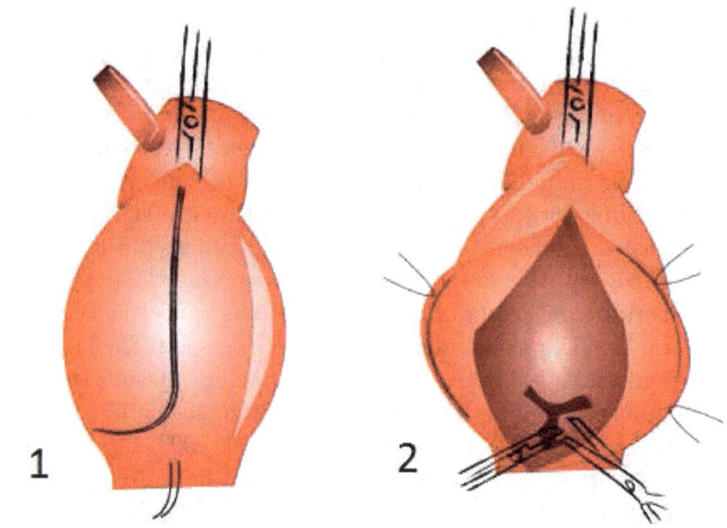

Fig. 6. "Waistcoat aortoplasty". The aorta is longitudinally incised, starting from the clamp towards the commissure between the right coronary sinus and the non-coronary sinus. At above 2 cm before reaching the commissure, the incision is deflected at an angle of 90° and continued towards the commissure between the left coronary and the non-coronary sinus (1). The native aortic valve is excised (2).

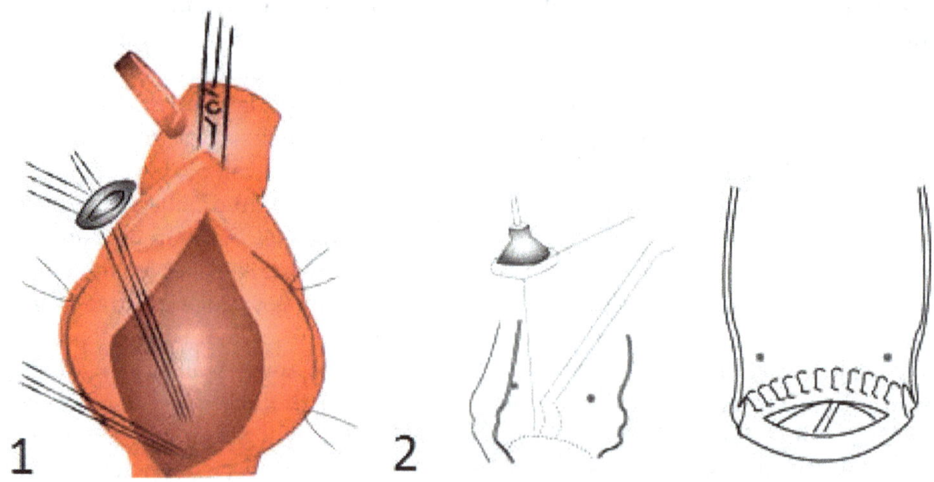

Fig. 7. The prosthetic valve is implanted (1). The sutures to anchor the aortic valve are driven in through the subcoronary aortic wall and out through the annulus. When implanting the prosthesis, there is a longitudinal plication of the sinuses (2).

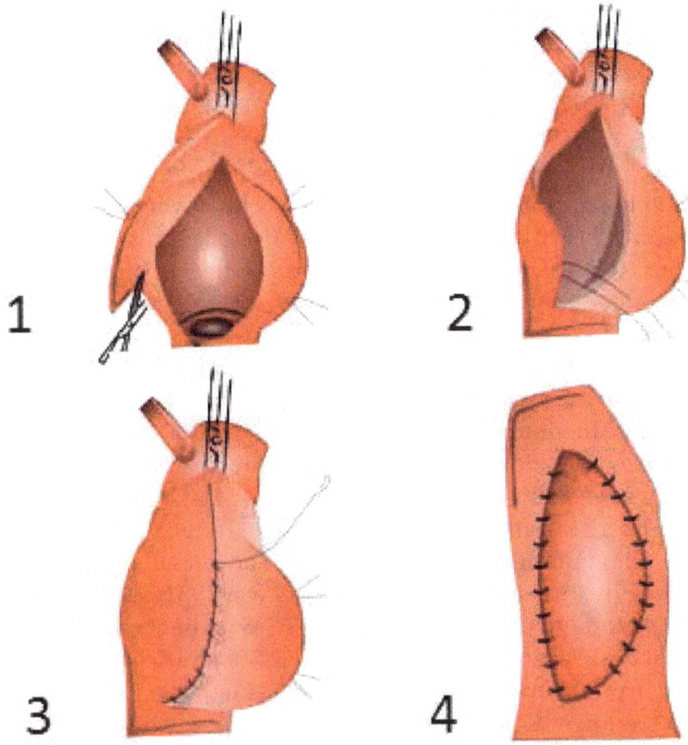

Fig. 8. A triangular resection of the dilated aortic wall is obtained by extending the incision from above the commissure to the distal end of the incision (1). The right edge of the aortotomy is sutured to the inner surface of the anterior wall with a suture line starting from the right coronary ostium (2). The suture line continues longitudinally leaving a 2 cm wide anterior lap (3). The remaining anterior lap is sutured to cover and to reinforce the aortic wall (4).

In 2004, Arsan (Arsan et al., 2004) reported on 62 consecutive patients that underwent treatment for ascending aorta aneurysm by reduction aortoplasty and external wrapping during cardiac concomitant procedures. The mean preoperative aortic diameter was 52.7±0.5 mm and the diameter of the ascending aorta was greater than 45 mm in all patients. Mean follow-up time was 39.6±18.0 months (range 8 to 78 months). No mortality was registered during a 30-day period. The hospital mortality was 1.6%, one patient died as result of septic multiple-organ failure. Comparing the aortic diameter before surgery (AD1), aortic diameter in early postoperative (AD2) and aortic diameter during the late postoperative period (AD3), reduction aortoplasty of the ascending aorta with external wrapping resulted in a significant reduction of the ascending aorta diameter in all patients (AD1 versus AD2 and AD3, p=0.000). There was also a statistically significant difference between the ascending aortic diameters measured during early and late follow-up (AD2 versus AD3, p=0.000). Although this increase was statistically significant, all measurements of the follow-up period in groups AD2 and AD3 were still within the normal range. The author concluded that external wrapping of the aorta offers excellent results with very low mortality and morbidity, and it can be regarded as a safe and effective method for the treatment of ascending aortic aneurysm in selected patients. However, the patients should be carefully monitored for redilatation after the procedure.

The same author (Arsan, 2004) reported as well on 4 high-risk patients who underwent off-pump reduction aortoplasty and concomitant myocardial revascularization. In these patients, the diameter of the ascending aorta was less than 6 cm and there were no calcification, atherosclerotic penetrating ulcers, or suspicion of dissection. The author routinely performs an external wrapping technique without incising or excising the diseased aorta, a "sandwich technique". The tubular graft is tailored to the diseased aorta longitudinally using separate, full-thickness U sutures. This technique can be performed easily even on the beating heart in high risk patients in order to prevent complications. According to the author, this technique could be the procedure of choice in selected high-risk cases for the treatment of borderline ascending aortic aneurysms in patients undergoing coronary revascularization.

Polvani (Polvani et al., 2006), in 2006, published a study where he evaluated the midterm follow-up of unsupported aortoplasty and determined predictors of redilatation. He reported on 68 patients with dilatation of the ascending aorta treated by unsupported reduction aortoplasty in combination with other cardiac procedures. Indication for surgery was an aortic diameter between 40 and 50 mm for younger patients and up to 60 mm for older patients or in high risk patients, with the aim to reduce aortic cross-clamp and perfusion times. Mean follow-up time was 2.9±1.7 years. The overall perioperative mortality rate was 1.5%. Overall survival estimates at 3 and 6 years were 93.3%±4.5% and 89.3%±5.9%, respectively. Ascending aorta redilatation occurred in 5 patients (7.5%). The actuarial freedom from redilatation at 3 and 6 years was 97.7%±2.3% and 79.8%±8.4%, respectively. The actuarial freedom from reoperation at 3 and 6 years was 100% and 86.3%±7.5%, respectively. Only preoperative diameter was a significant predictor of redilatation, using multivariate stepwise logistic regression analysis. In the author's experience, unsupported aortoplasty resulted in a safe and effective technique with low mortality, low morbidity, and few late complications for selected chronic aneurysm of the ascending aorta with diameters less than 55 mm. A diameter greater than 55 mm is an independent risk factor for redilatation, and it should be considered a contraindication to this procedure and may be considered an indication to the Dacron graft support.

Walker (Walker et al., 2007), in 2007, investigated the postoperative stability and preservation of the physiologic elasticity of the reconstructed ascending aorta (Windkessel function). He collected the results of 97 patients who underwent aortoplasty without external stabilization, for a moderate enlargement of the ascending aorta up to 5 cm, as a concomitant procedure during cardiac surgery. Patients with Marfan syndrome, aneurysms of the sinus of Valsalva, aneurysms of the aortic arch and patients with an infective origin of the aneurysm were excluded. Hospital mortality was 3%. At 32 months follow-up, fifty-four patients agreed to be examined by computed tomographic scan (determination of the aortic diameter) and transthoracic echocardiography (determination of the Windkessel function). Mean dilatation during the time from early postoperative measurement to follow-up was 0.17 cm (±0.27 cm; CI 0.09 to 0.25 cm). In six patients with a follow-up of 60 months who had both early and late postoperative diameter assessment, the mean postoperative dilatation was 0.04 cm (±0.15 cm; CI 0.11 to 0.20 cm). By transthoracic echography, the diastolic-systolic augmentation (Windkessel function) of the ascending aorta was confirmed, with a median amplitude value of 0.25 cm (range, 0 to 1.1 cm). These results were compared with data from patients who received a tubular graft on the ascending aorta. They had only minor diameter changes during systole and diastole: median 0.06 cm (range, 0 to 0.12 cm). The systolic augmentation of patients with aortoplasty was 250% in comparison with those who received a tubular graft on the ascending aorta (CI 157% to 375%). The author concludes that aortoplasty without external support is a valid treatment in patients with moderate dilatation of the ascending aorta and preserves the Windkessel function of the ascending aorta.

In 2007, Feindt (Feindt et al., 2007), in a retrospective study, analyzed the results of a cohort of 50 patients who underwent size-reducing ascending aortoplasty with external wrapping. The maximum diameter of the ascending aorta in this group was measured between 45 and 65 mm without dilation of the sinotubular junction and aortic arch. Aortoplasty was associated with other cardiac procedures such as aortic valve replacement in 47 cases. The procedure was performed with low hospital mortality (2%) and a low postoperative morbidity. Computer tomographic and echocardiographic diameters were significantly smaller after reduction (55.8±9 mm down to 40.51 (±6.2 mm (CT), p < 0.002; 54.1±6.7 mm preoperatively down to 38.7±7.1 mm (echocardiography), p < 0.002), with stable performance at follow-up (mean follow-up time: 70 months, complete in 31 patients). The authors concluded that ascending aorta aortoplasty with external reinforcement is a safe procedure with excellent long-term results and that it is a therapeutic option in patients with poststenotic dilatation of the aorta, without dilatation of the sinotubular junction.

Belov (Belov et al., 2009), in 2009, compared the early results and late outcome in two groups of patients. Group 1 had prosthetic ascending aorta replacement, while group 2 had reduction aortoplasty and external wrapping. All had a diameter of the ascending aorta ≥5 cm and a sinus of Valsalva diameter <4.5 cm. Group 1 had longer cardiopulmonary bypass time, higher reoperation for bleeding and higher mortality. None of the patients in group 2 needed reoperation due to ascending aorta redilatation nor significant enlargement of the Valsalva sinuses during the follow-up. According to Belov, the main criterion for performing or not performing an aortoplasty with external wrapping on the ascending aorta should only be the diameter at the level of the Valsalva sinuses, rather than the ascending aorta maximal diameter. He considered a diameter <4.5 cm at the Valsalva sinuses as an appropriate condition for performing a reduction aortoplasty. On the other hand, important enlargement of the ascending aorta usually leads to aortic root dilatation; reduction aortoplasty with external wrapping may be impossible in these circumstances.

In the same year, Zhang (Zhang et al., 2010) published his report of 71 patients with fusiform ascending aortic aneurysms and aortic valve disease who underwent reinforced reduction aortoplasty associated with aortic valve replacement (RRA group, n 32) or ascending aortic replacement combined with aortic valve replacement (AAR group, n 39). Patients requiring other concomitant cardiac procedures were excluded, as well patients with Marfan syndrome. The mean follow-up time was 3 years and 4 months. The cardiopulmonary bypass time, the aortic cross clamp time and the length of stay were higher in the AAR group than in the RRA group. The overall survival rate in all patients was 88.6%±4.5% at 5 years. The 5-year survival rate was 90.7%±6.4% in the RRA group and 87.0%±6.3% in the AAR group. There were no reoperations on the aorta or aortic valve in all patients during follow-up. In both groups, the aorta was studied at the level of the aortic sinuses and proximal aortic arch, and no significant differences between the postoperative and late follow-up diameters were found in the RRA and in the AAR groups.

In 2009, Haddad (Haddad et al., 2009) published an article in which he analyzed the results of 6 high risk patients, with a Euroscore between 11 and 19, with ascending aortic aneurysm and aortic valve disease, who underwent reduction aortoplasty with external wrapping associated with the aortic valve replacement. The inclusion criteria were: patients with aortic valve disease with surgical indication, ascending aortic diameter >5.5 cm, EuroSCORE >6 and age over 60 years; the mean diameter of the sinotubular junction was 36 mm. The exclusion criteria were: presence of dissections of the ascending aorta and Marfan syndrome. At follow-up (28 months), the actuarial survival rate was 100%, and none of patients needed reoperation. The author concludes that, despite the limitations of the study (small sample of patients, mid-term follow-up, selected and not random population), the reduction aortoplasty associated with external wrapping and aortic valve replacement is a therapeutic option with promising midterm results in high surgical risk patients with ascending aortic aneurysm and aortic valve disease.

In a recent article published in 2010, Hwang (Hwang et al., 2010), in his series of 88 patients, evaluates the long-term results of aortoplasty performed with aortic valve surgery and compared the results in patients with bicuspid aortic valve with those in patients with tricuspid aortic valve. Indication for aortoplasty was a moderately dilated ascending aorta with a diameter between 40–50 mm. Patients with combined aortic root dilatation (diameter of the sinus of Valsalva greater than 5 cm and/or displaced coronary ostia distal to the sino-tubular junction), and patients with systemic connective tissue disease were excluded. Operative mortality was 1.1%. The overall 10-year survival rate was 91.1%. No patients suffered from aorta-related complications such as aortic dissection, rupture or aortic reoperation. At follow-up of 74 months per patient, a CT scan was performed to evaluate the ascending aorta. The mean diameter of the repaired aorta was 37.8±4.3 mm and none had a diameter greater than 5 cm. The author assesses that the reduction ascending aortoplasty for a moderate ascending aortic aneurysm combined with aortic valve disease can be performed with low periprocedural risks and good long-term results.

Recently, Ang (Ang et al., 2010) reported on the early impact of aortic wrapping in patients undergoing aortic valve replacement with mild to moderate ascending aorta dilatation. An important finding of this study refers to "the reduction of the diameter and reversed remodeling of the aorta not only at the site of dilatation but also proximally and distally to the aortic wrapping". These results suggest that "correction of dimensions of a dilated ascending aorta at an early stage, and before irreversible anatomical changes take place, results in the rapid reversed remodeling of the rest of the aorta, probably due to the restoration of normal blood flow haemodynamics".

5. Discussion and conclusions

From the above mentioned studies we see that aortoplasty with or without external wrapping or simple wrapping alone may represent a surgical alternative for mild to moderate ascending aorta dilatation in high risk patients. However, some points should be addressed.

The aortoplasty reduces the diameter of the ascending aorta and therefore reduces the tension on the aortic wall, but it does not reinforce the wall in itself. Blood ejected by the left ventricle hits an area of the ascending aorta, which after aortoplasty is less elastic and rather more fibrotic due to the formation of a scar on the suture line. Areas of the ascending aorta previously involved in the dilatation are still weakened by the hemodynamic stress trauma (Mueller et al., 1997; Robicsek, 1995). This mechanism could explain aneurysm recurrence observed after "simple aortoplasty" (Mueller et al., 1997; Egloff et al., 1982). Therefore, aortoplasty, even if it eliminates the aneurysm, may sometimes prove insufficient to prevent recurrence.

Furthermore, simple aortoplasty may not be appropriate to treat patients with concomitant aortic root aneurysm (Mueller et al., 1997; Barnett et al., 1995). In order to reconstruct physiologically the ascending aorta, the wall of the ascending aorta is incised longitudinally and an elliptical portion of the aortic wall is then removed. From its nature, the edges of the elliptical shape progressively reduce their width at the extremities. Using this technique, it could be difficult to extend the reductive aortoplasty to the sinuses of Valsalva. These limitations are not overcome by the technique suggested by Baumgartner (Baumgartner et al., 1998); this technique is applicable to reduce the diameter of the ascending aorta, but it does not reinforce the aortic wall and it cannot be used to reduce a dilatation of the sinuses of Valsalva.

Not unanimous is the consensus regarding the "external grafting technique" suggested by Robicsek. Incertitude is raised by the use of a prosthetic graft to reinforce the aortic root (Cooley, 1982; Gott, 1994). Gott (Gott, 1994) has observed that this technique does not offer an adequate reinforcement of the aortic root, although Robicsek has indicated the dilatation of the sinuses of Valsalva and dilatation of the ascending aorta in patients with Marfan syndrome as pathologies treatable by external grafting.

The tubular prosthetic graft should be adequately positioned in order to not compress the coronary ostia and compromise cardiac perfusion (Robicsek & Thubrikar, 1994; Robicsek , 1982; Barnett et al., 1995). Often, when a dilatation of the aortic root is present, the coronary ostia are dislocated distally and away from the annulus (Bahnson, 1982; Barnett et al., 1995; Gott, 1994; Lewis et al., 1992). They take origin from the distal part of the aneurysm. The remaining section of the aortic root under the coronary ostia remains, in these cases, unsupported.

An adequate anchoring of the tubular graft is important to prevent complications. Neri and colleagues (Neri et al., 1999) reported on 2 patients who developed false aneurysm of the ascending aorta after 7 and 11 years, respectively. Histological examination of the aortic wall underlying the reinforcement cuff revealed extensive wall degeneration. Dhillon and associates (Dhillon et al., 1986) observed late ruptures after wrapping of aortic aneurysms. In all 3 cases, the aortic wall had been eroded. Usually the border between the wrapped segment and the native aortic wall might be under high pressure, resulting in dissection and erosion of the native intima, producing a weakening of the aortic wall both proximally and distally. Akgun (Akgun et al., 2010) reported an aortic root aneurysm in a patient who 7 years earlier underwent a reduction aortoplasty with external wrapping. Bauer (Bauer et al., 2003) found, in 1 patient, that the dacron wrapping had become dislocated by moving to the distal part of the ascending aorta, creating a sharp fold at the inner curve of the vessel. In this region he noted an extreme rarefaction of the aortic wall with impending rupture. To prevent late complications such as coronary compression, redilatation of the ascending aorta due to dislocation of the wrap, secure anchoring of the prosthetic wrap to the aorta is mandatory. Furthermore, to avoid alterations of the aortic wall, the prosthetic wrapping has to be well fitted to prevent the creation of folds, which may become areas of high mechanical stress.

Limitations of the wrapping technique without aortoplasty, the "sandwich technique", are that the available vascular graft prostheses may be insufficient in diameter to fit a large ascending aorta (Ergin et al., 1999; Carrel et al., 1991). The vascular prostheses have a crimped fabric, which allows the prostheses to be moderately bent without angulations. When trying to fit a straight prosthesis in a curvilinear aorta, the prosthesis develops wrinkles in the aortic concavity. The wrinkles of the prosthesis may be responsible for erosion of the aortic wall with a resulting risk of rupture. Thus aortic wrapping could become more dangerous than dilatation itself. Tappainer (Tappainer et al., 2007) suggested a new technique for wrapping of the ascending aorta in association with aortic valve replacement. Usually, the aortic wrap is constructed before aortic cross-clamping. The vascular dacron prosthesis is cut into two halves of 6 cm length. Both halves are opened longitudinally with a curved cut. Thus two dacron sheets are obtained from the prosthesis, each of them having one concave and one convex side. Finally, the sheets are joined by suturing the two convex sides together and the two concave sides together. A curved dacron hose 5 cm in diameter is obtained for external wrapping of the ascending aorta (Figure 9). After surgery on the aortic valve, the posterior aspect of the ascending aorta is freed completely from the pericardial reflection up to the innominate artery. In this way, the custom-built prosthesis is easily inserted for wrapping the ascending aorta. After closing the aortotomy and releasing the aortic clamp, the prosthesis is pulled down to cover the suture line and fixed with few adventitial stitches. No solid transmural stitches are usually needed with this technique because the curved prosthesis fits the curved ascending aorta. Similarly, after decannulation, the prosthesis is pulled up to cover the cannulation site. With this technique, the whole ascending aorta is covered by the prosthesis without wrinkles or bends.

Thus, reduction aortoplasty seems to be a safe procedure and to give good postoperative outcomes. It could be a viable alternative to conventional aortic root replacement or interposition tube grafting in some selected patients. The underground wall disorder should be an aortic valve stenosis. Patients with cystic medial necrosis, connective disorders and ascending aorta dissections are not candidates for reduction aortoplasty; furthermore no calcifications or atherosclerotic penetrating ulcers should affect the aortic wall; aneurysms with an infective origin are to be excluded from this type of treatment. The dilatation should be localized only on the ascending aorta, between the sinotubular junction and not extending beyond the innominate artery and the aortic arch. The ascending aorta should be moderately dilated with a diameter of up to 5.5 cm. Patients with an ascending aorta larger than 5.5 cm could benefit from a reduction aortoplasty if they are older and at high surgical risk. As an appropriate condition for reduction aortoplasty, the diameter at the sinus of Valsalva should be up to 4.5 cm. The intra-operative reduction of the aorta should be to <3.5 cm. The external wrapping should be anchored to minimize the risk of dislocation and it should be shaped anatomically on the ascending aorta.

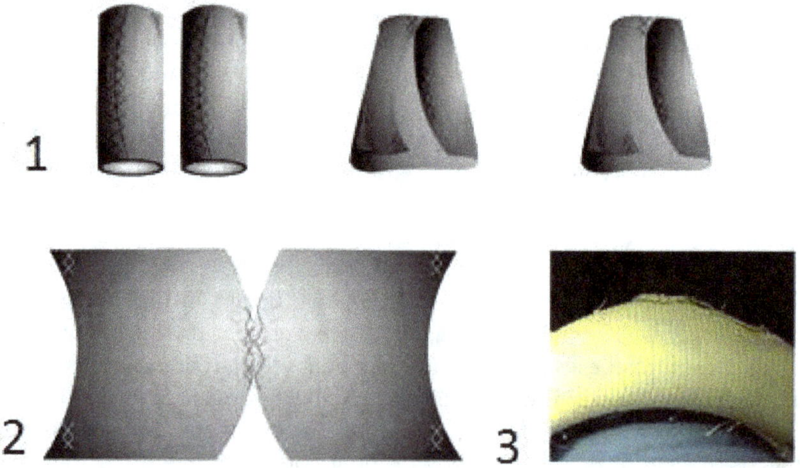

Fig. 9. Drawing of custom-made prosthesis preparation (1). Custom-made prosthesis before insertion (2).

6. References

Akgun S, Atalan N, Fazlioğullari O, Kunt AT, Basaran C, Arsan S. 2010. Aortic root aneurysm after off-pump reduction aortoplasty. *Ann Thorac Surg*. Vol 90, N 5, Nov 2010, pp 69-70.

Ang KL, Raheel F, Bajaj A, Sosnowski A, Galiñanes M. 2010. Early impact of aortic wrapping on patients undergoing aortic valve replacement with mild to moderate ascending aorta dilatation. *J Cardiothorac Surg*. Vol 6, N 5, Aug 210, pp 58.

Arsan S, Akgun S, Kurtoglu N, Yildirim T, Tekinsoy B. 2004. Reduction aortoplasty and external wrapping for moderately sized tubular ascending aortic aneurysm with concomitant operations. *Ann Thorac Surg*. Vol 78, N 3, Sep 2004, pp 858-61.

Arsan S. 2004. Off-pump reduction aortoplasty and concomitant coronary artery bypass grafting. *Ann Thorac Surg*. Vol 78, N 1, Jul 2004, pp 316-9.

Bahnson HT. 1982. The dilemma of the ascending aortic aneurysm. *Ann Thorac Surg*. Vol 34, N 2, Aug 1982, pp 115-6.

Barnett MG, Fiore AC, Vaca KJ, Milligan TW, Barner HB. 1995. Tailoring aortoplasty for repair of fusiform ascending aortic aneurysms. *Ann Thorac Surg*. Vol 59, N 2, Feb 1995, pp 497-51.

Bauer M, Pasic M, Schaffarzyk R, Siniawski H, Knollmann F, Meyer R, Hetzer R. 202. Reduction aortoplasty for dilatation of the ascending aorta in patients with bicuspid aortic valve. *Ann Thorac Surg*. Vol 73, N 3, Mar 2002, pp 720-3.

Bauer M, Grauhan O, Hetzer R. 2003. Dislocated wrap after previous reduction aortoplasty causes erosion of the ascending aorta. *Ann Thorac Surg*. Vol 75, N 2, Feb 2003, pp 583-4.

Baumgartner F, Omari B, Pak S, Ginzton L, Shapiro S, Milliken J. 1998. Reduction aortoplasty for moderately sized ascending aortic aneurysms. *J Card Surg*. Vol 13, N 2, Mar 198, pp 129-32.

Belov IV, Stepanenko AB, Gens AP, Savichev DD, Charchyan ER. 2009. Reduction aortoplasty for ascending aortic aneurysm: a 14-year experience. *Asian Cardiovasc Thorac Ann*. Vol 17, N 2, Apr, 2009, pp 162-6.

Bentall H, De Bono A. 1968. A technique for complete replacement of the ascending aorta. *Thorax*. Vol 23, N 4, Jul 1968, pp 338-9.

Cabrol C, Pavie A, Mesnildrey P, Gandjbakhch I, Laughlin L, Bors V, Corcos T. 1986. Long-term results with total replacement of the ascending aorta and reimplantation of the coronary arteries. *J Thorac Cardiovasc Surg*. Vol 91, N 1, Jan 1986, pp 17-25.

Carrel T, von Segesser L, Jenni R, Gallino A, Egloff L, Bauer E, Laske A, Turina M. 1991. Dealing with dilated ascending aorta during aortic valve replacement: advantages of conservative surgical approach. *Eur J Cardiothorac Surg*. Vol 5, N 3, 1991, pp 137-43.

Carrel T, Pasic M, Jenni R, Tkebuchava T, Turina MI. 1993. Reoperations after operation on the thoracic aorta: etiology, surgical techniques, and prevention. *Ann Thorac Surg*. Vol 56, N 2, Aug 1993, pp 259-68.

Cooley DA. Discussion on: Egloff L, Rothlin M, Kugelmeier J, Senning A, Turina M. 1982. The ascending aortic aneurysm: replacement or repair? *Ann Thorac Surg*. Vol 34, N 2, Aug 1982, pp 117-24.

Cotrufo M, Della Corte A, De Santo LS, De Feo M, Covino FE, Dialetto G. 2003. Asymmetric medial degeneration of the ascending aorta in aortic valve disease: a pilot study of surgical management. *J Heart Valve Dis*. 2003 Mar; Vol 12, N 2, Mar 2003, pp 127-33.

Crawford ES, Svensson LG, Coselli JS, Safi HJ, Hess KR. 1988. Aortic dissection and dissecting aortic aneurysms. *Ann Surg*. Vol 208, N 3, Sep 1988, pp 254-73.

Della Corte A, De Santo LS, Amarelli C, Romano G, De Feo M, Torella M, Scardone M, Cotrufo M. 2003. Surgical experience with "waistcoat aortoplasty": an update. *Ital Heart J*. Vol 4, N 12, Dec 2003, pp 875-9.

Dhillon JS, Randhawa GK, Straehley CJ, McNamara JJ. 1986. Late rupture after dacron wrapping of aortic aneurysms. *Circulation*. Vol 74, N 3, Sep 1986, pp 11-4.

Egloff L, Rothlin M, Kugelmeier J, Senning A, Turina M.1982. The ascending aortic aneurysm: replacement or repair? *Ann Thorac Surg*. Vol 34, N 2, Aug 1982, pp 117-24.

Ergin MA, Spielvogel D, Apaydin A, Lansman SL, McCullough JN, Galla JD, Griepp RB. 1999. Surgical treatment of the dilated ascending aorta: when and how? *Ann Thorac Surg*. Vol 67, N 6, Jun 1999, pp 1834-9.

Feindt P, Litmathe J, Börgens A, Boeken U, Kurt M, Gams E. 2007. Is size-reducing ascending aortoplasty with external reinforcement an option in modern aortic surgery? *Eur J Cardiothorac Surg*. Vol 31, N 4, Apr 2007, pp 614-7.

Gaeta R, Savasta M, Tancredi F, Monaco F, Lentini S. 2009. Resection and end-to-end anastomosis for ascending aortic aneurysm: surgical technique. *Minerva Chir*. Vol 64, N 6, Dec 2009, pp 665-8.

Ggoves LK, Effler DB, Hawk WA, Gulati K. 1964. Aortic insufficiency secondary to aneurysmal changes in the ascending aorta: surgical management. *J Thorac Cardiovasc Surg*. Vol 48, Sep1964, pp 362-79.

Gott VL. Invited commentary on: Robicsek F, Thubrikar MJ. 1994. Conservative operation in the management of annular dilatation and ascending aortic aneurysm. *Ann Thorac Surg*. Vol 57, N 6, Jun 1994, pp 1672-4.

Haddad R, Fagundes WV, Pinheiro BB. 2009. Reduction aortoplasty with external wrapping associated with aortic valve replacement in high-risk patients. *Rev Bras Cir Cardiovasc*. Vol 24, N 2, Jun 2009, pp 194-9.

Hirst AE, Gore I. 1976. Editorial: Is cystic medionecrosis the cause of dissecting aortic aneurysm? *Circulation*. Vol 53, N 6, Jun 1976, pp 915-6.

Hwang HY, Shim MS, Park EA, Ahn H. 2011. Reduction Aortoplasty for the Ascending Aortic Aneurysm With Aortic Valve Disease. *Circ J*. Vol 75, N 2, Feb 2011, pp 322-8.

Imaizumi T, Orita Y, Koiwaya Y, Hirata T, Nakamura M. 1982. Utility of two-dimensional echocardiography in the differential diagnosis of the etiology of aortic regurgitation. *Am Heart J*. Vol 103, N 5, May 198, pp 887-96.

Jarchow BH, Kincaid OW. 1961. Poststenotic dilatation of the ascending aorta: Its occurrence and significance as a roentgenologic sign of aortic stenosis. *Proc Staff Meet Mayo Clin*. Vol 18, N 36, Jan 1961, pp 23-33.

Klima T, Spjut HJ, Coelho A, Gray AG, Wukasch DC, Reul GJ Jr, Cooley DA. 1983. The morphology of ascending aortic aneurysms. *Hum Pathol*. Vol 14, N 9, Sep 1983, pp 810-7.

Kouchoukos NT, Marshall WG Jr, Wedige-Stecher TA. 1986. Eleven-year experience with composite graft replacement of the ascending aorta and aortic valve. *J Thorac Cardiovasc Surg*. Vol 92, N 4, Oct 1986, pp 691-705.

Laske A, Jenni R, Maloigne M, Vassalli G, Bertel O, Turina MI. 1996. Pressure gradients across bileaflet aortic valves by direct measurement and echocardiography. *Ann Thorac Surg*. Vol 61, N 1, Jan 1996, pp 48-57.

Lawrie GM, Earle N, DeBakey ME. 1993. Long-term fate of the aortic root and aortic valve after ascending aneurysm surgery. *Ann Surg*. Vol 217, N 6, Jun 1993, pp 711-20.

Lewis CT, Cooley DA, Murphy MC, Talledo O, Vega D. 1992. Surgical repair of aortic root aneurysms in 280 patients. *Ann Thorac Surg*. Vol 53, N 1, Jan 1992, pp 38-45.

Massetti M, Veron S, Neri E, Coffin O, le Page O, Babatasi G, Buklas D, Maiza D, Gerard JL, Khayat A. 2004. Long-term durability of resection and end-to-end anastomosis for ascending aortic aneurysms. *J Thorac Cardiovasc Surg*. Vol 127, N 5, May 2004, pp 1381-7.

McCready RA, Pluth JR. 1979. Surgical treatment of ascending aortic aneurysms associated with aortic valve insufficiency. *Ann Thorac Surg*. Vol 28, N 4, Oct 1979, pp 307-16.

Milano A, Pratali S, De Carlo M, Borzoni G, Tartarini G, Bortolotti U. 1998. Ascending aorta dissection after aortic valve replacement. *J Heart Valve Dis*. Vol 7, N 1, Jan 1998, pp 75-80.

Mueller XM, Tevaearai HT, Genton CY, Hurni M, Ruchat P, Fischer AP, Stumpe F, von Segesser LK. 1997. Drawback of aortoplasty for aneurysm of the ascending aorta associated with aortic valve disease. *Ann Thorac Surg*. 1997 Mar; Vol 63, N 3, Mar 1997, pp 762-6.

Natsuaki M, Itoh T, Rikitake K, Okazaki Y, Naitoh K. 1998. Aortic complications after aortic valve replacement in patients with dilated ascending aorta and aortic regurgitation. *J Heart Valve Dis*. Vol 7, N 5, Sep 1998, pp 504-9.

Neri E, Massetti M, Tanganelli P, Capannini G, Carone E, Tripodi A, Tucci E, Sassi C. 1999. Is it only a mechanical matter? Histologic modifications of the aorta underlying external banding. *J Thorac Cardiovasc Surg*. Vol 118, N 6, Dec 1999, pp 1116-8.

Perrotta S, Lentini S, Rinaldi M, D'armini AM, Tancredi F, Raffa G, Gaeta R, Viganó M. 2008. Treatment of ascending aorta disease with Bentall-De Bono operation using a mini-invasive approach. *J Cardiovasc Med (Hagerstown)*. Vol 9, N 10, Oct 2008, pp 1016-22.

Perrotta S, Lentini S. 2009. Ministernotomy approach for surgery of the aortic root and ascending aorta. *Interact Cardiovasc Thorac Surg*. Vol 9, N 5, Nov 009, pp 849-58.

Polvani G, Barili F, Dainese L, Topkara VK, Cheema FH, Penza E, Ferrarese S, Parolari A, Alamanni F, Biglioli P. 2006. Reduction ascending aortoplasty: midterm follow-up and predictors of redilatation. *Ann Thorac Surg*. Vol 82, N 2, Aug 2006, pp 586-91.

Prenger K, Pieters F, Cheriex E. 1994. Aortic dissection after aortic valve replacement: incidence and consequences for strategy. *J Card Surg*. Vol 9, N 5, Sep 1994, pp 495-8.

Robicsek F. 1982, A new method to treat fusiform aneurysms of the ascending aorta associated with aortic valve disease: an alternative to radical resection. *Ann Thorac Surg*. Vol 34, N 1, Jul 1982, pp 92-4.

Robicsek F, Thubrikar MJ. 1994. Conservative operation in the management of annular dilatation and ascending aortic aneurysm. *Ann Thorac Surg*. Vol 57, N 6, Jun 1994, pp 1672-4.

Robicsek F. Invited commentary on: Barnett MG, Fiore AC, Vaca KJ, Milligan TW, Barner HB. 1995. Tailoring aortoplasty for repair of fusiform ascending aortic aneurysms. *Ann Thorac Surg*. Vol 59, N 2, Feb 1995, pp 497-51.

Roman MJ, Devereux RB, Kramer-Fox R, O'Loughlin J. 1989. Two-dimensional echocardiographic aortic root dimensions in normal children and adults. *Am J Cardiol*. Vol 64, N 8, Sep 1989, pp 507-12.

Schlatmann TJ, Becker AE. 1977a. Histologic changes in the normal aging aorta: implications for dissecting aortic aneurysm. *Am J Cardiol*. Vol 39, N 1, Jan 1977, pp 13-20.

Schlatmann TJ, Becker AE. 1977b. Pathogenesis of dissecting aneurysm of aorta. Comparative histopathologic study of significance of medial changes. *Am J Cardiol*. Vol 39, N 1, Jan 1977, pp 21-6.

Stein PD, Sabbah HN. 1976. Turbulent blood flow in the ascending aorta of humans with normal and diseased aortic valves. *Circ Res*. Vol 39, N 1, Jul 1976, pp 58-65.

Svensson LG, Crawford ES, Hess KR, Coselli JS, Safi HJ. 1992. Composite valve graft replacement of the proximal aorta: comparison of techniques in 348 patients. *Ann Thorac Surg*. Vol 54, N 3, Sep 1992, pp 427-37.

Tappainer E, Fiorani V, Nocchi A, Likaj E, Memishaj S, Zogno M. 2007. Safe wrapping of the borderline dilated ascending aorta during aortic valve replacement. *J Cardiothorac Surg*. Vol 22, N 2, Feb 2007, pp 15.

Viganò M, Rinaldi M, D'Armini AM, Boffini M, Zattera GF, Alloni A, Dore R. 2002. Ascending aortic aneurysms treated by cuneiform resection and end-to-end anastomosis through a ministernotomy. *Ann Thorac Surg*. Vol 74, N 5, Nov 2002, pp 1789-91.

Walker T, Bail DH, Gruler M, Vonthein R, Steger V, Ziemer G. 2007. Unsupported reduction ascending aortoplasty: fate of diameter and of Windkessel function. *Ann Thorac Surg*. Vol 83, N 3, Mar 2007, pp 1047-53.

Wheat MW Jr, Wilson JR, Bartley TD. 1964. Successful replacement of the entire ascending aorta ad aortic valve. *JAMA*. Vol 25, N 188, May 1964, pp 717-9.

Yearwood TL, Misbach GA, Chandran KB. 1989. Experimental fluid dynamics of aortic stenosis in a model of the human aorta. *Clin Phys Physiol Meas*. Vol 1, N 1, Feb 1989, pp 11-24.

Zhang H, Lu F, Qu D, Han L, Xu J, Ji G, Xu Z. 2011. Treatment of fusiform ascending aortic aneurysms: A comparative study with 2 options. *J Thorac Cardiovasc Surg*. Vol 141, N 3, Mar 2011, pp 738-43.

6

Aortic Valve Sparing Operation

Júlia Čanádyová and Aleš Mokráček
Department of Cardiac Surgery, Regional Hospital České Budějovice, Czech Republic

1. Introduction

A standard approach in the surgical treatment of severe aortic regurgitation and/or aortic root dilatation is Bentall procedure, it means replacement of the aortic valve and ascending aorta with a composite graft including mechanical or biological valve. The original technique described by Bentall and De Bono in 1968 (5). This is a „safe" method with low mortality, but patients have to accept the disadvantages of lifelong anticoagulation and comercial valvular prosthesis, such as higher risk of tromboembolic complications, bleeding, endocarditis and also rapid degeneration of biological prosthesis (28).
The alternative technique for the patients with aortic root dilatation and/or ascending aorta aneurysm and aortic valve incompetence, causing by outward displacement of the commissures is the aortic valve-sparing operation (24). The technique of aortic root remodeling first described by Sarsam and Yacoub and technique of aortic valve reimplantation first described by David and Feindel in 1993 (33,9). The both techniques preserve the native aortic valve and partialy dynamic native aortic valve annulus, which may have hemodynamic benefits over a rigid prosthetic valve stent. The major benefits are freedom from anticoagulation treatment, relative resistance to infection compared with prosthetic valves and maybe better resistance against the premature degenerative changes of the bioprosthesis (multifactorial etiology). A major drawback is the increased risk of early failure of reconstructed valve cause the valve incompetence and needing the early reoperation (24).
Aortic valve sparing operations were developed to preserve native tricuspid aortic valve without gross structural defects and absence of severe cusp prolapse or assymetry (9). In recent years, surgeons gaining more and more experience and skills and indications were liberally expanded to include older and also younger patients, patients with bicuspid valves, aortic valves with cusp prolapse, Marfan patients, patients with acute type A dissection, endocarditis and reoperation (1,14,26,19,18). Future and longer follow up will show us the best solutions for each of these categories.

2. Operative technique

For choosing the right type of valve sparing operation is important to assess the pathology of the leaflets, aortic root and asending aorta. Our approach based on the functional classification of aortic regurgitation linked to the pathophysiologic mechanism and desribed by El Khoury (tab. 1, tab. 2) (6,16).

Type I	**Normal appearing cusps with FAA dilatation**
Ia	Ascending aorta dilatation (starting at the sinotubular junction)
Ib	Valsalva sinuses and sinotubular junction dilatation
Ic	Funcional aortic annulus dilatation
Id	Cusp perforation
Type II	**Cusp prolapse**
Type III	**Cusp retraction and thickening**

Table 1. Functional classification of aortic regurgitation.

Aortic root is functional unit consist with two major components: the leaflets and the functional aortic annulus (FAA). It is a classification of the different mechanism of aortic insuficiency that allows the surgeons to define and categorize pathological findings and apply the appropriate repair technique. (6,16,26).

AI class	**TYPE I** Normal cusp motion with functional aortic annulus dilatation			**TYPE II** Cusp prolapse	**TYPE III** Cusp restriction
	Ia	Ib	Ic		
Mechanism	Ascending aorta dilatation (starting at the sinotubular junction)	Valsalva sinuses and sinotubilar junction dilatation	Funcional aortic annulus dilatation	Excess of cusp tissue, or commisural disruption	Cusp retraction and thickening
Repair techniques (primary)	**STJ remodeling** *ascending aorta graft*	**Aortic valve sparing** *Reimplantation or Remodeling with SCA*	**SCA**	**Prolapse repair** *Plication* *Triangular resection* *Free margin resuspension* *Patch*	**Leaflet repair** *Raphe shaving* *Decalcification* *Patch*
(secondary)	SCA		STJ annuloplasty	SCA	SCA

Table 2. The functional classification of aortic regurgitation linked to the pathophysiologic mechanism. (STJ- sinotubular junction; SCA- subcommissural annuloplasty).

Echocardiographic examination

Crucial and very important is echocardiography examination. All patients underwent preoperative transthoracic (TTE) and transesophageal echocardiography (TEE) and intraoperative TEE. Severity of aortic regurgitation was classified according to four grades using semiquantitative criteria. Leaflets morphology and motion were described in order to determine which leaflet was prolapsing. Also the quality of the cusp tissue (the presents of sclerosis or calcification, cusp damage), the level of coaptation, the length of the free margin of the leaflets, hight of the cusp and the anatomy of the aortic root were assessed. (Fig. 1, Fig. 2., Fig. 3.)

For long-term durability is important to respect some echocardiographic signs :

- preoperative the leaflet coaptation is minimally 6 mm above the annulus

- the length of free margin is maximal 50% longer than diameter of the annulus (Fig. 1.)
- after the operation the coaptation area is completely above inferior edge of prosthesis (type A, Hannover classification)

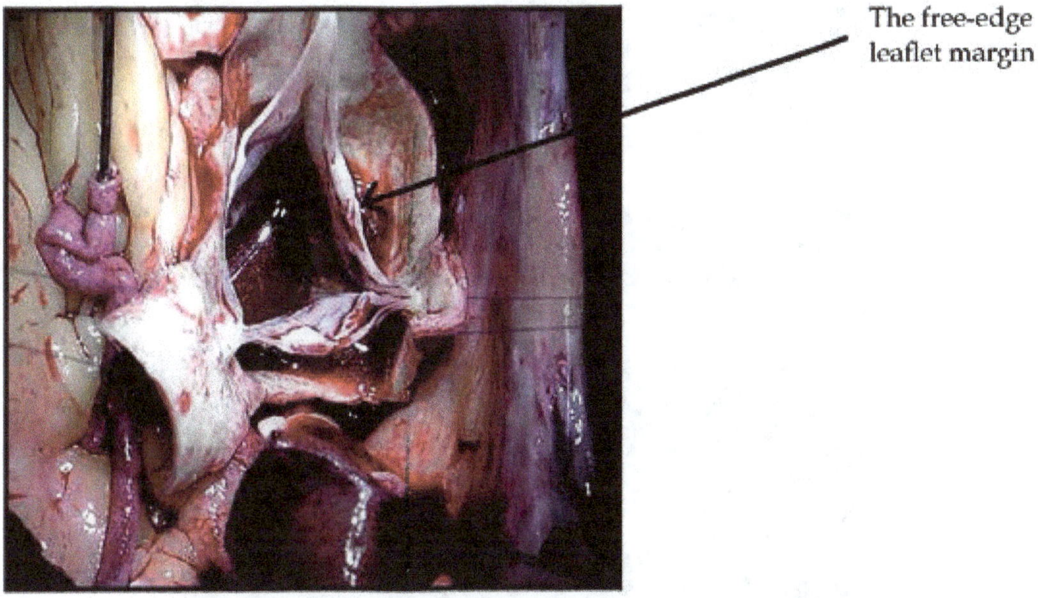

Fig. 1. The free-edge leaflet margin is maximal 50% longer than annulus diameter.

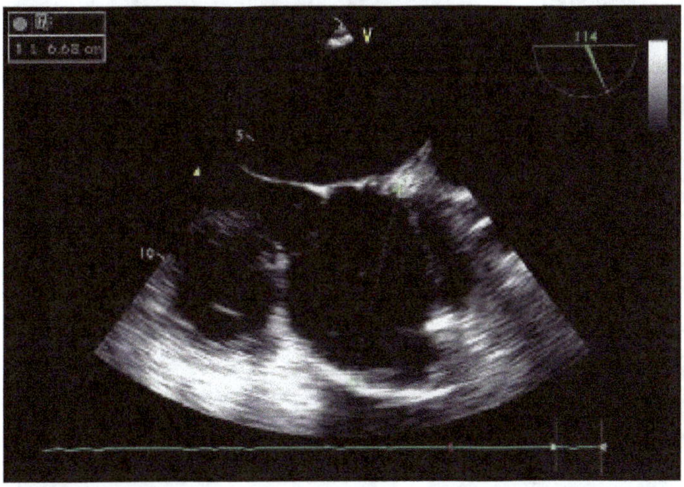

Fig. 2. Annulus, Valsalva sinuses and STJ dilatation.

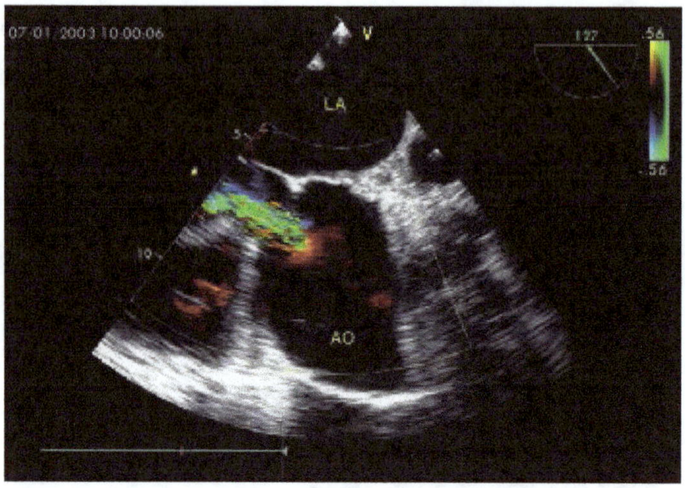

Fig. 3a. Aortic regurgitation.

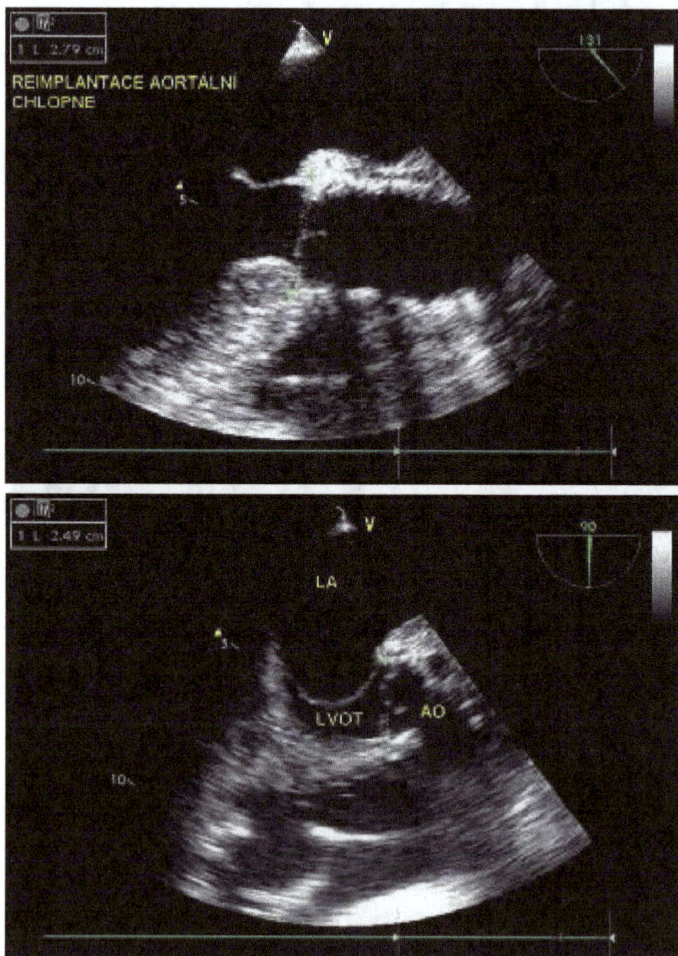

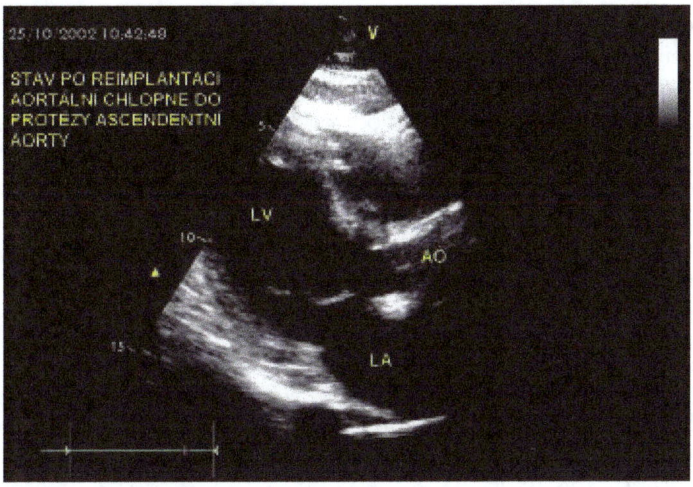

Fig. 3b. Condition after aortic valve reimplantation.

2.1.1 Ascending aorta replacement

Supracommisural ascending aorta replacement with tube dacron prosthesis is indicated in patients with isolated dilatation of sinotubular junction (STJ) and ascending aorta, where the severe aortic insuficiency is due to changes in root geometry and outward displacement of the commissures. Restoration of a normal diameter of STJ is important and obviosly enough to correct the aortic incompetence. (Fig. 4.)

We prefer to use 10% (2 or 3 mm) bigger diameter of prosthesis than native aortic annulus measured by echogardiographic examination (in diastola) and by Hegar dilator during the procedure. (Fig. 6.)

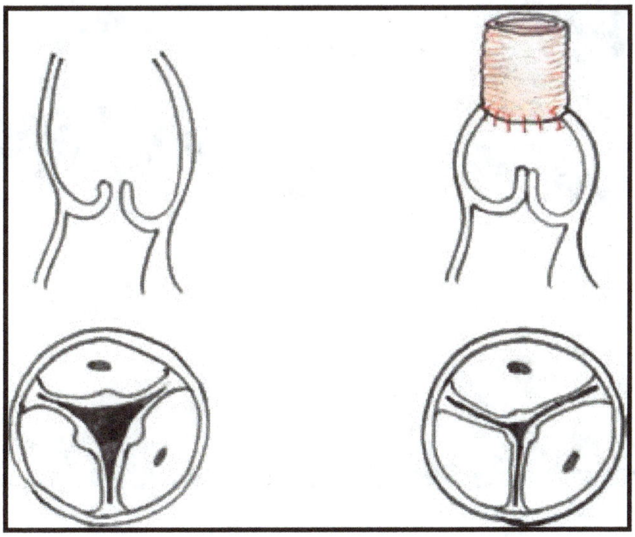

Fig. 4. Ascending aorta replacement.

2.1.2 The remodeling technique (Yacoub)

Remodeling is physiologic reconstruction of the aortic root. This approach preserves the anatomy and the function of the Valsalva sinuses. According to our opinion and experience of other surgeons, it is not a suitable method for patients with dilated annulus, because of lack of annulus support and there is a tendency toward progressive aortic insuficiency. (34)
Remodeling (sec operation. Yacoub) - aortic bulbus, diseased sinuses, including the ST junction and necessary part of the ascending aorta were trimming, leaving only 4-5 mm of the aortic wall at the base of aortic leaflets and annulus. The coronary arteries were prepared for a button reimplantation in standard manner. Subsequently, vascular prosthesis was prepared - Gelweave Valsalva prosthesis (Vascutec Ltd., UK) by trimming to obtain three tongue-shaped extensions (neosinuses) that are then sutured to the aortic annulus at the line of the attachment of the cusps. (Fig. 7.) Prosthesis size was derived from the size of annulus measured by echogardiographic examination and also we used a Hegar dilator or the size of the graft is based on the diameter of sinotubular junction (STJ). The prosthesis was subsequently chosen by 10% higher compared to the native annulus or equal to the diameter of STJ. The prosthesis was fixed to the rim of the sinuses with three running polypropylene 4-0 stitches. Stitches were placed up to the base of leaflets – that we consider crucial for long-term durability. We use of stentless valvular sizer (Toronto SPV) for measurement of extent of circumference for each sinus and after that we individualizate the extent of each neosinus on vascular prosthesis. (Fig. 5.) Coronary arteries buttons were sewn end to side into the prosthesis with polypropylene 6-0 stitches and the prosthesis was anastomosed to the distal aorta. (33,34). We don´t use a glues.

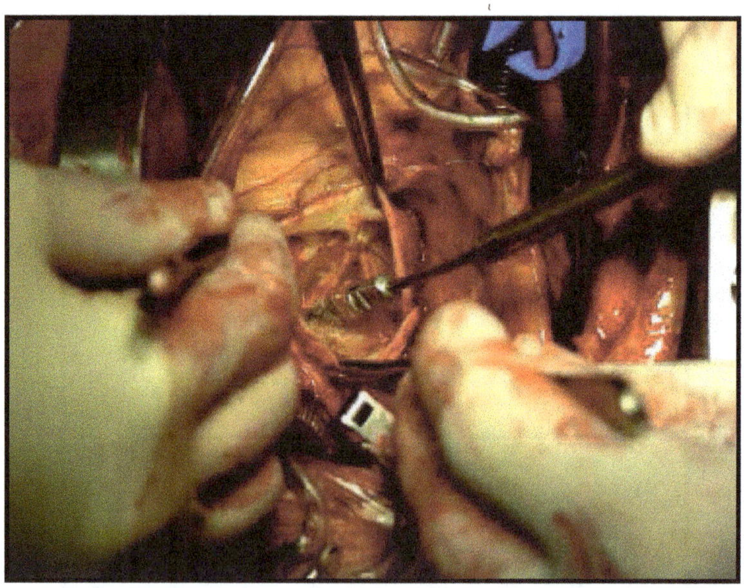

Fig. 5. The use of stentless valvular sizer (Toronto SPV).
(Photo is from the author´s archive)

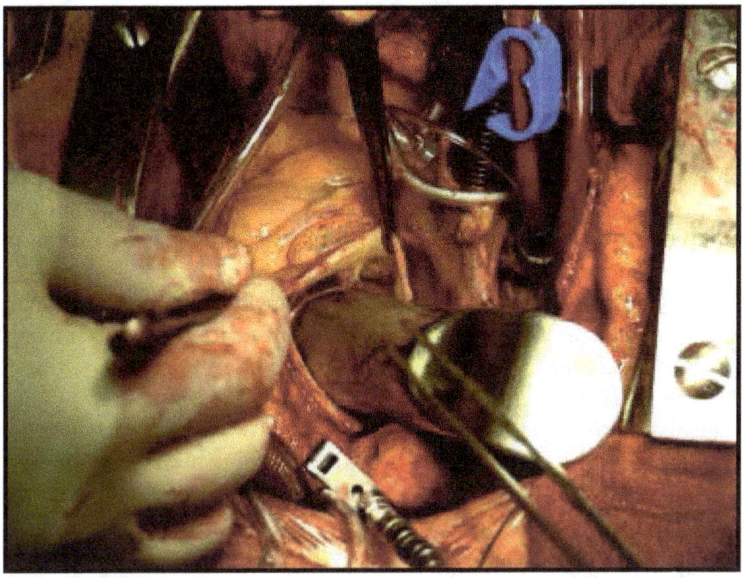

Fig. 6. The measurement of diameter annulus by Hegar dilator.
(Photo is from the author´s archive)

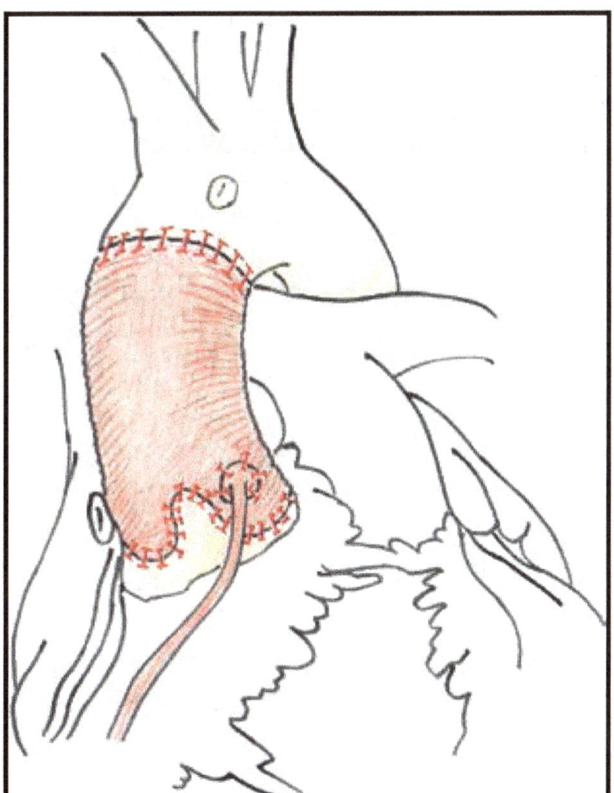

Fig. 7. Remodeling of the aortic root.

2.1.3 The reimplantation technique (David)

Reimplantation (surgery sec. David I) – the surgical procedure followed the steps originally described by David and Feindel. (9).

Detailed description of the techniques (aortotomy and exposure, aortic root preparation, prosthesis sizing, proximal suture line, prosthesis preparation and fixation, valve reimplantation) mentioned Boodhwani et al. (6).

Briefly the aorta is transected 1 cm above the sinotubular junction starting above the non-coronary sinus. Three full-thickness 4-0 polypropylene traction sutures are placed at the level of the three commissures. Very important is to externally dissect the aortic root as low as possible, started along the non-coronary sinus and continued towards the left and right commissures and leaflet with respect the external anatomical limitations (insertion of the root into the ventricular muscle). The diseased sinuses of Valsalva are then resected leaving approximately 3-5 mm of the aortic wall attached. Then the coronary buttons are prepared. (Fig. 9.)

We prefer the Valsalva prosthesis with neo-sinuses (13), which was prepared by „scaloping" in areas of commissures to the depth 1 cm according to valve anatomy.

The diameter of the graft was about 50% smaller than the average length of the free margins of the aortic cusps. If there is some discrepancy, we could repare a leaflets too.

Then the coronary arteries buttons and aortic valve were prepared in the same manner as in remodeling.

Proximal anastomosis is bilayer. The first layer of multiple horizontal mattress sutures of 2-0 polyester are passed from the inside to the outside of the left ventricle outflow tract circumferentially below the nadir of aortic annulus and following the scalloped shape of the aortic annulus along the muscular interventricular septum. The second layer of the stitches attached the remaining sinuses into the graft using three 4-0 polypropylene sutures. Important is to achieve correct cusp geometry and sufficient height of commissural resuspension within the prosthesis at the level of the new sinutubular junction. (Fig. 8., Fig. 9., Fig. 10.) Than the coronary arteries were implanted and the distal anastomosis between the graft and the native ascending aorta was performed using running 4-0 Prolen suture. (Fig. 11., Fig. 12., Fig. 13., Fig. 14.)

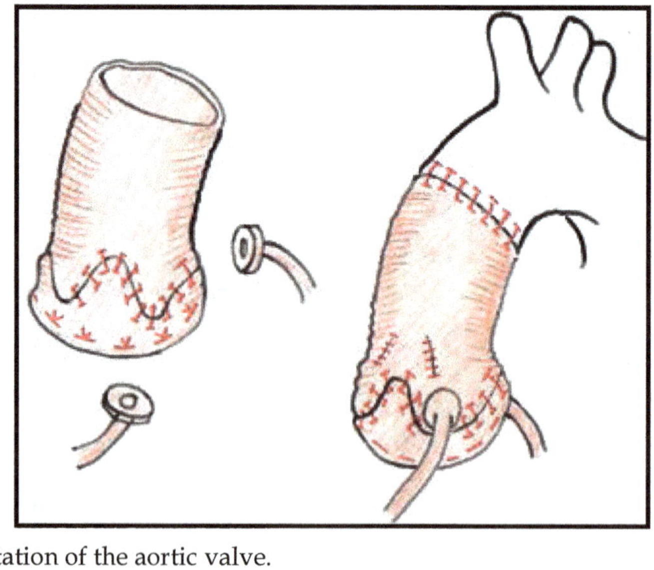

Fig. 8. Reimplantation of the aortic valve.

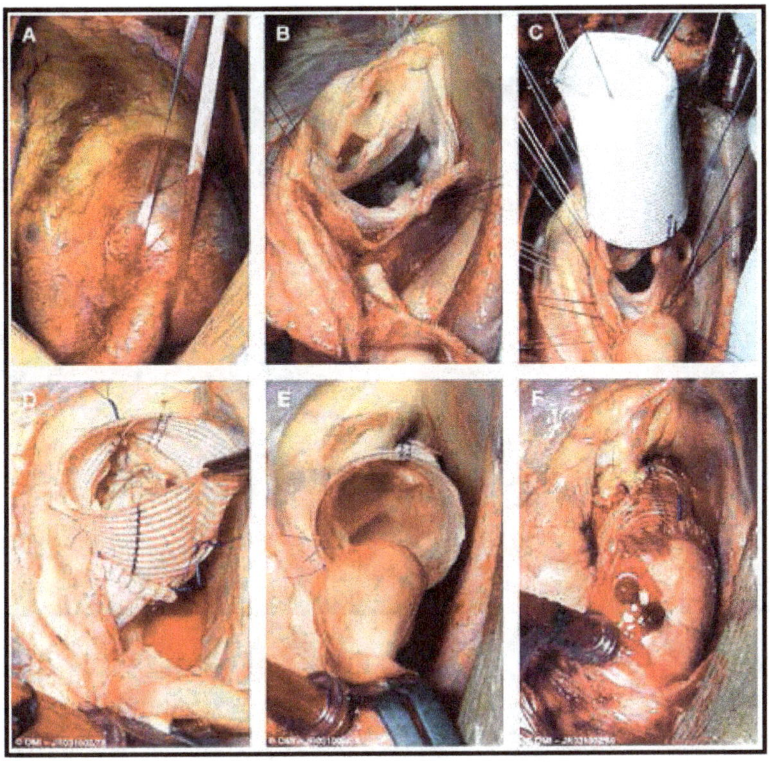

Fig. 9. A-root dilatation, B-resection of diseased Valsalva sinuses with preparing coronary artery buttons. C, D-reimplantation of the aortic valve into the prosthesis, E, F- distal anastomosis between the graft and the native ascending aorta.

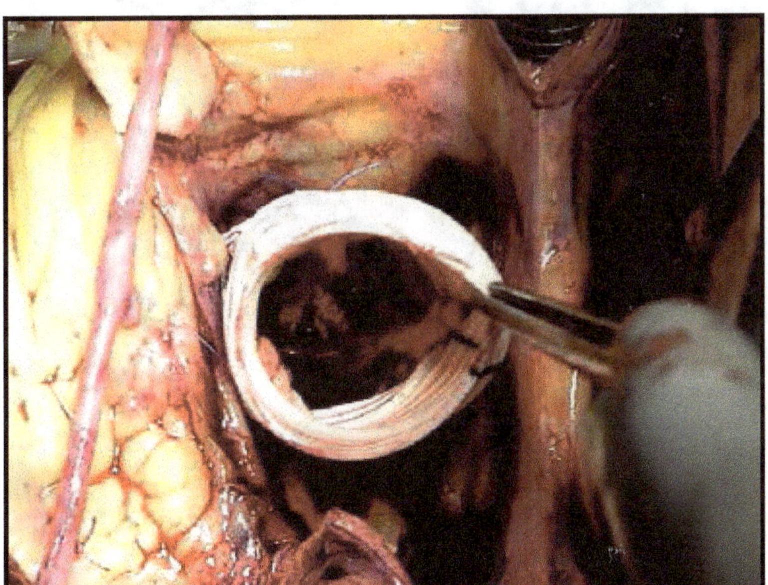

Fig. 10. Reimplantation of the valve into the prosthesis. (Photo is from the author´s archive)

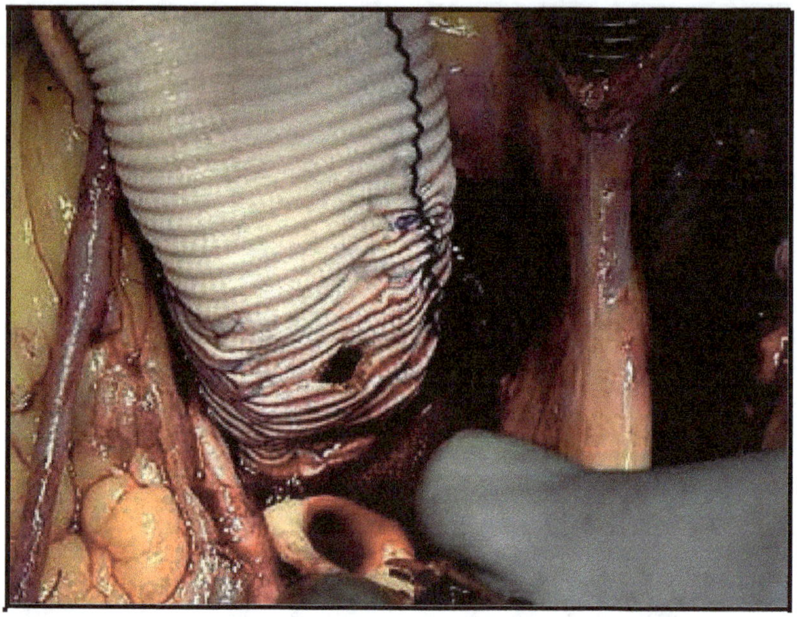

Fig. 11. Hole preparation by electrocautery for coronary artery button reimplantation. (Photo is from the author´s archive)

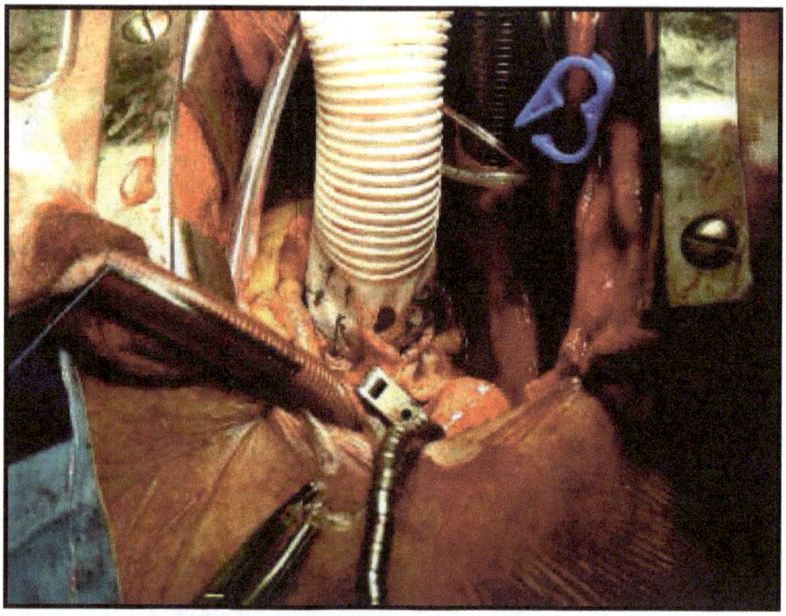

Fig. 12. The implantation of the coronary artery button end to side into the prosthesis. (Photo is from the author´s archive)

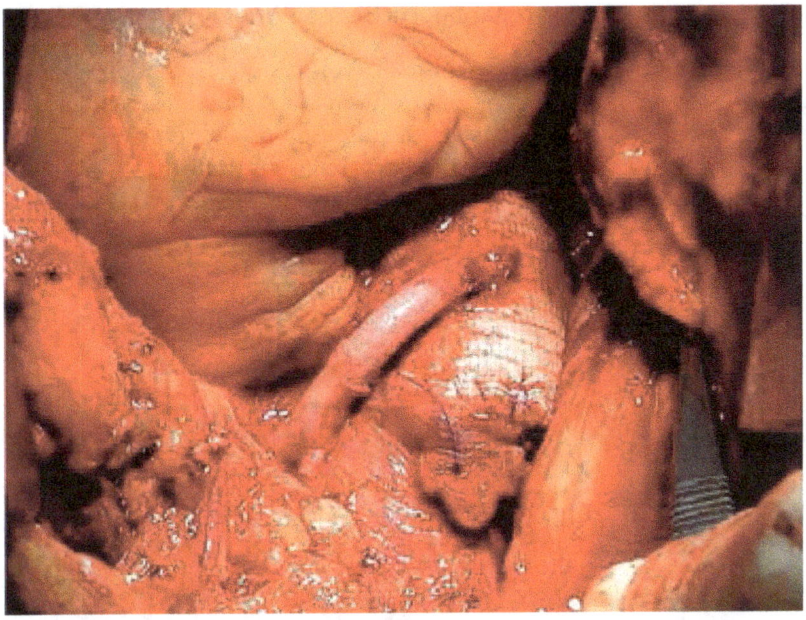

Fig. 13. Venous graft sewn into the prosthesis.
(Photo is from the author´s archive)

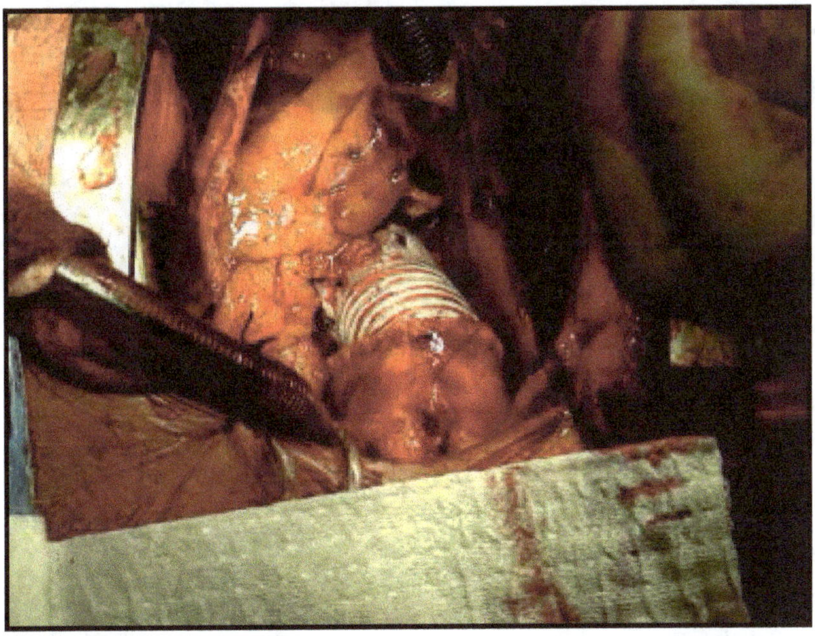

Fig. 14. The distal anastomosis between the graft and the native ascending aorta.
(Photo is from the author´s archive)

2.1.4 Replacement of the non-coronary aortic sinus (Wheat)

Indicated in patients with isolated non-coronary aortic sinus dilatation (exceptionally two sinuses). In our practise is the non-coronary sinus the most diseased sinus in case of nondegenerative diseases (atherosclerosis). The diseased non-coronary sinus and ascending aorta were replaced by a scalloped shape dacron tubular graft. (Fig. 15.)

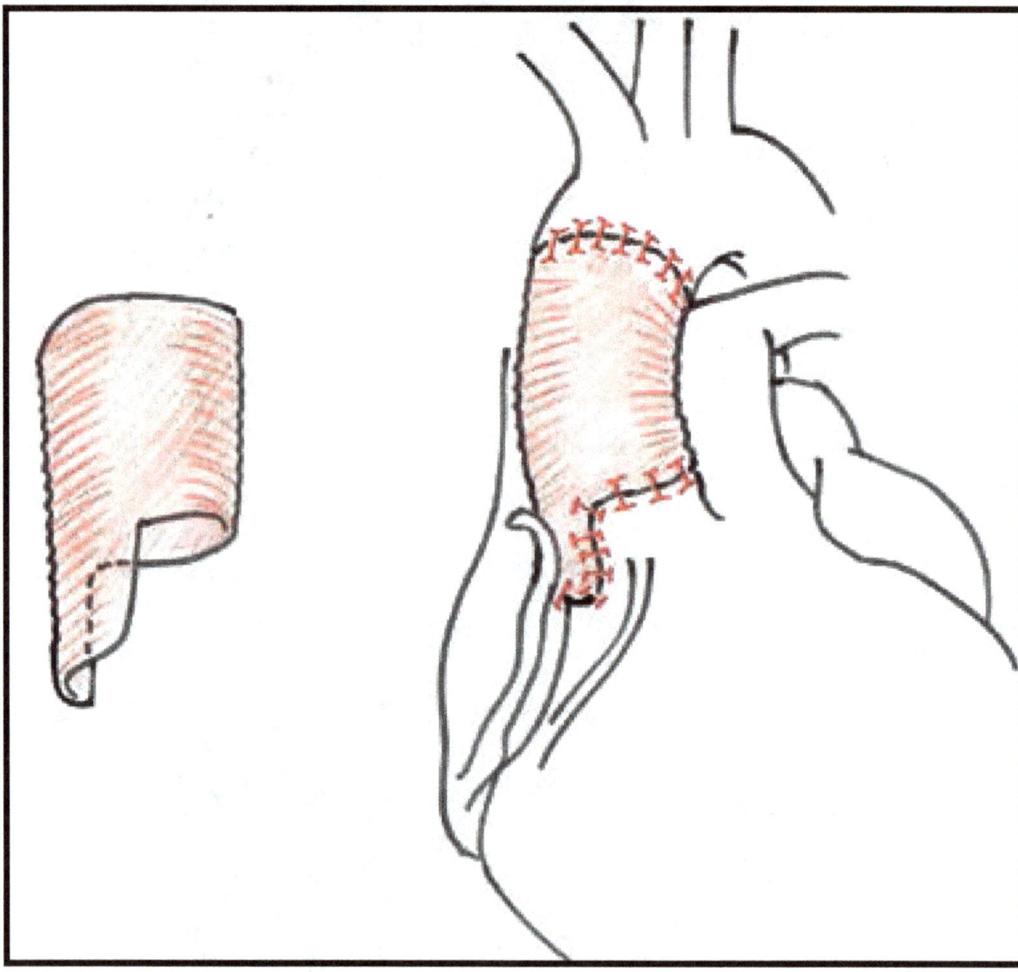

Fig. 15. Replacement of the noncoronary aortic sinus.

2.1.5 Cusp repair technique

Cusp perforation

When the leaflet defect is too large for direct closure with a running locked suture of 6-0 polypropylene, an autologous pericardial patch is used. The patch size is larger than the defect area to avoid any restriction of the repaired leaflet (26,15,27,10). (Fig. 16.)

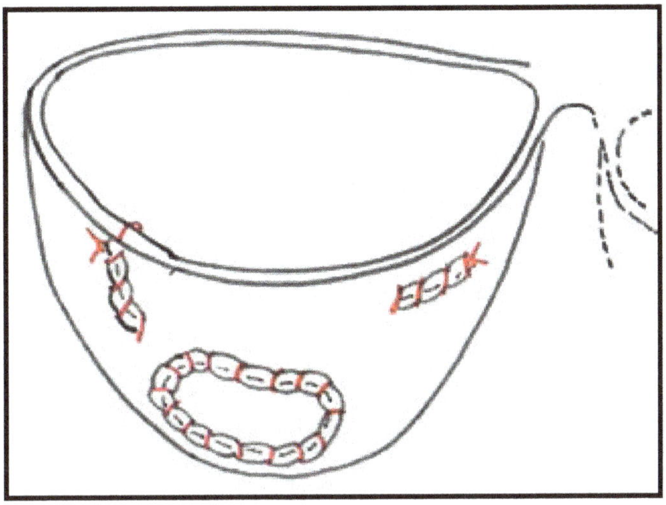

Fig. 16. Patch repair.

Stress fenestration

Caused by dilatation of the sinutubular junction (STJ) and increased mechanical stress on the free margin of the cusp. Most often located in the commissural areas and may be repared with a double layer of 6-0 PTFE suture along the free margins or by pericardial patch (11). (Fig. 17., Fig. 18.)

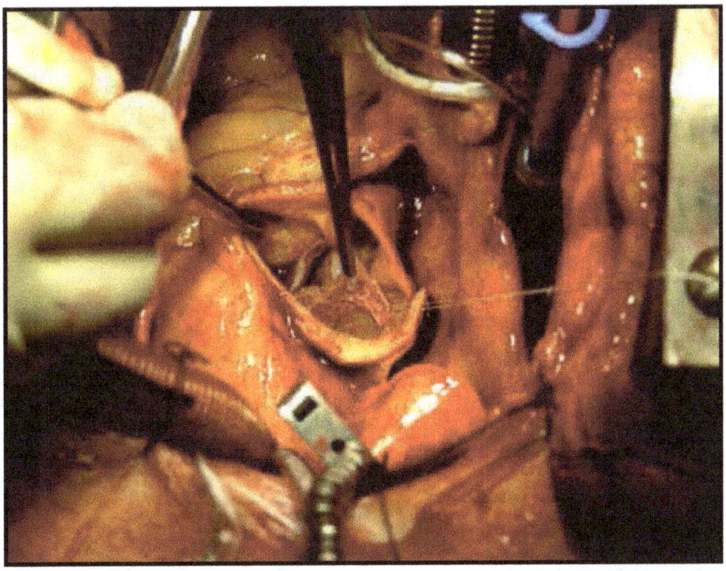

Fig. 17. Pericardial patch repair of the defect located in the commisural area.
(Photo is from the author´s archive)

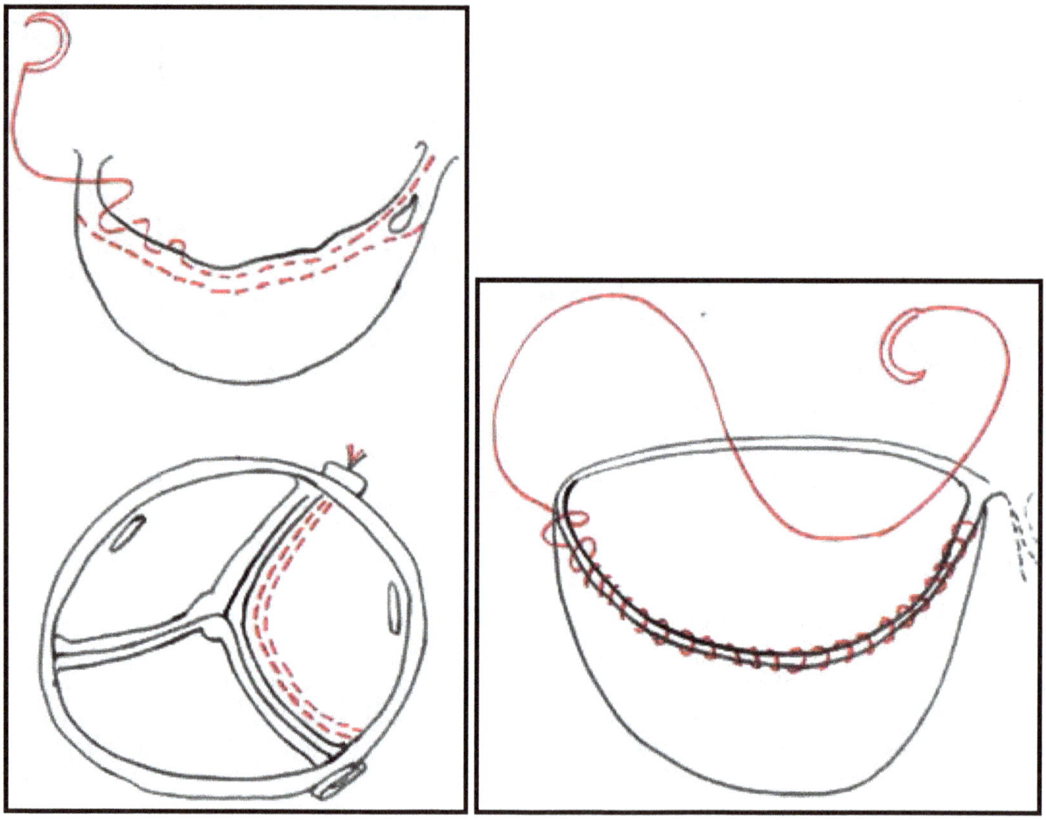

Fig. 18. Free margin reinforcement.

Leaflet prolapse

Is frequent cause of aortic insuficiency. The etiology is multiple-is frequent in bicuspid aortic valve, in patients with connective tissues diseases (Marfan syndrome), in chronic aortic root aneurysm. Acute leaflet prolapse can occur in patients with acute type A dissection, trauma. El Khoury et al. detaily desribed 4 different techniques of leaflet prolapse repair. (15,16,27).

- Central leaflet plication with 6-0 polypropylene suture
- Triangular resection

This two techniques are indicated when the leaflets are thin and flexible.

- Free margin resuspension with running suture of Gore-Tex 7-0 (Fig. 18.)
- Autologous pericardial patch repair

This techniques are prefered in case of poor quality of leaflets with thickening.

Kerchove et. al had a very good results with 146 patients with cusp prolapse corrected with this technique. During the initial hospitalization only two patients required reoperation for reccurent aortic insuficiency (AI). At 4 years freedom from reoperation and from reccurent AI (grade >2) was 94 ± 5% and 91 ± 7% respectively. (26)

3. Discussion

For long term durability and good results of the operation is essential to achieve a coaptation cusp area type A. Harringer et al. confirmed a direct correlation between early development and progression of aortic regurgitation and the type of coaptation area after the reconstruction of the valve on transthoracic echocardiography - tab. 3. (21). The authors confirmed the association between type B and C coaptation area and faster progression of aortic regurgitation compared with patients who had the type A of coaptation area. (p<0,05, C versus A in early postoperative period, p<0,001, C versus A and B after 1 year). Fig. 19. (21)

Type A	Coaptation area completely above inferior edge of prosthesis
Type B	Coaptation area at inferior edge of prosthesis
Type C	Coaptation area >= 2 mm below lower edge of prosthesis

Table 3. Type of coaptation area (Hannover classification).

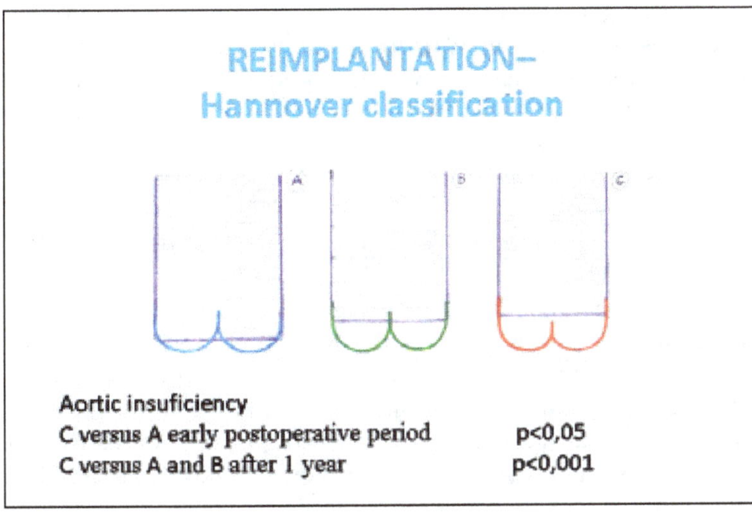

Fig. 19. Significance of aortic insuficiency.

If we decided to perform a reconstructive surgery of the aortic valve we have to answer 3 basic questions. Which **type of surgery** we perform, which **type** and **size of prosthesis** we use.

In the case of a limited expansion and dilatation of sinuses and ascending aorta the remodeling technique described by Yacoub is chosen. This technique seems more physiological. Restoration of the aortic sinuses provide a proper opening and closing velocities of the valve leaflets, with reducing their mechanical stress. (13). On the other hand remodeling is associated with higher risk of early reccurence of aortic regurgitation. The reason is lack of annular support.

If the dilatation affects the sinuses, including the annulus, we prefer reimplantation technique described by David, which provide more effective stabilization and external support of the annulus and better long term durability.

If one or maximum two sinuses are affected our decision is a created a neo-sinus by tailoring the graft with a tongue of tissue that is sutured directly to the aortic annulus replacement this part of aortic root with prosthesis.

Furthermore, we must decide what type of prosthesis we use-Dacron tube graft or prosthesis with neo sinuses. Aybek et al. showed that the tubular graft should have a greater rate of opening and closing of the valve and shorter times compared with native root and reimplantation into the prosthesis with neo sinuses. Similarly the distance between the cusps and graft wall during the systole was smallest. (9).

Also Leyh et al. (28) observed that near normal opening and closing characteristics can be achieved by a technique that preserves the shape and independent mobility of the sinuses of Valsalva. There is a theoretical assumption that neo sinuses (created by any method) will extend the durability of valve. But clinical differences in the intermediate term follow-up were clearly demonstrated.

De Paulis et al. introducing modified Dacron conduit (Gelweave Valsalva, Sulzer Vascutek, Renfrewshire, Scotland) that on implantation recreates sinuses of Valsalva of normal shape and dimension, providing a sufficient gap that should avoid any contact between the open leaflet and the Dacron wall. (34,13).

On the other hand, very good results with reimplantation technique into the Dacron tube graft achieve colleques in Hannover (24). In the 11 year interval a total of 284 patients operated on with an average follow up was 44 months (0-130 months). The number of reoperations for recurrent significant aortic regurgitation was only 11 patients. Only Marfan syndrome be considered as a risk factor for reoperation.

We also prefer the Vascutek Valsalva prosthesis which we prepare by parcial or complete scalloping.

For the good result of the operation is also important the size of prosthesis. Most authors derived it from the diameter of the annulus and length of the free margin of the leaflets in a relationship and in relation to type of valve preserving technique (remodeling or reimplantation). An interesting insight provides Maselli et al. (29), which is based on the consideration that in the case of native valve even when fully valve open in a systole remains space several millimeters between the leaflets and the wall of the aorta. Results of their simulations suggest that the ideal graft oversizing in respect the final aortic annulus diameter is +7 mm for a standard graft and +3 mm for the Valsalva grafts. It is very simply solution, available in every situation. We prefer to derive the size of prosthesis measured preoperatively by echocardiographic examination and perioperatively by Hegar dilator. Prosthesis is chosen by 10% greater for remodeling. For reimplantation technique in patients with severe dilatation of the annulus the free-edge length of the leaflet was measured in the short-axis view by tracing the leaflet outline. The parameters were determined in the closed valve and in the open valve. The size of the prosthesis was chosen by 50% less.

From 2002 to 2009, 37 patients underwent aortic valve sparing operations in our department. Mean age was 58 ± 9 (range 21 to 77) years. Of the 37 patients, 24 were male (64.8%) and 13 female (35.2%).

The average degree of aortic regurgitation was 2.9 ± 0.5, ejection fraction of the left ventricle was 56% ± 9. The average size of aortic annulus was 26,4 ± 2,6 mm, aortic root 50,6 ± 7,4 mm, sinotubular junction was 43,7 ± 5,1 mm and the ascending aorta 51,2 ± 6,8 mm. 32 (86,5%) patients underwent the reimplantation of the aortic valve according to the technique described by David, 2 (5,4%) patients underwent the remodeling procedure and 3 (8,1%) patients had a replacement of the noncoronary sinus descibed by Wheat.

Chronic ascending aortic aneurysm was present in 23 patients (62.2%), acute aortic dissection type A in 13 patients (35.1%) and chronic type A dissection in 1 patient (2.7%). 4 patients (10.8%) had Marfan syndrome and bicuspid aortic valve was present in 2 patients (5.4%).

Reoperation of the reconstructed vlave was required in 4 patients. One patient (with chronic aneurysm of the ascending aorta) has coaptation area type B in perioperative TEE and anatomical effects of the operation was not therefore prognostically optimal. In another patient, with Marfan syndrome, operated on for acute dissection, there was an abrupt aortic regurgitation 2 years after primary surgery because tearing one of the commissure. Second patient with Marfan syndrome and chronic ascending aorta aneurysm was reoperated after 4 years. The last patient with chronic aneurysm, and copatation area type A was reoperated after 3 years. It is considered that this type of procedures in carefully selected patients is safe and the mild-term follow-up is satisfactory.

3.1 Specific acces in the management of selected group of patients

3.1.1 Marfan syndrom

Composite replacement of the aortic valve and ascending aorta (Bentall procedure) is a standard approach in patients with Marfan syndrome associated with excellent long term outcomes. The major disadvantage are complications related to long-term anticoagulation treatment in young individuals. This is the main reason for increasing interest for preserve the native aortic valve.

Karck and associates (25) compare the results of aortic valve sparing reimplantation (45 patients) and aortic root replacement with mechanical valve conduits (74 patients) in patients with Marfan syndrome. The results during the mean follow up of 30 months (range 1-94 months) for patients undergoing aortic valve reimplantation and mean follow up 114 months for patients undergoing composite grafting were comparable. Freedom from reoperation and death after 5 years postoperatively was 84% and 96% in patients after vlave reimplantation and 92% and 89% in patients after Bentall procedure.

De Oliveira et al. (30) examine the long-term results of surgery for aortic root aneurysm in patients with Marfan syndrome. 44 patients underwent aortic root replacement and 61 patients underwent aortic valve sparing operations (remodeling/reimplantation). Freedoms from reoperation on aortic valve in patients with Marfan syndrome after aortic valve sparing operations was 100% et 5 and 10 years and in patients after aortic valve replacement 92±5% and 75±9% at 5 and 10 years.

Kallenbach from Hannover, Germany (23), did not observe any difference in short-term outcomes in patients with Marfan syndrome between the reimplantation technique and replacement with composite conduit.

A great supporter of the operation by the Bentall is Hagl from New York (20). He evaluates the results of 142 patients younger than 65 years (32% younger than 40 years, 58% between 40-60 years and 10% 60-65 years old) operated on by Bentall technique. Event-free interval was observed in a set of 0.85/5 years and 0.78/8 years. The gold standard in this age group the authors consider surgery by Bentall and prefer it before valve sparing operations.

3.1.2 Bicuspid aortic valve

A particular problem is the valve sparing operations for bicuspid aortic valve associated with aortic regurgitation, particularly in young patients.

Alsoufi and coworkers (2) presents the results of 71 patients with bicuspid valves and aortic regurgitation who were treated by remodeling, reimplantation or isolated aortic leaflets repair. Risk of reccurence of aortic regurgitation was greater in isolated leaflets repair as compared to remodeling/reimplantation. However, the risk of aortic regurgitation and the risk of reoperation and aortic valve replacement (in case of bicuspid aortic valve) is higher than the remodeling/reimplantation of the tricuspid valve in the same workplace. The risk of bleeding or thromboembolic complications are minimal, but the risk of significant aortic regurgitation (3+/4) is 56% 8 years.

The largest published series on aortic valve repair for aortic insufficiency due to prolapse of bicuspid aortic valve came from Cleveland Clinic. Casselman and colleagues reported on 94 patients with a mean age of 38 years. The freedom from reoperation was 84% at 7 years. (7). The only risk factor predictive of reoperation was residual aortic insufficiency at the time of repair.

Aicher and associates (3) reported a 5year freedom from recurrent aortic insufficiency of 96%, and a freedom from reoperation of 98% after the remodeling procedure in patients with incompetent bicuspid aortic valve and dilated aortic root.

Our insitutional approach in patients with bicuspid valves is very cautious. From our own experience we know that they are technically feasible very often. It is even possible to say that the correction of prolapse in bicuspid valve is simpler than the tricuspid valve. The problem we see in long term durability.

Robicsek et al. (32) showed that in bicuspid valve is never possible to achieve physiological flow and is always greater stress on the cusps in comparison with symmetrical tricuspid aortic valves. Therefore, very often we prefer a valve replacement. But this is a controversial topic with many opinions both for and against.

3.1.3 Aortic dissection type A

Acute dissection of the ascending aorta (Stanford classification type A) requires emergent surgical intervention to prevent life-threatening complications. The valve sparing techniques are innovative approach for patients in whom the aortic leaflets and annulus does not involved. Minor extension of the dissection into the aortic root with near normal size of the sinuses led to conventional valve sparing techniques using Teflon felts and glue. Severe extension of dissection including fragile tissue or aneurysmatic dilatation of more than 4,5 to 5 cm diameter of the dissected root favour valve sparing root replacement by the remodeling or reimplantation techniques. (17,18,19,8,31). Advantages of preservation of the native aortic valve are avoidance of a life-long anticoagulation treatment in mechanical valve replacement and facilitating the thrombotic obliteration of the false lumen. Persistent patency of the false lumen leads to the aneurysm formation, which has been associated with reduced late survival.

Erasmi et al. (19) reviewed 36 patients with acute aortic dissection type A who underwent aortic valve sparing operations. Only 3 patients required reoperation during the mean follow up 7,3 years (after remodeling technique) upon for redetachement of one commissure. All 3 reoperations have been associated with the use of GRF glue (at reoperation they found the necrotic and fragile tissues, which led to anastomotic dehiscences).

Also Casselman et al. (8) revealed the use of fibrinous glue and presence of an aortic valve annulus more than 27 mm as independent risk factors for aortic root reoperation.

Kallenbach et al. presents (24) excellent results in 53 patients with acute aortic dissection type A and valve sparing operations, only 2 patients required reoperation of the reconstructed aortic vlave, both because endocarditis.

Preliminary results of valve sparing techniques for type A dissection in a small series were encouraging with low hospital mortality, and aoutcome is comparable to patients treated with a Bentall procedure. But follow up is short and we have to wait for long term results.

4. Conclusion

Aortic valve sparing operations extend the spectrum of treatment options for aortic regurgitation. They provide excellent results and are associated with very low rates of valve-related complications. However, as they are technically demanding operations, only surgeons with extensive experience in aortic surgery should perform them.

The reimplantation technique with the Gelweave Valsalva prosthesis is our procedure of choice for patients with aortic root aneurysm, including the annulus dilatation with absence or minimal damages of aortic leaflets.

Long-term follow up of more number of patients are needed to confirm the eligibility of using this method in our daily practise.

5. References

Albes J. M. Aortic valve reconstruction: why, when, and how? Thorac Cardiovasc Surg 2010,58:61-68.

Alsoufi B. et al. Results of valve reservation and repair for bicuspid aortic valve insufficiency. The J Heart Valve Disease 2005,14:752-759

Aicher D. et al. Valve-sparing aortic root replacement in bicuspid aortic valves. A reasonable option? J Thorac Cardiovasc Surg 2004,128:62-668

Aybek et al. Valve opening and closing dynamics after different aortic valve operations. J Heart Valve Disease 2005,14:114-120

Bentall H., De Bono A. A technique for complete replacement of the ascending aorta. Thorax 1968,23:338-339.

Boodhwani M., Kerchove L, El Khoury. Aortic root replacemnt using the reimplantation technique: tips and tricks. Interact Cardio Vasc Thorac Surg 2009,8:584-586

Casselman F. P. et al.: Intermediate-term durability of bicuspid aortic valve repair for prolapsing leaflet. *Eur J Cardiothorac Surg* 1999; 15:302.

Casselman F. et al. Durability of aortic valve preservation and root reconstruction in acute type A aortic dissection. Ann Thorac Surg 2000,70:1227-1233

David T. E., Feindel C. M. An aortic valve-sparing operation for patients with aortic incompetence and the aneurysma of the ascending aorta. J Thoracic Cardiovasc Surg 1992,103:617-622.

David T. E. et al. Aortic valve sparing operations: an update. Ann Thorac Surg 1999,67:1840-1842

David T E. et al. Long-term results of aortic valve sparing operations for aortic root aneurysm. J Thorac Cardiovasc Surg 2006,132:347-354

David T. E. Aortic Valve Repair and Aortic Valve - Sparing Operations. Cohn Lh, ed. Cardiac Surgery in the Adult (third edition). New York: McGraw-Hill, 2008:935- 948.

De Paulis et al. Opening and closing characteristics of the aortic valve after valve- sparing procedures using a new aortic root conduit. Ann Thorac Surf 2001,72:487- 489

El Khoury G. et al. Reconstruction of the ascending aorta and aortic root: experience in 45 consecutive patients. Ann Thorac Surg,2000;70:1246-1250.

El Khoury G. et al. Repair of aortic valve prolapse: experience with 44 patients. Eur J Cardiothorac Surg 2004,26:628-633.

El Khoury G. et al. Functional classification of aortic root/valve abnormalities and their correlation with etiologies and surgical procedures. Curr Opin Cardiol 2005,20:115- 21

Erasmi A. W. et al. In vitro hydrodynamics, cusp-bending deformation, and root distensibility for different types of aortic valve - sparing operations: Remodeling, sinus prosthesis, and reimplantation. J Thorac Cardiovasc Surg 2005,130:1044 - 1049.

Erasmi A. W. et al. Remodeling or Reimplantation for Valve-Sparing Aortic Root Surgery? Ann Thorac Surg 2007;83: S752 - S756.

Erasmi A. W. et al. Up to 7 years´ experience with valve-sparing aortic root remodeling/ reimplantation for acute type A dissection. Ann Thorac Surg 2003,76:99-104

Hagl C. et al. Is the Bentall procedure for ascending aorta or aortic valve replacement the best approach for long-term event-free survival? Ann Thorac Surg 2003,76:698-703

Harringer W. et al. Ascending aortic replacement with aortic valve reimplantation. Circulation. 1999,100:II-24.

Jeanmart H. et al. Aortic vlave repair: the functional approach to leaflet prolapse and valve sparing surgery. Ann Thorac Surg 2007,83:S746-51

Kallenbach K. et al. Valve sparing aortic root reconstruction versus composite replacement. Eur J Cardiothorac Surg 2001,20:77-81

Kallenbach K. et al. Decade of aortic valve sparing reimplantation. Circulation. 2005,112:I-253-I-259).

Karck M. et al. Aortic root surgery in Marfan syndrome: comparison of aortic valve-sparing reimplantation versus composite grafting. J Thorac Cardiovasc Surg 2004,127:391-398

Kerchove L. et al. Repair of aortic leaflet prolapse: a ten-year experience. Eur J Cardiothorac Surg 2008,34:785-791.

Kerchove L. et al. Cusp prolapse repair in trileaflet aortic valves: free margin plication and free margin resuspension techniques. Ann Thorac Surg 2009,88(2):455-461

Leyh G. R. et al. Opening and closing characteristics of the aortic valve after different types of valve preserving surgery. Circulation.1999,100:2153

Maselli et al. The ideal graft oversizing in valve sparing aortic operations. Eur J Cardio Thorac Surg 2005,28:845-849

De Oliveira N. C. et al. Results of surgery for aortic root aneurysm in patients with Marfan syndrome. J Thorac Cardiovasc Surg 2003,125:789-796

Pessotto R. et al. Preservation of the aortic valve in acute type A dissection complicated by aortic regurgitation. Ann Thorac Surg 1999,67:2010-2013

Robicsek F, Thubrikar MJ, Cook JW, Fowler B. The congenitally bicuspid aortic valve: how does it function?. Why does it fail? *Ann Thorac Surg*.2004;77:177-185.

Sarsam M. A, Yacoub M. Remodeling of the aortic valve anulus. J Thoracic Cardiovasc Surg 1993,105:435-443.

Settepani F. et al. Aortic valve sparing operations in patients with aneurysm of the aortic root or ascending aorta: preliminary results. Interact Cardio Vasc Thorac Surg 2005,4:137-139

Part 3

Anesthetic and Radiation Management in Aortic Surgery

7

Endovascular Repair: Radiation Risks

John A. Kalef-Ezra
University of Ioannina, Medical School,
Greece

1. Introduction

Abdominal aortic aneurysms (AAA) occur when weakened areas of the abdominal aortic wall result in a ballooning of the vessel. Endovascular repair of AAA (EVAR) has rapidly been integrated into clinical care worldwide as an alternative to open surgical repair. However, such a management is coupled with extended exposure to X-rays for intervention planning, manipulations of catheters and endovascular devices and documentation of the repair, as well as for long-term postoperative surveillance. The energy absorbed in the human body by X-rays causes ionizations triggering biochemical changes that may lead to death or modification of cells. Although many patients derive great benefit from such repairs, some may suffer radiation - induced harm (e.g. skin injuries and increased risk for future cancer), mainly due to the use of inappropriate equipment and, more often, due to poor operational practices (International Commission on Radiological Protection [ICRP], 2000). The three key principles of radiological protection, justification and optimization and application of dose limits, have to be applied in AAA management, as in any practice related to use of ionizing radiations. The radiological burden to both patient and staff has to be assessed at each facility, and if required, the employed practice has to be modified, to keep the risks as low as reasonably achievable, commensurate with the medical purpose.

2. Dosimetric quantities

The medical use of ionizing radiations has the potential to cause harm, as well as provide benefit. Most of the energy emitted from of the X-ray unit during aorta imaging is absorbed non-uniformly in the imaged sections of the patient's body. The patient's bed and the image receptor absorb another fraction of the emitted energy. An additional fraction, usually of the order of 20%, is scattered towards other directions, such as non imaged sections of the patient's body and the staff present in the operation room.

The estimation of the probability of induction of radiobiological effects, either acute or delayed, requires the assessment of quantity absorbed dose, D, at any point in the human body, i.e., the quotient of the energy imparted by ionizing radiation to a volume to the mass in the volume. This quantity is measured in grays, Gy (J/kg). Direct dose measurements at any point are impractical for most organs and tissues. Therefore, simulations of clinical practices are often carried out using physical or mathematical anthropometric phantoms coupled with the following quantities that are assessed in real-time during AAA repair:

- dose at the interventional reference point, D_o , i.e., the procedure cumulative absorbed dose in air at a specific point in space along the central beam axis, with no patient in place, i.e., this quantity, sometimes also referred as cumulative air kerma. does not include backscattering from the human body
- dose area product, i.e., the cumulative product of the absorbed dose in air with the beam cross sectional area (this quantity is often referred as kerma area product, KAP, due to the marginal differences between the physical quantities kerma and absorbed dose in low energy X-ray radiation fields). This distance invariant quantity is related to the entire amount of energy delivered to the patient during the procedure.

C-arm units used for fluoroscopically guided vascular interventions should to be equipped with a device called DAP (or KAP) meter, that tracks and displays dosimetric quantities on or near the operator's imaging monitors both in real-time and cumulatively (FDA regulations enacted on June 2006, require all new fluoroscopic equipment to be equipped with a DAP meter, that is integrated into the unit, Conference of Radiation Control Directors [CRCPD], 2010). The meter consists of a large parallel plate ionization chamber located close to the exit window of the fluoroscopic head and connected with an electrometer. A rough estimation of D_o and DAP can be obtained alternatively in some units using a build-in software (in practice, the software does not take into account possible temporal changes in the X-ray tube output per mA during its working life). The thus obtained dosimetric data as well as procedural and anatomical data, are often introduced off-line to software that allows the assessment of the mean value of absorbed dose in the various organs and tissues of the human body, but not on the spatial distribution of the dose in each of them.

3. Radiobiological aspects

The various biological effects that can be induced by ionizing radiations are divided in two groups, stochastic and deterministic. The former can be induced even after irradiations at low doses of irradiation; on the contrary, the latter can be induced only by high doses (International Commission of Radiological Protection [ICRP], 2007). However, controversy exists today regarding the risk of exposure to X-ray doses less than 100 mGy. Many mechanisms operated in cells and tissues are still evasive in this dose range. Some radiobiologists claim that extrapolation of high-dose to the low-dose region of the dose-effect relationship may overestimate the risk (Feinendegen, el al, 2011). However, the current strategy to quantify the radiological risks in daily practice, assumes that both radiogenic cancer induction in exposed individuals attributed to mutations of somatic cells and heritable effects in their offspring attributed to mutations of reproductive cells, may occur at low doses. Risks of other non-cancer diseases following low dose irradiations, such cardiovascular disorders and vision impairment, still remain uncertain (ICRP, 2007).

3.1 Stochastic effects

Stochastic effects are those for which the probability of induction, but not their severity, is regarded as a function of dose without threshold. More specifically, epidemiological data on subjects irradiated with -X of -γ rays at doses >100 mGy indicate a linear relationship without threshold between the mean absorbed dose in a number of irradiated organs and tissues and the probability of cancer induction to them. Therefore, an increment of absorbed dose induces a proportional increment in risk at low doses. So far only two effects are considered to be stochastic, induction of malignant disease and heritable effects. In radiation

protection the quantity called effective dose, E, expressed in Sv (J/kg), is widely used as an estimator of the health detriment at low doses.
The probability of induction of stochastic effects is related to the quantity effective dose, i.e., the weighted sum of the doses absorbed in a number of organs and tissues specified by ICRP, that their exposure may induce cancer or heritable effects. This quantity takes into account the fact that the induction probability and severity of radiobiological effects per unit dose are not identical in various parts of the body by weighting individual organs and tissues by the relative detriments. Nowadays, most countries base their legislation on the 1990 ICRP recommendations (ICRP, 1990), that take into account the absorbed doses to gonads and to 21 organs or tissues. More specifically, a 0.20 organ weighting factor was assigned to gonads (testes or ovaries), 0.12 to red bone marrow, lung, stomach and colon, 0.05 to five organs (urinary bladder, breast, liver, esophagus and thyroid), 0.01 to bone surface and skin, and 0.005 to ten organs or tissues (adrenals, brain, upper large intestine, small intestine, kidney, pancreas, spleen, thymus, uterus or prostate and muscle). ICRP assigned a nominal risk coefficient of 7.3% per Sv for the whole population and 5.6% per Sv for adult workers (18-64 years old).
According to 1990 ICRP recommendations, the detriment-adjusted risk to patients that undergo a CT examination of the aorta, that results to a 14 mSv effective dose, is about 0.1% (=14 10^{-3} x 7.3%). Let's assume that the examination has to be repeated three times. Taking into account that the fact that the risk increases linearly with dose and the hypothesis often made that that the time period over which the dose is given does not modify the risk, the three examinations result in a 0.3% risk. Similarly, the occupational radiological risk of an interventionist that gets an effective dose of 100 mSv due to his occupation over a 25 year period (4 mSv annually on the average) is estimated to be almost 0.6% (~100 10^{-3} x 5.6%).
Recently ICRP updated its recommendations (ICRP, 2007). Among others, the number of organs/tissues that are taken into consideration for cancer induction was increased from 21 to 27, the weighting factors were modified (for example, the nominal risk for heritable effects in adult workers up to second generation was reduced by a factor of eight) and the nominal risk coefficients for the whole population and for adult workers were reduced to 5.7 % and 4.2% per Sv, respectively. Taking into account that most EVAR patients are past reproductive age and have serious underlying health problems, i.e., with life expectancy shortened as compared to whole population, deterministic injuries in patients are usually of greater concern than those of stochastic effects.

3.2 Deterministic effects

Deterministic effects, or tissue reactions, can be induced by X-ray doses of a few Gy from X-rays to ovaries, testes, red bone marrow, skin, carotid arteries, brain and the eye lens (ICRP, 1984, 2007). However, recently ICRP stated that "although uncertainty remains, medical practitioners should be made aware that the absorbed dose threshold for circulatory disease may be as low as 0.5 Gy to the heart or brain". Doses higher than few Gy are required to induce deterministic effects to other organs, such as lungs, intestine and kidneys.
The incidence of radiation induced injuries in patients is small when compared with the large number of fluoroscopy - guided procedures carried out world-wide, but their consequences can be devastating (Balter & Moses, 2007; ICRP, 2000). Therefore, practitioners should apply methods to avoid the induction of such effects and know how to recognize their signs. In addition, they have to communicate the radiation risk information to patients and provide them the opportunity to ask questions, whenever they deliver doses that could potentially induce them.

Early tissue reactions (on time scale less than about two months after irradiation) usually are the result of either inflammatory type reactions occurring as a result of cell permeability changes or sterilization of stem and progenitor cells. On the contrary, late tissue reactions (on time scale from months to many decades) may occur as a result of either the direct injury to the target tissue, or as a result of severe of early reactions (e.g., dermal necrosis as a result of epidermal denudation) or/and chronic infection. Late tissue reactions, such as excess cardiovascular disease that becomes clinically apparent only 10 to 20 years post-irradiation, have a long and dose-dependent latency period before their clinical expression, reducing thus the probability of induction in elderly patients.

Although deterministic effects may appear in all body areas, the various tissues and organs have different tolerances. Once a threshold dose has been exceeded, the probability of induction and the severity of the effect increases with increasing dose. The threshold dose, TD_1, i.e. the amount of radiation that is required to cause a specific observable effect in 1% of the exposed individuals, depends on a number of factors, such the irradiated tissue or organ, the type of response and the time over which the dose was given. TD_1 usually increases with increase of the time over which the dose is given, or by dose fractionation, due to cellular repair and even repopulation. Therefore, increase of the interval between medical procedures that require "heavy" exposure of the same body region, if clinically acceptable, modifies the dose response relationship.

The TD_1 currently used values, such as those on skin reactions (Table 1) refer to healthy adults. No specific data have been proposed to be used for children and subjects with mutations in important DNA damage sensing or repairing genes (the homozygous form of ataxia telangiectasia gene, Fanconi anemia, and Bloom syndrome are typical examples), patients with diabetes, active connective tissue diseases (scleroderma, lupus erythematosus, etc), autoimmune disorders, and patients with disrupted skin due to surgery or burns.

In most tissues and organs, responses are greater when the irradiated volumes are greater. This volume effect means that the threshold dose increases as the volume of the irradiated organ/tissue decreases. Cell migration, proliferation and differentiation of progenitor cells from the margins to the heavily irradiated tissue volume may explain this effect (Dilmanian et al., 2007). Paired organ, such as the kidneys, and organs with functional subunits arranged in parallel, such as elements in the liver, rather in series, such as elements in the spinal cord, can sustain partial inactivation without clinical signs of injury.

3.2.1 Skin reactions

Since the early 1990s reports of radiation-induced skin injuries to patients due to fluoroscopically guided medical procedures have steadily increased. The skin is the only organ, which is always exposed to primary radiation during X-ray imaging (the skin region of beam entrance is the region that gets the highest dose). Relative to other organs, skin is less liable to develop fatal cancer after irradiation (ICRP 1991, 1992, 2007). However, the thresholds for mild deterministic effects are relatively low compared other organs (International Atomic Energy Agency [IAEA], 1998). Therefore, only five months after the discovery of X-rays, serious skin damage was documented, three weeks after imaging the head of a child (Daniel, 1896; Tarbell et al., 1981). Since then, a vast literature has been published on skin injuries that may evolve slowly over time, extending from hours to years after irradiation, often with periods between them of none or few symptoms (Table 1).

A minimum number of adjacent cells must be damaged by radiation to elicit skin injury (Peel & Hopwell, 1984; Dilmanian, et al., 2003). The dose-response relationship for each type of skin damage due to X-ray irradiation (Table 1), as well as the kinetics of healing, depend on a large number of factors, such as protraction of irradiation or dose fractionation (potential of partial or full repair between fractions), size and location of the exposed area (the skin in the back of the trunk is considered to be of medium radiosensitivity), obesity, skin hydration status and coloration (light-colored skin is regarded to be most sensitive). The dose-response relationship is often modified in patients given some medications that may modify skin response, before, during, or even years post irradiation (Burris & Hurtig, 2010; Camidge et al., 2001; Hymes et al., 2006).

In general, the earlier the onset of clinical changes (Table 2) the more severe the pathology of the skin lesion (Muller & Meineke, 2010). Following skin irradiation some basal cells are destroyed. The remaining cells shed more quickly. Mitotic inhibition appears about 30 minutes after a single 4 to 5 Gy X-ray irradiation, followed by decrease in the proliferation of the germinal layer of the endothelium. No clinically observable skin reactions are expected to be induced following a single acute dose up to 2 Gy of X-rays (higher total doses can be tolerated following prolonged or fractionated irradiations). Pain, if occurs, does not occur immediate (as in thermal burns), but when it appears, it is sever and resistant to drugs (its evolution is regarded as a good indicator for the prognosis and prediction of local skin atrophy and even necrosis (Rojas-Palma, et al., 2009). Therefore, although skin injuries are not usually life threatening, the more severe lesions may result among others in chronic intractable pain and permanent disability, such as that related to amputation (IAEA, 1998, 2002).

The earliest visible skin response that may appear is a transient skin erythema, (reddening), at the entrance site of the X-ray beam. It resembles to sunburn with no hair loss at this stage, in contrast to thermal burns, where early hair and tissue loss is observed (Table 2). The first wave of erythema may be accompanied by sensation of heat and itching. It may be seen from a few hours up to 48 h after irradiation at single X-ray doses above 2 Gy, when the exposed skin area is relatively large (as in EVAR where ~250 cm^2 is a typical field area), and fades after few hours to two days. This injury is attributed to inflammation due cytokine activation and capillary dilation, thus increasing blood volume beneath epidermis and vascular permeability. This stage is followed by a latent one during which there are no apparent skin reactions, despite the subcellular processes that may take place. In daily clinical practice, the isolated or confluent prodromal patches in the skin of EVAR patients that received high local doses may go unnoticed, because they are anticipated to occur at the patient's back, an area that patients could no easily see. However, if observed, they can serve as an alarm for possible more serious radiation reactions. In this case, the use of dermatoprotector creams is recommended (IAEA, 2002).

effect	TD_1 (Gy)	effect	TD_1(Gy)
early transient eryrhema	2	dry desquemation	14
temporary epilation	3	late erythema	15
main erythema	6	dermal necrosis	>15
permanant epilation	7	moist desquamation	18
dermal atrophy	10	ischemic dermal necrosis	18
telangiectasia	10	secondary ulceration	24

Table 1. Threshold acute X-ray doses (ED) for skin reactions in 1% of the subjects (protraction of dose over a period of 1-3 weeks results in higher TD_1).

stage	latency	persistence	symptoms
prodromal	minutes-hours	0.5 – 36 h	erythema, pruritus
manifestation	3 weeks	1- 2 weeks	erythema, pruritus, bullae, ulcer
subacute	16 weeks	months	erythema, ulcer
chronic	years	unlimited	ulcer, keratosis, fibrosis, epidermal atrophy, teleangiectasia, angioma, alterations in pigmentation
late	>10 years	unlimited	angioma, basal and squamous, cell carcinoma

Table 2. Clinical stages of skin reactions (IAEA, 2002).

If the dose is sufficient, inflammatory processes prevail and a second hyperemic phase of more sustained erythema (second wave of erythema), may appear at two to four weeks after dosing of at least 3 to 6 Gy in adults, usually lasting 20 to 30 days (ICPR, 2007). The severity of erythema and the latent period are dose dependent. This erythema phase may appear even one week after an acute dose above 15 Gy, often accompanied by subepidermal blister formation due to apoptosis and necrotic destruction of the epidermis (Muller & Meineke, 2010), heat sensation, itching, tenderness in the irradiated skin area and changes in pigmentation. However, if the dose is not much a greater than the threshold, the erythema fades after about 4 weeks (Koening et al., 2001). The third phase of erythema (third wave of erythema) may also be seen with an onset of about 8 to 20 weeks post-irradiation following a single irradiation of at least 15 Gy. This phase may vary in severity, but at its maximum is characterized with a dusky / mauve appearance. Recently, Rahimi et al. (2011) associated to radiation damage a square shaped burn observed in the back of a patient with abdominal aortic aneurysm during the second post-repair visit to the hospital.

Two to three weeks after an acute X-ray dose exceeding the 4 Gy threshold (ICRP, 2007), epilation may occur due to damage in the base of the hair follicles (in some anatomic locations the TD_1 could be higher than 4 Gy). Single acute doses from X-rays in excess of 7 to 10 Gy may irreversibly reproductively sterilize or lead to apoptotic death the stem cells in hair follicles, resulting in permanent epilation (Koening et al., 2001; Kim et al., 2003). However, epilation is temporary following low radiation doses. Survival of basal and germinal matrix cells in the hair follicles may allow for hair re-growth (Geleijns et al., 2005) about 1.5 to 4 months post-irradiation. At the initial stage of re-growth, hair may be thinner (up to 30% reduction in diameter) and sparse, differing occasionally in pigmentation and structure from that before irradiation.

Alopecia has been reported in literature to be induced in patients who underwent endovascular treatments for various clinical conditions, such as aneurysm (Foroozan et al., 2008; Lee et al., 2004; Marti et al., 2008) and arteriovenous malformations (Fellman, 2011; Wen, et al., 2003) mainly in the skull, as well as in practitioners, such as hair loss reported at the lower legs of cardiologists (Wipper et al., 2005). Taking into account the locations of the X-ray entrance ports used in patients with aortic aneurysm and their age distribution, radiation induced hair loss is not as stressful as in other patients, such as those in young patients with malformations in the head or those with radiotherapy.

The rate of gradual decline in cell density in the basal layer depends on the rate of epidermal turnover at the irradiated site. A 50% reduction of the normal basal cell density appears to provide a stimulus to the remaining viable colonogenic stem cells to proliferate starting about 3 weeks post irradiation in pig skin, the model historically assumed to be the best one for human skin (Van de Aardeg et al., 1988). At relatively low doses the number of developing colonies will be adequate to unite into a single group, thus leading 3 to 6 weeks to dry desquamation, an atypical keratination of the skin (ICRP, 1992). If the X-ray dose exceeds 18 Gy, the reduced number of developing colonies may not cover the entire damaged area and cell loss will continue, leading to moist desquamation, i.e., loss of the epidermis. At this stage dermis is denuded, allowing serum from the deep cutaneous layers to be excreted (Koening et al., 2001) often responding with marked inflammation (the use of glucocorticoids and hydrocolloid dressings might be considered, as well as local infection prophylaxis and treatment). When the area of the irradiated skin is completely denuded of clonogenic epithelial cells, healing must occur totally as a result of division and migration of epithelial cells from the edges of the irradiated skin area. For all, but the very small radiation fields, the repopulation progresses slowly, thus exposing the skin to risk of secondary ulceration, at least 6 weeks post-irradiation (ICRP, 1992; Balter et al., 2010). Some radiation ulcers that were healed over time have a tendency to recur in the following months and years (Koenig et al., 2001). Other ulcers never heal completely even years after fluoroscopically guided interventions.

In general, dermis presents clinically its response at a later stage than epidermis and may not reach its peak even after some years (Geleijns et al., 2005). Cutaneous reactions are attributed to complex interactions between antiproliferative and proinflammatory processes, involving a variety of cytokines, adhesion molecules, growth factors and their receptors (IAEA, 2002). Dermal ischaemia and necrosis may appear 6 to 8 weeks post-irradiation at doses of at least 20 to 25 Gy. These effects were preceded by loss of endothelial cells, microvascular damage, reduction in capillary density, edema and impaired lymphatic clearance (ICRP, 1992). Late skin damage is characterized by dermal atrophy, dermal tissue thinning, long-lasting telangioectasia (it appears at least 1 year after an acute X-ray dose of at least 10 Gy), cutaneous fibrosis characterized by an increase of collagen fibers, keratosis, and often by reduction in the linear dimensions of the irradiated area. The use of interferon gamma as an inhibitor of collagen can be considered.

The various techniques for diagnosis and medical management of localized radiation injuries were reviewed by various organizations and investigators (IAEA, 2002; Rojas-Palmas et al., 2009; Muller et al., 2010). For example, moist desquamation may require surgical intervention to remove irradiated dermal and subcutaneous tissue (Rojas-Palmas et al., 2009).

3.2.2 Eye reactions

The eye lens is one of the most radiosensitive tissues of the human body, not with respect to cancer induction but mainly to the induction of lens opacity. The potential of X-rays to produce cataracts was suggested only two years after their discovery (Merriam & Worgul, 1983). Lens transparency depends on proper differentiation of fibre cells from a layer of epithelial cells in the lens anterior surface near its equator. The earliest lens change is the visualization of granular opalescent on the posterior lens capsule observed by slit lap examination followed by the appearance of small vocuoles (ICRP, 2007; Merriam & Worgul, 1983), which, over time, aggregate to form larger opacities of great impact in vision. The time between irradiation and the clinical manifestation of eye damage varies from half a year after "heavy" exposures to many decades.

In the past, induction of vision-impairing cataract was considered as a deterministic effect with threshold of 5.0 Gy following a single brief exposure to X-rays and higher than 8 Gy following highly fractionated exposures (ICRP, 2000). Based on knowledge available on 2007, ICRP reduced the TD_1 for cataract formation to 1.5 Gy, stating, however, that "the Committee can not ultimately exclude cataract induction at even lower doses". Recent studies indicated a significant association between exposure to lower doses and increased risk of cataract formation (Ainsbury et al., 2009; Chodick et al .,2008; Ciraj-Bjelac et al., 2010; Jacob, et al.; Shore et al., 2010, Worgul et al., 2007). For example, some investigators reported on increased cataract rate even after ~0.5 Gy, acute or fractionated; others found detectable lens changes even after only 0.1 Gy doses and some even proposed the use of a linear non-threshold model (Chodick et al., 2008; Nakashima et al., 2006). Based on evidence available on April 2011, ICRP further reduced the threshold dose for the eye lens to 0.5 Gy.

Those occupationally exposed during fluoroscopically guided procedures are at a risk of radiation-induced eye damage. For example, Vano et al. (2010) found a 3.2 relative risk of posterior subcapsular opacities in 116 interventional cardiologists versus unexposed individuals. Ciraj- Bjelac et al. (2010) found a 5.7 relative risk of posterior subcapsular opacities in 56 interventional cardiologists of average age 42 y, that received a mean cumulative dose to the lens 3.7 Gy versus unexposed matched individuals (prevalence 52% vs 9%). Therefore, precautions, such as protective glasses and X-ray tube positioning, have to be taken to protect the eyes of staff heavily involved in fluoroscopically guided interventional procedures, delaying thus opacity propagation and limiting future cumulative lens dose (Vano et al., 2008).

3.2.3 Effects of antenatal exposure

Embryo and fetus are highly radiosensitive during the entire gestation period. The possible biological effects due to prenatal irradiation were reviewed in ICRP Publication 90 (ICRP, 2003). The type and the severity of the damage depend on the time of exposure relative to conception (ICRP, 2003, 2007; Brent, 2007). Chronic or fractionated irradiations to X-rays at a specific total dose are usually assumed to be four to ten times less risky than single acute doses.

The life-time cancer risk after prenatal irradiation is assumed to be at most few times that of the population as a whole and not greater than that following exposure in early childhood (ICRP, 2007). For example, following an 100 mGy fetal dose there is a 99% chance that the exposed fetus will not develop childhood cancer or leukaemia. Animal experiments indicate higher radiosensitivy for cancer induction in females than in males and at late than early gestation periods (ICRP, 2003). However, it is not clear if these findings hold for humans. In addition, it is not possible to determine tissue/organ weighting factors of the conceptus, based on the currently available data.

The risk for lethality of the developing organism is assumed to be highest during the first post-conception days (pre-implantation period). At this period the number of cells in humans increases from one, the zygote, to about 200. No observations are available at this gestational period in humans, as conception in not noticed at that time. Therefore, the current knowledge is based on animal models. At doses of few tens of mGy lethal effects are very infrequent. However, lethality reaches 50% for 1 Gy X-ray doses given at stages from the zygote to expanded blastocyte (ICRP, 2003). The currently available data provide no reason to believe that, if death does not occur at this stage, significant health effects may occur after birth, except if there is genetic predisposition for malformations (ICRP, 2007).

Human epidemiological studies and animal studies indicate that the *in utero* radiosensitivity for malformations (defects visible at birth) depends on gestation age and that the regenerative capacity decreases as differentiation of tissues and cells progresses It is currently believed that there is a dose threshold of about 100 mGy for malformation during the most radiosensitive period for such an effect, the period of major organogenesis (3 to 7 weeks post-conception). Studies on rodents indicated the existence of a dose threshold for induction of intrauterine growth retardation of about 0.25 Gy following an X ray irradiation within a short time period during the most sensitive period that is advanced stages of organogenesis and 0.5 Gy during the less sensitive stages (ICRP, 2003). Therefore, for stage of peak sensitivity for fetal underweight differs from those for lethality and malformations. Nakasima, et al (1994) analyzing body habitus of age 18 years of *in utero* exposed atomic-bomb survivors found a clear radiation effect on standing height, however in a later study (Nakashima, et al., 2005) they failed to find dependence of the effect on the gestational period at exposure, particularly among males. Neurobehavioral studies of animals exposed *in utero* demonstrate a threshold for behavioral effects at the same dose as for other teratological effects, i.e. 0.2 Gy (Brent, 2007).

High radiation doses (1 to 2 Gy) of ionizing radiation to the developing human fetus may induce mental retardation and microcephaly (Brent, 2007). The susceptibility of the developing human to injury from prenatal exposure was clearly shown by Schull and Otake (1984, 1999). The human data related mainly to those exposed to radiation from the use nuclear weapons in Hiroshima and Nagasaki are in good agreement with data on animal models. Severe mental retardation may occur following prenatal irradiation. When the cases assumed to have non-radiation aetiology at the two Japanese towns were excluded (e.g. Down's syndrome), threshold dose values of 0.55 Gy (95% confidence interval 0.3 to 0.6 Gy) and 0.87 Gy (95% confidence interval 0.3 to 1.1 Gy) were proposed for irradiations 8-15 and 16-25 weeks post-conception, respectively, i.e. the major neuronogenetic periods of the developing human neocortex during which the developing brain expands very fast (ICRP, 2000; Nowoakowski & Haeys, 2008). In addition, a decline in IQ values of about 25 IQ points per Gy was observed due to irradiation 8 to 15 weeks post-conception, resulting in very small detriment at X-ray doses less than 0.1 Gy. Irradiations 16 to 25 weeks pos-conception resulted in lower IQ decrement, 13 IQ points per Gy. From the other hand, there is no data supporting a similar damage, when the dose is given at a later gestation stage (ICRP, 2003, 2007).

4. Radiation protection in aneurysm repair

Radiation dose and image quality strategies are important for ensuring a balance between cost and benefit. The question to ask in daily clinical practice is not "is this radiation-related procedure safe?" but "is this procedure needed to help the physicians provide the best medical treatment?" The practitioner has the responsibility to order / carry out the appropriate tests and interventions when justified by the presenting symptoms or concerns with the lowest cost consistent with the medical aim.

In EVAR, as in any other type of fluoroscopy guided vascular intervention, both patient and staff radiation exposures are related to the dose at the interventional reference point (D_o) or/and the dose area product (DAP) value. Patient data related to over AAA 1000 repairs are summarized in Table 3. The corresponding studies indicated that the vast majority of the patients were male with mean age 70 to 75 years and that the mean fluoroscopic time

reference	n	mean age (years)	mean fluoroscopy time (min)	mean DAP (Gy cm^2)	median DAP (Gy cm^2)	Dose (mGy)	PSD (mGy)	type of fluoroscopic unit
Geijer, et al., 2005	24	72	28	72±45	60.1		390	mobile
Kalef-Ezra et al., 2009	62	74	23	42.5±25.6	37.4		227	mobile I
Lipsitz, et al., 2000	47		39				360	mobile
Present study	142	70	22	30±24	24.4		205	mobile II
Weerakkody, et al., 2008	96*	73	21*,++		150*		850*,++	mobile
Weiss, et al., 2008	12		21	152			750	mobile
Farrar, et al., 2005	121	74	24++					not specified
Jones, et al., 2010	64	75	23	54±34				not specified
Jones, et al., 2010	320	75	29	47 ±28		1187		not specified
Bannazadeh, et al., 2009							729	stationary
Blaszak, et al., 2009	61	71.5	23	381±285	355			stationary
Geijer, et al., 2005	24+				600 +	2900+		stationary
Kalef-Ezra, in press	6	72	12	192	205		1050	stationary
Kuhelj, et al., 2010	152	71	21		154		440**	stationary
Panuccio, et al., 2011++	47	75	83	782	697	6300	2590	stationary

* excluding data on seven patients, ** median rather than mean value,
PSD: peak skin dose, + simulated procedures, ++ thoracoabdominal aneurysms

Table 3. Demographic data, fluoroscopy time and dosimetric quantities related to AAA repairs.

per repair was about 20 min, with two exceptions, the studies by Lipsitz er al, and by Panuccio et al. (2011) who treated thoracoabdominal aneurysms. On the other hand, the spread of the DAP and the mean peak skin dose, (D_{peak}) values were also large, even excluding the study by Pannuccio, et al. In addition, as in other types of vascular interventions, the spread of values at each facility was also large (65% is a typical value of the coefficient of variation) and their distributions were not Gaussian (the median is typically about 15% lower than the mean value). In the following paragraphs some of the factors related to the spread of the mean DAP values between facilities and between repairs carried out at each facility are discussed, as well as, some means to control the radiation burden.

The currently acceptable errors in D_o and DAP measurements are quite large, ±35% by the Food and Drug Administration (FDA) and ±50% by International Electrochemical Commission (IEC). In addition, there is no unique definition on the place of the interventional reference point along the central beam line. IEC defines it to be at 15 cm distance on the X-ray tube side (IEC, 2000), while FDA defines it at 30 cm distance from the image receptor, leading a factor of four difference in the displayed D_o values in systems with 100 cm focus to distance. An additional source of error is the angular dependence of the X-ray beam attenuation on the patient's bed (the calibration of the DAP meter is often carried out at a geometry that differs from that used during AAA repair). Therefore, spatial attention is required when comparing values presented in various studies and/or correlating the displayed quantities with the mean or the peak doses in an organ or a tissue.

4.1 Assessment of stochastic risk to patient

The assessment of the effective dose related to AAA management is required to weigh the potential stochastic risks against the anticipated medical benefits. However, direct dose measurements are impractical for most organs and tissues. Thus, the assessment of mean doses absorbed by the organs and tissues of interest is usually made by introducing to a software some repair-related parameters (DAP, field size, data on patient's body habitus, the anatomic location of the lesion, X-ray tube high voltage and filtration, etc.). The dose corresponding to each radiation field has to be assessed separately and then summed-up to calculate E (most investigators so far assumed that the location and the size of the X-ray beam and spectral distribution remained unchanged throughout repair, and neglected the influence of body shape and composition on dose distribution). Various investigators reported mean E to DAP ratios ranging between 0.14 and 0.25 mSv/Gy cm^2 (Table 4) using the 1990 definition of E by ICRP. On the other hand, the mean E values shown in Table 4 differ up to two orders of magnitude, with the lower ones being comparable to the effective dose resulting from three years of exposure to natural background radiation.

Reference	E / DAP (mSv/Gy cm^2)	mean E (mSv)	median E (mSv)
Badger, et al., 2010	0.25	12	
Bannazadeh, et al., 2009	0.14		109
Ho, et al., 2007		12.7	
Geijer, et al., 2005	0.14	10.5	8.7
Kalef-Ezra, et al., in press	0.23	5.8 *	4.6
Kalef-Ezra, et al., in press	0.23	6.6 **	
Kalef-Ezra, et al., in press	0.21	40 ***	
Weerakody, et al., 2008	0.18		27

* mobile C-arm unit I, ** mobile unit II, *** stationary C-arm unit

Table 4. Repair related effective dose.

The excess life mortality after exposure to ionizing radiations at low doses decreases with increasing age (ICRP, 1991). It is about 4.8% per Sv in men exposed at age of 65 years, 2.6% and 1.1% per Sv in men exposed at 75 and 85 years, respectively, and slightly lower in women (3.9%, 2.9% and 0.9%, respectively). In case of uniform irradiation, leukemia is anticipated to be the main cause of death (almost 50% in men exposed at age of 70 years). Taking into account the age and sex distribution of EVAR patients (Table 3), an excess life mortality of 3.5% per Sv can be assumed. Therefore, the radiological health detriment of a repair requiring an effective dose of 10 mSv is about 3.5 10^{-4}.

Combining dosimetric data on 91 repairs carried out at Ioannina University Hospital (IUH) using a Pulsera mobile C-arm unit with a PC-based Monte Carlo software (Kalef-Ezra in press), it was found in that:

- the mean E/DAP ratio was 0.23 mSv/Gy cm^2 (range 0.17 to 0.31 mSv/Gy cm^2),

- the red bone marrow and colon were the main contributors to E in male patients,
- the image registration contribution to E was only 20%,
- the effective dose was linearly correlated with fluoroscopy time, t_{fl}, and body mass index (BMI), i.e.,

$$E\ (mSv) = -7.24 + 0.298\ t_{fl}\ (min) + 0.237\ BMI\ (kg/m^2)$$

The effective dose related to the repair itself is often lower than that related with the other aspects of AAA management. For example, a typical two-phase CT abdominal/pelvic angiography often requires about 20 mSv, i.e. few times higher than that of a repair itself carried out using a mobile unit. Therefore, various protocols for diagnostic / planning and postoperative follow-up imaging have been proposed to reduce both radiological and renal function deterioration risks. Dose reducing protocols related to post-operative imaging can be divided in three main groups:

- application of less intensive follow-up procedures, including an optimized temporal spacing between CT scans (Dias, et al., 2009; Go, et al, 2008; Verhoeven, et al., 2011; White & McDonald, 2010; Zhou, 2011),
- optimization of the CT scanning parameters (Diehm et al., 2008; Iezi et al, 2006,2009; Kalef-Ezra et al., in press; Kirby et al., 2007; Macari et al., 2006; Nakayama, et al., 2006; Sommer, et al., 2010; Wintersperger, et al., 2005),
- replacement of CT imaging with alternative imaging / assessment techniques, that require lower or even no radiation dose, such as ultrasound or MRI imaging (Elkouri et al.; 2004, Manning, et al, 2008.; Sternbergh, et al., 2008; Ten Bosch, et al.; 2010; Tomlinson, et al, 2007, 2009; Truijers, et al., 2009).

The application of the life-long protocol for AAA management at IUH with optimized post-operative CT parameters resulted in a cumulative effective dose of almost 60 mSv (Kalef-Ezra, in press), which leads to a 0.2% excess life-time mortality, using the 3.5% per Sv risk factor. However this value has be divided by a factor of two according to the current ICRP recommendations (ICRP, 2007) due to dose fractionation over many years, resulting in a life-time mortality of 0.1%.

4.2 Assessment of deterministic effects to patient

On contrast to radiation-induced cancer that can be observed clinically after many years, deterministic reactions are often near-term radiation effects. In CT imaging the X-ray spectrum is harder than that used in AAA repair and the X-ray source rotates around the human body, dispersing thus the imparted energy to the body more uniformly and over larger volumes. Therefore, the induction of deterministic effects in AAA patients is mainly related to the repair itself and not to CT.

If such effects occur, the most probable location is the skin at the patients' back (Table 3). Damaging skin levels can be reached in a short time especially when obese patients are treated using short focus-skin distance, non-optimized fluoroscopic units and/or high image magnification factors. Therefore, each medical facility has to develop techniques to assess peak skin dose, PSD, and control it at levels below the threshold for induction of deterministic effects (Tables 1 and 2), taking into account that the same skin area may absorb additional doses due to other imaging procedures made within a relatively short time period.

Skin dose mapping shows the overlapping fields and allows the accurate determination of PSD. Recently some manufactures of stationary fluoroscopic units introduced the use of software to calculate PSD combining the readings of the DAP meter with geometrical data related to bed movements during the procedures, focus to table distances, beam angulations, etc. High sensitivity self-developing radiochromic films, such as reflective-type dosimetric gafchromic XR type films and arrays of thermoluminescent dosimeters (TLDs) have been used for direct 2D dose skin mapping by placing them between the surgical bed and patient's back (Table 5). The extent of polymerization of the films, and thus the changes in their optical properties, are influenced by their dosing. TLDs emit light upon heating at any time after irradiation. Other types of dosimeters could be used, such as the scintillating ZnCd dosimeters and diodes. Slow photographic film, such as those use in radiation therapy, do not allow accurate determination of the dose distribution due to the large dependence of their response to X-ray spectrum. Currently there is no perfect dose mapping system available and each facility should use the best available indicator.

TLD handling and processing are complex and time consuming and the cost of the equipment to process is high. In addition, there is a risk to miss with TLDs the region with the peak skin dose. On the other hand, one has to consider the cost of the radiochromic films, that can be used only once, the substantial dependence of their response on the X-ray spectrum and the fact that they cannot be read accurately until after their use, because they must undergo a time-consuming stabilization process (Kalef-Ezra et al., 2008, 2010). However, if concern is raised over skin dose, the radiochromic film can be removed from the bed during repair and examined by bare eye in normal light at the operation room for a rough dose assessment.

Kuhelj, et al. (2010) analyzing the dosimetric data on 179 patients treated using a suboptimal mobile C-arm unit found a 0.44 Gy median PSD (range 0.12 to 2.7 Gy). Investigators at Cabridge reported a 0.85 Gy median PSD on 96 repairs (Weerakkody, et al. 2008; Walsh, et al., 2008). About 1/4 of their patients received PSD higher than 3.75 Gy and the maximum dose was 8.8 Gy (the authors excluded from the analysis data on seven additional repairs because the "values were orders of magnitude greater than typical values recorded"). Pannuccio, et al. (2011) reported on 47 patients that undergone thoracoabdominal aneurysm repair a 2.5 Gy mean PSD (in ten patients the dose was higher than 4.0 Gy, and the maximum value was 6.5 Gy). The most heavily irradiated areas were of 4 cm^2 size and located at the central part of the back close to the kidneys. Despite the high PSDs found, no skin reactions were reported. On the contrary, Rahimi et al. (2011) related to radiation the acute gastrointestinal complications (nausea, diarrhea and abdominal pain) reported by an EVAR patient during the first post-repair visit. These symptoms were coupled with skin color alterations observed during the second visit. According to the authors "the procedure required about 56 min of fluoroscopic imaging time resulting in 6.8 Gy total radiation exposure".

Lower mean PSD values were reported by other investigators (Table 3). For example, Weiss et al. (2008) measured a 0.75 median value (range 0.27 to 1.25 Gy) in twelve repairs. Geijer, et al. (2005) analyzing data on 24 procedures calculated a 0.33 Gy median value (range 0.08 to 1.1 Gy). Among the 204 patients treated with EVAR at IUH using mobile C-arm units, no patient received a peak dose exceeding 1.1 Gy. Therefore, in none of the repairs presented in these studies using mobile fluoroscopic units, PSD approached the threshold for any skin reaction.

In daily clinical practice direct 2D dose skin mapping in all patients is considered to be a time and money consuming procedure. In addition, it does not provide real-time guidance to the operator on accumulated dose to adjust the employed techniques during repair, such as the use of dose spreading techniques, i.e. change of the X-source angle, while the intervention site is kept in the centre of the field of view (Johnson et al., 2001).

An empirically determined relationship between indications of meter and PSD obtained by direct measurements in a subgroup of patients in each facility can be used for this purpose (Kalef-Ezra, et al., 2009, 2010). This approach bypasses the accuracy limitations of the DAP indicators and many of the differences in employed imaging strategies. If no direct data is available at a facility, data from other facilities could be used as a rough estimation, keeping in mind that the relationship depends on a larger number of factors. The currently available data on the PSD to DAP ratio for AAA repairs vary between 3 and 7 mGy per Gy cm^2 (Table 5). Assuming a 6 mGy / Gy cm^2 value, the restriction of the DAP below 333, 667 Gy cm^2 keeps PSD below the threshold for temporary erythema and epilation (Tables 1 and 2), 1.0, 1.15 and 2.3 kGy cm^2 below the threshold of main erythema reaction, permanent epilation and dry desquamation respectively, provided that no other imaging with X-rays is carried out within a short time period. Based on such findings a warning level (called also as triggering level) of 250 Gy cm^2 can be used for the operator to consider modification of the imaging strategy during the repair of the specific patient. In practice the operator could be notified by the technical staff present in the room when the 150, 250, 350, 650 and 1000 Gy cm^2 levels were reached. However, it is up the interventionist in charge to decide how to proceed, when a significant dose level has been crossed.
To avoid the induction of skin injuries, practitioners should always seek to establish before repair whether the patients had previous imaging procedures or radiotherapy sessions, together with the estimated skin doses and the beam entrance sites (ICRP, 2000). In addition, monitoring and tracking of radiation doses in endovascular AAA management should to be carried out after repair (CRCPD, 2010). More specifically, the dose indications should to be recorded in the machine's log book (physical or electronic) and reviewed immediately after repair to determine if the patient is at risk to develop skin injuries. The dosimetric data have to be recorded to the patient's medical record, indicating the beam entry site. If some threshold is exceeded, such as 150 Gy cm^2 (the level depends on national legislation and the local rules), the medical (or health) physicist in charge of the unit has to assess more accurately the doses and the associated risks. The facility radiation safety committee/ officer should periodically check the distribution of the dosimetric parameters, compare them over time and review one by one all repairs that exceeded some dose value, such as a PSD of 3.0 Gy. In departments with "heavy" duty, the data have to be also analyzed according to the interventionist in charge.

References	C-arm unit	operation bed	D_{peak}/DAP (mGy/ Gy cm^2)	dosimetric method
Geiger, et al., 2005	mobile	angiographic	5.5	calculated
Kalef-Ezra, et al., 2009	mobile I	surgical	5.0	LiF:Mg,Ti TLD
Kalef-Ezra, et al., 2011	mobile II	angiographic	6.8	LiF:Mg,Ti TLD
Kalef-Ezra, et al., 2011	mobile II	angiographic	6.7	gafchromic XR-RV2
Kuhelj, et al., 2010	stationary	angiographic	3.5	gafchromic XR
Panuccio, et al., 2011	stationary	angiographic	~3	gafchromic
Weiss, et al., 2008	mobile	-	~5	gafchromic
Weerakkody, et al., 2008	mobile	surgical	~6	calculated

Table 5. Skin peak dose and its relationship with DAP.

All patients who potentially received a skin dose higher than some predetermined value, usually set at 3.0 Gy, should be closely monitored for potential serious skin injuries. The practitioner should arrange for the patient to be reviewed about two weeks after repair. The patient and family should to be informed of the possible symptoms and signs and instructed to check the patient's skin during the first 48 h procedure (in case of out-patients) and once a week over the following five weeks. If radiation cannot be ruled out as the cause of skin lesion, the patient has to be referred to either a dermatologist or a radiation therapist, experienced in managing radiation injuries. In addition, patient's personal physician should be informed to avoid procedures during subsequent two months, which could result in a substantial dose to the same skin area. Such actions are important because radiation injuries are often misdiagnosed and treated inappropriately.

4.3 Determinants of patient's radiation risks

The potential risks of medical exposures to ionizing radiation must be balanced against the potential medical benefits of the procedures. Limiting potential radiological risk is essential, remembering the currently applied working hypothesis that there is no dose below which there is zero risk. In general radiation burden, besides the age and general clinical conditions of the patient, is influenced by a number of anatomical and technical factors, as well as to the education and training of the interventional team. Radiation protection can be ensured by appropriate design, procurement and commissioning of equipment, optimal operational technique and quality assurance backed by quality audit. In particular, the choice of the fluoroscopic unit to be used and the irradiation modes to be selected, have to be based primarily on the required level of image quality, ergonomic factors, financial costs, and associated radiological risks. The analysis of the influence of the various factors and the analysis of the accumulated experience may allow the selection of the optimum repair strategy.

4.3.1 Equipment related factors

Repairs can be carried out using angiographic units equipped with either low power generators, such as mobile C-arm fluoroscopic units widely used in operation theaters, or with high power stationary generators, such as those designed primarily for guidance in coronary artery interventions and located at radiology / cardiology suites. According to data shown in Table 3, the mean DAP per repair carried out using mobile units ranged between 30 and 152 Gy cm^2. On the other hand, higher mean (192 to 782 Gy cm^2) and median values (154 to 697 Gy cm^2) were reported on repairs carried out using stationary units.

To exclude the possible influence of the use of different protocols, few AAA repairs were carried out at IUH using a stationary 100 kW unit, an Allura 9C by Philips, at the lowest available mode (12.5 p/s fluoroscopy and registration rate 12.5 images/s and 11 mm Al equivalent filtration). The dosimetric data of these repairs was compared with those of repairs carried using a much cheaper mobile unit, a 7.5 kW Pulsera unit by the same manufacturer, selecting a registration rate of 3 images/s, and 50% of its maximum power during fluoroscopy in the majority of the patients, and avoiding magnified views. The repairs carried out with the stationary unit required on the average lower fluoroscopic time than those using the mobile one (Table 3). However, the use of the stationary unit resulted in an increase in both patient and personnel dose by a factor of about seven (this finding dictated the early stop of repairs using the stationary unit). The increase was related in large part to the five-fold higher mean DAP rate during fluoroscopic imaging with the stationary unit and to the fact that registration contributed about 50% to total DAP, rather than only 20% when the mobile unit was used, indicating the importance of the rate of registered images. Similarly to the present study (Table 3), Geijer et al. (2005) simulating a typical repair using a stationary high-power unit, reported that the replacement of the mobile unit with a stationary resulted in an eight-fold increase in DAP.

Radiological burden, purchase and operation costs are not the only factors against the use of high power stationary units. AAA repairs performed at surgical theaters with mobile angiographic units are carried out in a more sterile environment, do not require the transfer of surgery and anesthesia equipment as well as staff to an often remote location in the hospital. In addition, repairs carried out under such conditions, could be easily changed during the procedure from enovascular to open repair, if required. Taking into account that AAA repairs are often time consuming, when such procedures are carried out in angiographic suite, an extra suite has to be kept free to carry out urgent cardiac procedures. Therefore, AAA repairs carried out using units designed for interventions in vessels of small diameter, such as the coronary arteries, have to be avoided. Hybrid units designed for interventions in both cardiac and non-cardiac vessels could be used, only if it is possible to adapt the operating parameters to the needs of AAA repair.

Some mobile units may not meet the required criteria (e.g. adequate anode cooling rate, image quality, image processing capabilities). For example, two units made by the same manufacturer were tested at IUH under clinical conditions, a 3.15 kW Libra unit equipped with a stationary anode made of tungsten (W), two foci (0.6 and 1.4 mm, respectively), and a 9″ CsI/CCD image intensifier and a Pulsera unit equipped with a rotating W/Rh anode, foci 0.3 and 0.6 mm in diameter and a 12″ CsI/CCD image intensifier (Kalef-Ezra, et al., in press). The mean fluoroscopic times per AAA repair were similar (Table 3), however, the superior image quality of the Pulsera unit allowed its operation at lower mean power during fluoroscopy (120 versus 250 W on the average) leading to a mean skin dose reduction by a factor of about two and to a 15% reduction in the mean effective dose. In addition, most of the procedures carried out in obese patients with the Libra unit, had to be interrupted for few minutes to let the non-rotating anode to cool down, increasing thus the overall procedure time.

The machine output depends on the mode selected by the operator. For example, Vano et al. (2008) simulating PA projection found in eight C-arm units that the use of the low dose fluoroscopy mode rather the high dose one, decreases the dose rate by a factor of about 2.5 on the average (range of values 1.5 to 4.5), while the image registration increased the rate by a factor of 4 on the average (range 2 to 8). In addition, the high voltage and the X-ray tube current are automatically selected according to the distance between the focus and the image receptor, and the X-ray beam attenuation (in the patient's body and in any supporting material, such as the bed).

In general EVAR is carried out with the X- ray tube located below the bed. In this geometry, beam attenuation in the bed is anticipated to have a marginal influence on the patient's dose, but not on the staff. Scattered radiation to staff is proportional to the X-ray machine output. To test the influence of bed attenuation thirty AAA repairs were carried out at IUH using a conventional surgical bed (Marquett Alphamaxx) and sixty with an angiographic table with carbon table-top and bed-suspended side shielding. The use of the latter reduced the mean DAP per repair by ~30% and personnel dose at chest level by about 40%.

4.3.2 Patient related factors

Analyzing data on 140 patients treated at IUH over a 3 year period using a mobile unit, it was found that DAP values were positively correlated fluoroscopy time (r=0.78), a parameter that is related with the complexity of the repair. Similar correlations were observed by Blaszak, et al. (2009), Jones, et al. (2010), and Kuhelj, et al. (2010), but not by Pannucio (2011). Badger (2010) found that the radiation burden is also influenced by the operative strategy chosen by the surgeon, that depends on the clinical presentation. Studies at Belfast City Hospital on possible correlations between the DAP values of 320 elective AAA repairs and lesion-related morphological parameters, revealed weak positive correlations between DAP and proximal neck, sac and distal diameters, but no statistically significant correlation with neck length, and sagittal or coronal neck angles (Badger, et al.; 2010, Jones, et al., 2010). In addition, they failed to find a statistically significant difference in the DAP values of urgent and those of elective repairs (Table 3). Panuccio, et al. found that type II or II thoracoabdominal repairs require higher mean DAP values than those of type IV repairs (1006 and 642 Gy cm^2, respectively).

Obese patients appear in particular to benefit from EVAR over open repair (Johnson 2010). However, DAP was found be positively correlated with the patient's body mass index (BMI) (Kalef-Ezra, et al.; 2009, Panuccio, et al., 2011). Therefore, the risks for induction of radiobiological effects are increased in obese patients. In addition, higher mean DAP values are anticipated in male than in female patients, mainly due to differences in body built and body composition.

4.3.3 Staff related factors

Aneurysm repairs are complex and demanding procedures performed according to the operator's education, training and practical skills. The number of initial repairs required to achieve the optimal surgical result was the subject of a number of studies (Forbes, et al., 2007). Another factor to be considered is the potential for radiation-induced damage to patients and clinical staff. Therefore, medical and non-medical staff related to AAA management should receive appropriate theoretical and practical training in both clinical technique and radiation protection.

All medical students should receive basic training on radiation physics, radiation biology, instrumentation, and radiation protection with emphasis on justification and optimization as part of the basic curriculum. Additional training on the span and impact of all factors that modify the radiological risks is required for those who intend to perform fluoroscopically guided vascular interventions (EC, 2000; Hirshfeld, et al, 2005; ICRP, 2011). For example, according to the European Union guidelines and the International Commission on Radiological Protection, medical doctors involved in interventional cardiology should get an accredited 20 to 30 h - long training program on radiation protection, which should include among other things, practical exercises and practical sessions (EC, 2000; ICRP, 2011). Specific additional training on the safe use of new radiation-related equipment / techniques should be provided at each medical facility before commissioning and during the initial stages of use and to all new personnel before the initiation of the clinical work (Dimitriou, et al., 2011). Such programs of initial and continuing education and training should be established at national, regional or institutional level, approved by the Regulatory Authority of the country/state, and carried out in collaboration with academic institutions and appropriate professional bodies.

4.4 Assessment of staff radiological risk

Staff exposure has to be assessed on a regular basis. In busy facilities trunk dosimeters may be combined with extremity dosimeters, such as ring and eye dosimeters. They can be of either passive or active type, such as solid state electronic dosimeters. Passive dosimeters, such as thermoluminescent badges, are typically used for one month before submitted for processing. On the other hand, active personal dosimeters (APDs) that often provide real-time readings, may introduce substantial errors when used in fluoroscopy. Most of the currently commercially available APDs may not have appropriate characteristics for use in pulsed X-ray fields, such as those observed in EVAR, due to the dependence of their response on dose rate, X-ray pulse frequency and duration, as well as on angle of incidence (Clairand, et al., 2011). For example, APDs of the type used by surgeons that carried out EVAR (Panuccio, et al., 2011) were found to have substantial energy dependent response, that varies up to a factor of two in the spectral region of interest and saturates at dose rates above 30 mGy/min. Irrespective of the type of dosimeter used, the readings have to be analyzed by an experience medical (health) physicist.

If a single personal trunk dosimeter is used, it can be located either above or below the protective apron, usually at the waist level, the chest or the base of the neck, depending on local regulations The effective dose to professionals due to fluoroscopically guided interventions will be numerically much lower than the dose registered by their dosimeter, if worn below the apron, and higher, if worn above. Therefore, in some departments, two dosimeters are routinely used, one above and the other below the apron. For example, the doses registered by personnel dosimeters worn above the protective apron at IUH catheterization laboratories, are 15 times higher than the doses registered by dosimeters worn below the apron.

Various algorithms have been developed to correlate the readings of the trunk dosimeters with the worker's effective dose. However, quite often these algorithms provide very different results for the same configuration. In those countries, that a specific algorithm is not posed by legislation, one may estimate the effective dose simply by dividing the reading of a dosimeter worn above an apron of lead equivalence of at least 0.35 mm (section 4.4) by the factor of 12 and 8, depending on the use or no use of a protective collar. Therefore, if the dose registered by such dosimeters during a single year is 24 mSv, the occupational effective dose is 2 mSv, if the worker used a protective collar and 3 mSv, if he does not use it, irrespective of the exact type of the apron used.

The probability of induction of stochastic effects to staff present in an operation room during AAA repair is related to the collective effective dose (staff presence is required, as far as robotic techniques are not used). The collective dose increases with increasing DAP and kV, and decreases with increasing distance between staff and the centre of the irradiation port. The mean collective dose registered by TLD badges worn by the IUH staff outside the apron at chest level per to DAP ranged between 2.1 and 2.5 μGy per Gy cm^2, depending on the type of the C-arm unit used (Kalef-Ezra, in press). About 58% of the collective dose from repairs carried out using a mobile unit. Corresponded to the chief surgeon, 24% to the surgeon that stood at the opposite side of the bed and 18% in the remaining staff present in the room. The relative contribution of the chief surgeon decreased by a factor of two in procedures carried using a stationary unit. This difference was mainly attributed mainly to a ceiling-suspended radiation shield available only in the room equipped with the stationary unit. The replacement of the surgical bed used with an angiographic table with a table suspended radiation shield reduced the collective dose by about 40% (Section 4.3.1).

Assuming a 0.1 ratio between personnel effective dose and the dose registered by a badges worn at chest level outside apron for the IUH staff, that used 0.5 mm Pb equivalent wrap-around aprons and thyroid collars, the mean collective effective dose per repair carried out with the mobile and the stationary units coupled with angiographic beds (Table 3) were about 6 and 48 μSv, respectively. These values were lower than the 170 μSv value calculated by Panuccio, et al. (2011), i.e., 130 and 230 μSv per type IV thoracoabdominal repairs and type II or III repairs, respectively.

The mean "chest" dose to the chief surgeon at IUH that used a mobile Pulsera unit was ~35 μGy per AAA repair using an angiographic table with table-suspended side protection. The registered mean dose per repair increased to 50 μGy by the use of a surgical bed and to almost 200 μGy by the use of a stationary unit. Liptsiz et al. (2000) and Panuccio et al. (2011) reported mean "chest" doses 300 and 560 μGy per repair, respectively. Ho et al. (2007) measured eye and left index finger doses to the first surgeon 6 and 33 μGy, respectively. However, Liptsiz at al. measured 165 and 380 μGy mean eye and finger doses per repair. Similarly, Saether, et al. (2005) analyzing data on fifteen repairs, found a mean dose at the middle phalanx of the middle finger of the first surgeon of 350 μGy per repair (the maximum value was 1.18 mGy). The main reason for such a large spread of values is attributed in large part to the interrelationship between staff and patient exposures.

The number of repairs that a surgeon may perform to reach a predetermined radiation level is related to the mean DAP per repair and the means used to control personnel exposure. According to ICRP recommendations (ICRP, 1990, 2007) any of the following annual limits must not be exceeded in those exposed to low energy X-rays due to their occupation (additional limits refer to pregnant worker)

- effective dose: 20 mSv,
- eye lens dose: 150 mGy,
- dose to any skin area that exceeds 1 cm^2: 500 mGy.

The 20 mSv annual effective dose could be reached at IUH by the first surgeon in case that he was carrying out annually repairs with a total DAP of ~160 kGy cm^2 (20 mSv divided by the experimentally determined 0.125 μSv / Gy cm^2 factor), under that assumption that he is not occupationally exposed to any other radiation source. This value corresponds to about 5330 AAA repairs using the Pulsera mobile unit and the angiographic table and 830 repairs using the Alura stationary unit (Table 3, Section 4). However, one has to consider also the other two limits. The dose to the lens of the eye is closely related to the dose registered by the badge worn out side the apron (Lie et al., 2008). In case that no eye protection is used, the maximum number of AAA repairs has to be reduced by 25% (3800 and 580, respectively) assuming an eye lens dose equal to the one measured above apron (Kim, et al., 2008). Early in 2011 ICRP modified its recommendations and reduced eye lens dose limit from X-rays from 150 to 20 mSv, averaged over defined periods of 5 years, with no single year exceeding 50 mSv. The application of the new limit restricts the maximum number of AAA repairs down to 533 and 83 respectively, if no eye protection is used.

In the case that adequate eye protection is used and one of the surgeon's legs is close to the imaged region, the maximum annual number of repairs could be dictated by skin dose. Simulations of repairs carried out at IUH were made to assess the absorbed dose at 35 cm horizontal distance from the central beam axis of the X-ray tube operated at 83 kV and located below the angiographic table. The dose to DAP ratio increased with increasing height from the floor, from 10 μGy/Gy cm^2 at ~3 cm height, up to 50 μGy/Gy cm^2 at ~80 height (~15 cm below the lower surface the bed), and reduced at higher heights, (e.g., ~20

Gy cm^2 at 110 cm height, i.e., at the horizontal level of the centre of the patient's body). Assuming the operator's leg is unprotected by his apron up to a 60 cm height from the floor, i.e. at a height where the dose to DAP ratio is ~40 μGy/ Gy cm^2, an annual total DAP of only 12.5 kGy cm^2 results in 500 mGy skin dose, thus reducing the maximum annual number of repairs to about 415 or 65, depending on the type of fluoroscopic unit used. This example indicates the need to increase the distance of the operator's leg from the X-ray source and the importance in the use of bed mounted drapes (Section 4.5). In case that a member of the operating team is a pregnant woman specific measures have to be carried not to exceed the limits related to the conceptus dose (section 4.6).

4.5 Determinants of personnel radiation risks

Those present in the room during AAA repair are irradiated from scattering radiation from the patient's body and the operation table, and to a lower extent from radiation leaking from the X-ray head. Staff exposure can be limited by using various techniques. The most obvious techniques to reduce patient radiation burden are the reduction of the number of workers present in the room to minimum required for the procedure, shielding, and the appropriate positioning of the workers relative to the X-ray tube and the area of the patient's body where the beam enters his body.

The ratio of the scattered dose to the incident dose decreases with increasing distance from the center of the area where the beam enters the scattering material, increases with increasing beam area and kV and depends on the scattering angle. Therefore, one has to increase the staff distance from the location where the beam enters in the patient's body and reduce the radiation field to the needs of the repair, i.e., "collimate tightly and view only what has to be seen, not more". In addition, the higher the photon energy, the higher is the transmission of the primary X-ray beam. However, the increase of the mean photon energy by either kV increase or beam hardening (e.g. addition of a 0.2 mm Cu filter), usually reduces staff exposure. Forward scattering ratio is less than the backwards scattering ratio (the maximum value of the ratio in AAA repairs occurs usually at ~120° scattering angle). Therefore, if the X-ray beam has to be vertical, or near vertical it is preferable to keep the X-ray tube under the patient. On the other hand, if the beam has to be horizontal or almost horizontal, staff should stand close to the detector and not close to X-ray tube.

The interposition of a suitable barrier between the source of radiation and staff reduces the exposure by an amount that depends on its nature and its thickness, the photon spectrum and the angle of incidence of the photons to the barrier. Shielding requirements depend among other things on the type and location of the equipment in the room, the types of procedures performed, room design work habits and workload. Lead is the most widely used shielding material in rooms where fluoroscopically guided procedures are carried out. Shielding properties are often expressed by the thickness of lead that provides the same protection when irradiated with an X-ray beam (usually a 100 kV broad x-ray beam). The types and thickness of the barriers to be used are specified by the radiation protection adviser during the design or the re-design of the room, bearing also in mind ergonomic factors and the anticipated workload. The various types of shielding can be divided to structural stationary shields, or movable shields inside the room and personal protective equipment.

Structural shielding, usually made of lead sheets of total thickness 0.25 to 2.0 mm with no gaps or holes, is built into the walls and doors of the room (the concrete thickness of the floor and the ceiling usually provide adequate shielding). Optically clear lead glass windows of adequate dimensions are often used to protect those outside the room, who may have to observe the procedure. In rooms with heavy fluoroscopic load, it may be advisable to provide a separate protected area inside the room for anesthesiologists in the form of protective cubicles.

As a "golden rule" mobile barriers used in the room should be placed as close to the radiation source as practicable, casting the biggest shadow. Free-standing mobile radiation shields with or without visible screens, which rest on the floor are particularly well suited for the protection of the nurses, the technicians and the anesthesia personnel as well as other medical staff possibly present in rooms with heavy work load. Protective drapes suspended from the operation bed and ergonomically designed optically clear shields suspended from the ceiling are often used to protect the lower and the upper body of the practitioners respectively. For example, in the framework of collaborative project sponsored by EU, it was found that when drapes and ceiling mounted screens were used, the dose to the eyes of the first operator was reduced by a factor of five (Dommienick, et al, 2011).

Bed-mounted shields, such as drapes made of flexible lead vinyl with attenuation characteristics similar to those of at least a 0.5 mm thick lead layer, measuring at least 60 cm by 80 cm (height), are often used. It is preferable that such drapes be attached to the accessory side rail of the table, with double joins to allow movement along the table side and swiveling away from the patient's body forming two protective wings. Bed shields with an extra removable separate high top shielding section of similar equivalent thickness, were found to be very useful.

Ceiling-suspended shields are usually made of clear leaded plastic with lead thickness equivalence of at least 0.5 mm, mounted either on a ceiling column or in a ceiling track and moved partially over the patient's body. Such pull-down shields can be rotated and tilted until the ideal angle is obtained to protect the upper trunk, the neck and the head of the practitioners (the operator should only see the imaged area by looking through the shield to decrease lens exposure). Larger shielding area allows some degree of movement by the practitioner without having to reposition the shield and even protect more than one worker. In some cases, additional protection can be achieved by attaching a flexible lead-vinyl drape at the lower part of the transparent shield.

Sterile disposable, protective surgical drapes that contain elements of high atomic number, Z, such as bismuth and tungsten, usually attenuate X-rays similar to that of a 0.25 mm thick lead layer and can be placed on the patient to be submitted to EVAR to reduce the dose from scattered radiation (Germano, et al., 2005). However, their use adds some cost to the procedure and in case that during manipulations such drapes are accidentally exposed in the primary beam, the output of the machine is automatically increased dramatically, thus increasing both patient and staff doses.

Personal protective equipment, PPE, protect specific body regions, such as the trunk and the upper legs (aprons), the thyroid (collars), the eyes (protective glasses) and the hands (protective gloves). The typical flexible material for protective clothing is lead-impregnated vinyl or rubber. There is also lead-free clothing, that provides adequate shielding with the use of a combinations of elements with a high Z, such as tungsten (Z=74), barium (Z=56) antimony (Z=51) and tin (Z=50) at slightly reduced weight (Christodoulou et al. 2003; Finnerty & Brennan 2004; Zuguchi et al., 2008).

Maximum protection will only be obtained by ergonomic PPE that fits well to the worker's body and maintained to the standards specified by the manufacturer's tests (IAEA, 2004).

Taking into account that PPE is expensive, it should be kept in good condition. The shielding material can develop cracks and holes over time. Therefore, folding and lying over a pointed object must be avoided. A visual inspection for obvious tears, rips, cuts, thickness variations, etc, should be carried out monthly and fluoroscopic inspection on initial receipt and at least once a year (Lambert & McKeon2001; Stam, et al., 2008). If defects are found, practical rejection criteria have to be applied. For example, if the sum of the areas of the holes or cracks in an apron exceeds about 5 cm^2 (about 2.5 cm in radius, in case of a circular hole) it should be replaced. However replacement has to be carried out at an earlier stage, if the unprotected area over testes and the thyroid exceeds 0.2 and 0.1 cm^2, respectively.

Aprons with 0.5 mm nominal Pb equivalent thickness reduce staff effective dose by a factor of about eight, when an 87 kilovolatge is selected (von Boetticher, et al., 2009). Higher kV, such as those used on obese patients, sharply reduces the shielding benefit. When procedures are performed that require individuals to turn away from the radiation beam, wraparound protective aprons should be used. Taking into account that wraparound 0.5 mm Pb aprons weigh about 7 kg, their use in lengthy procedures may result in fatigue, back pain and other more serious orthopedic complications (Klein, et al., 2209). Aprons made of two pieces (vest - skirt) as well as aprons with a belt to transfer the weight to the hips and off the shoulder, help to reduce the mechanical load on the cervical and lumbar spines (Fadl, et al.; 2007). Wraparound aprons with lead equivalent protection of 0.5 mm in the front and the sides of the trunk and 0.25 or 0.35 mm in the back could be also used. Lighter aprons, such as those of 0.25 lead equivalence, reduce the mechanical load on the neck, shoulders and the back of the user, as well as reducing the shielding benefit. However, in general, it is better practice to always use an apron with smaller lead equivalence than using no apron in some procedures. Those having to stand close to the beam entrance area during AAA repair are recommended to use 0.5 mm thick apron, while those at longer distances, such as the anesthesiologist, may wear a lighter PPE. Whatever apron design is selected, it is important to use an apron of appropriate size to body-build falling below the knees with adequate coverage at the armpits, balancing between radiation risk and the risk of induction of orthopedic complications associated to its use (Klein et al.; 2009). When aprons are not in use, they should be hung vertically by the shoulders, or in approved apron rounded hangers to prevent cracks and holes.

Similar considerations to the use of protective aprons hold true on the use of collars or shields which mainly protect the upper oesophagus and the thyroid; the later organ is of high importance mainly in female workers younger than ~40 years, due increased radiosensitivity (ICRP, 2007; Kuon, et al., 2003). It was found that the use of 0.5 mm Pb thyroid collars in catheterization laboratories in combination with 0.35 mm Pb equivalent aprons, result in an effective dose per procedure lower than that using 0.5 mm Pb equivalent aprons without thyroid protection, despite the 20% reduction in total weight (von Boerricher, 2009).

The protective eyeglasses must have additional side panels and fit properly for both protection and comfort (protective glasses can be worn over traditional prescription glasses, while others can be specially made and worn instead of regular ones). In addition, they have to provide protection equivalent to that of at least a 0.5 mm of lead. For example, the use eyeglasses with lead equivalence of 0.75 mm in interventional radiology suites was found to provide a reduction of the eye lens dose by a factor of 3 to 10 (Challa et al.; 2009; Thornton, et al., 2010).

The physician's hands must often be in close proximity to the X-ray beam during repair. Therefore, in case of heavy duty, radiation ring monitors must be worn, if possible, on the middle phalanx of the hand likely to get the highest dose with the sensitive element facing the oncoming beam. Disposable protective gloves containing elements of a high Z, such as tungsten and bismuth, that pose less health and environmental problems than lead, could be used for hand protection from scattered radiation. However, the requirement of tactile sensitivity and dexterity restrict drastically the dose reduction (Kesley & Mettler, 1990). For example, 0.2 to 0.3 mm thick gloves with 30 to 40 μm Pb equivalent attenuation reduce the dose rate of the scattered radiation from a 80 kV beam by 35% to 50%. However, the use of such gloves not only increases the financial cost of the procedure, but also poses the risk of false feeling of radiation safety, that may even result to direct exposure of the hand in the primary beam, i.e. at dose rates many orders of magnitude higher than those outside the beam. In addition, the insertion of the "protected" hand in the direct field triggers the Automatic Brightness Control of the X-ray unit to increase the machine output usually by increasing the kV, decreasing the image quality and increasing the patient's dose. In general, if fingers or a hand appear on the monitor, they should always be pulled back from the imaged area unless necessary for the safety of the patient.

4.6 Radiation protection of the pregnant healthworker

Taking into account the age and the sex distribution of patients with AAA, pregnancy is a matter for concern on workers but not on patients. According to ICRP (2000b, 2207), a pregnant worker can continue her work with unnecessary discrimination, as long as there is reasonable assurance that the conceptus dose can be kept below 1 mGy during the remaining pregnancy period after declaration of pregnancy, eirther verbally or in writing, to the radiation protection officer or the management (the 1 mGy dose is similar to the one that all persons receive annually from penetrating natural background radiation). Pregnancy declaration is voluntary in most countries and can be withdrawn by the employee at any time (Schreiner-Karaussou, 2009).

In some countries other limits are used. For example, in USA, the conceptus dose should not exceed 5 mGy due occupational exposure during the 9 months of pregnancy, under condition of exposure uniform in time (US DOE, 1999), i.e., in practice not exceeding monthly the 0.5 mGy limit after pregnancy declaration. In some countries additional limits are used, such as 0.2 mGy and 0.5 mGy between 1-5 weeks and 5-7 weeks respectively, on top of the limit of the 1 mGy during the remaining gestation period after the pregnancy declaration.

The various limits enforced by legislation do not mean that is necessary for pregnant worker to avoid work with radiation completely, or that she must be prevented from entering or working in designated radiation areas. It does, however imply that the employer should carefully review her exposure conditions (ICRP, 2007).

There is great disparity in the polocies on the protection of the conceptus in different countries and even in different regions of the same country (Best, et al, 2011; Schrewiner - Karoussou, 2009). For example, in some countries supervisors are prevented by law from removing an employee from work area simply on the basis of information that the worker is pregnant (Clark, 2003), while in an other country the pregnant worker is automatically placed in another department (Schrewiner-Karoussou, 2009).

Following the confidential preganacy decalration to the licensee along with the estimated date of conception, preferably in writing, the radiation officer of the facility has to review the radiation history of the worker. In addition, it is desirable to discuss with the pregnant healthworker the associated radiological risks and the options proposed by the management, pointing out that fetal dose for most women who work in fluoroscopy guided intervantional precedues are extremely low (Best, 2011) and reminding her the contribution of natural background radiation and the risks to the conceptus that are unrelated to her occupation. In other words the radiation expert has to put the radiological risk into prospective with the objective of having the pregnant worker's attitude on neither extreme (Clark, 2003).

In practice there are three options to be considered:

1. change to a job that has essentially no radiation,
2. modification of work assignments,
3. no change in assigned working duties with an upgrade of protective means used, if required.

The first option is sometimes requested by pregnant healthworkers who realize that risks may be small, but do not wish to accept any increased risk (ICRP, 2000b). The employer may arrange for this in order to avoid future difficulties in case the employee delivers a child with a spontaneous congenital abnormality (which occurs at a rate of about 3 in every 100 births). This approach is not required on a radiation protection basis, and it obviously depends on the facility being sufficiently large and flexibility to easily fill the vacated position.

Modification of job assignments and locations relative to radiological hazards is a widely emplpoyed option, ensuring that these recommendations are mutually satisfactory. For example, some intervenionists prefer to avoid to act as the first surgeon during pregnancy, because this assignment is related to the highest exposure in the team of surgeons that perform AAA repairs, as shown in section 4.4. Others prefer to modify the order of the topics to be trained, during their training as vascular surgeons, postponing thus their training on fluoroscopy guided porcedures after delively. Another example, is the change of the position of a radiation technician or a nurse from fluoroscopy suites to another position in the same department, such as the mammography suite, where exposure to ionizing radiations is considered unlike. An extra ethical consideration involved in choosing the most appropriate option for the pregnant healthworker is the fact that if the first two options are chosen, another radiation worker will get higher radiation exposure.

There are situations that the anticipated doses are very small (such as the doses of the anesthesiologist that is present during AAA repairs, departments with low workload), situations in which the pregnant worker wishes to continue doing the same job, or the employer may depend on her to continue in the same job in order to maintain the level of patient care. From a radiation protection point of view, this is perfectly acceptable providing the conceptus dose can be reasonably accurately estimated and falls within the recommended limit (ICRP, 2000b). In this case, the radiation protection officer has to evaluate her workplace, watch closely the worker's practices and the dose registered monthly by her personnal dosimeters (a supplementray dosimeter, a "baby's badge", could be issued to be worn at the waist height, under the protective apron - this practice is obligatory in some country).

Sometimes, the conceptus dose can be substantially reduced by wise choise of the position of the worker in the fluoroscopic suite (such as one or two extra steps away from the location where the beam enters the patient), the use of movable radiation shileding and protective aprons of appropriate fit and lead equivalence. For this purpose maternity aprons are commercially available that are adequately wide and have extra lead in the area of the abdomen. However, the use of a heavy apron, especially an wraparound apron that is not divided to two pieces (vest, skirt), in combination with the susbsantial incerase in body weight during the last trimester of pregnency, may result in fatigue, back pain and other orthopedic complications. A possible solution is the use an apron with non-uniform lead equivalence arround her trunk. However, in this case the wearer needs to ensure that her patrially or totally unshielded back is not facing the patient (if it happens, not only there is no adequate shileding, but her personal dosimeter is going to measure a dose tens of higher lower than the dose absorbed by the concetpus). Therefore, the type of apron to be used by the pregant healthworker has to been optimized on individual base.

The proposed options for those working in suites where fluoroscopy guided interventional procedures are carried out, have to take into account that the recommended dose limits apply to the conceptus dose and differ from the dose assessed by the worker's personell dosimeter. For example, Osei and Kotre (2001) found that during the first few months of pregnancy, the ratio of the conceptus dose to the dose registered by the dosimeter worn over a 0.33 mm Pb thick protective apron depends on the high voltage used, incerasing from 1% at 74 kV to 5.4% at 112 kV in the undercouch X-ray tube geometry. These values are increased by a factor of about two, when the lead equivalent thickness is reduced from 0.33 to 0.25 mm. In case that the personal dosimeter is worn below the apron, the conceptus to dosimeter dose ratio is slighlty infleunceed by high voltage, ranging between 36% and 40%. In addition, Damilakis, et al. (2005) found that the conceptus dose in pregnant cadiologists that carry out fluoroscopically guided electrophysiological procedures, depends on the gestation period, ranging from 32% of the value of the air kerma during the 1st tremester to 20% during the 3rd tremester, when a 80 kilovlotage is used. These values, as expected, also depend on kV, beeing at 60 kV 26% and 16%, respectively, and 40% and 27% at 110 kV.

Factors other than radiation exposure should be also considered in choosing the optimum options for work assignments. For example, there are often requirements for lifting patients and for stooping or bending below knee level. Non-radiation related guidelines for such activities at various stages of pregnancy have to be applied. Supervisors have often the tendency to be overptotective of the pregnant worker. However, if he moves her from the usual work assignmenents without her permission, this action can be interpreted as discriminatory (Clark, 2003). Therefore, decisions about working in a radiation enviroment during pregnancy is preferable to be made by both the employer and the pregnant healthworker.

In conclusion, a pregnant health worker can continue working in rooms were endovascular AAA repairs are carried out on a voluntary basis, as long as the there is reasonable assurance that the conceptus dose can be kept below the recommended levels and ALARA principles are enforced. Sex discrimination should be avoided based on radiation risks during pregnancy. If the pregnant woman prefers to continue her work, it has be reensured that she is adequately trained on radiation biology and practical methods to reduce her occupational dose and that she is controling her workload in fluoroscopically guided interventions.

5. Conclusions

Radiological risks associated with fluoroscopically guided vascular interventions are related to patient characteristics, the available infrastructure and staff. The practical actions to control radiological risks were given at various national and international guidelines (American Society for Gastrointestinal Endoscopy, 2010; Balter & Moses, 2007; Chambers et al.; 2011, CRPD, 2010; Hirshfeld, et al., 2005; Johnson et al. 2001; IAEA, 2010; ICRP, 2000;

Society of Interventional Radiology Device Forum, 2003). These actions, as exemplified in AAA repairs can be divided in three groups, general, patient and staff related actions.

5.1 General actions

- Interventions should be carried out by appropriately trained staff taking into account the risks and the benefits to the individual patient.
- Each facility should include in the local clinical protocol, a statement on the strategy to be followed before, during and after repair including the equipment maintenance and quality assurance programs.
- A low-power C-arm angiographic unit (10 to 20 kW) equipped with a ~30 cm detector and rotating anode is to be preferred over high power unit units (~100 kW) designed for coronary interventions.
- The fluoroscopic unit must provide a real-time display of dosimetric quantities (DAP, DAP rate, fluoroscopy time, mode of operation, focus to image receptor distance, etc.) on or near the operator's imaging monitors (duplication of the indications in the control room is advisable).
- The fluoroscopic unit has to be coupled with an angiographic bed and not with a surgical one.
- Reduce fluoroscopy time and the number of registered images to the absolute minimum compatible with the task and take the advantages offered by the last image hold and road mapping capabilities, if available.
- Image size and quality have to be adjusted as low as compatible with the task t (e.g., 3 to 5 pulses or images per second, rather than 12 to 15 per second, avoid - image magnification, beam collimation closely to the area of interest, i.e., "image only the aorta length of interest").
- High exposure levels can be reached in a short time, when obese patients treated using short focus-skin distance or/and image magnification.
- Advice should be available on patient and staff dosimetry, equipment selection and commissioning, and quality assurance by a radiation protection adviser, usually by a qualified medical radiation physicist.

5.2 Patient related actions

- Patient medical file has to be reviewed before procedure, for possible recent "heavy" exposure of the section of the body to be imaged.
- The patient should be counselled on radiation risks,
- Keep the detector (image receptor) as close to the patient as possible.
- Use thick filters to harden the X-ray beam, provided that the power of the fluoroscopic unit and the anode heating allow their use.
- In complex repairs, consider alternative imaging projections, to avoid the induction of deterministic effects to heavily irradiated skin areas.
- Record the dosimetric data of each procedure and correlate the indications of the DAP meter to PSD and effective dose. In case of an anticipated dose to a skin region exceeding a predetermined level, inform the patient's personal physician and avoid radiological procedures with high doses at the same skin region for up to 2 months post-exposure. If the anticipated dose to a skin region exceeds a higher limit, such as 3 Gy, the patient should be counselled and his skin followed-up to two weeks after repair.

- The operator should audit and review the outcomes of the repair, including the potential of radiation injuries with the aim of modifying the selection of patients, the method and the operational procedures to improve clinical outcomes and reduce complication rates.

5.3 Staff-related actions

Personnel exposure is in general proportional to DAP. Additional actions that can be made to control radiological risks are:

- Carry out AAA repairs only in rooms with shielding adequate to the task.
- Reduce the staff present in the room to the minimum required for the task and the needs of the individual patient.
- Distribute the staff in an ergonomic and safe way (room dose mapping is a useful tool for optimization).
- Extremities have to be kept far away from the X-ray beam.
- Dose rate during image registration is much higher than that during fluoroscopy. Therefore, take more aggressive measures during image registration, such as increase staff distance from the area of entry of the beam to the patient's body, if practical.
- If the beam is vertical, or near vertical, keep the X-ray tube under the bed.
- Avoid, if possible, horizontal and almost horizontal radiographic projections. However, if carried out, personnel should stand close to the detector and not close to X-ray tube.
- Take into account that the increased kV automatically selected in obese patients, increases the ratio of scattered dose to DAP.
- Use appropriate physical protection (protective aprons, thyroid shields, protective eye-glasses, viewing screens, table-mounted shields, portable personal shields, etc.).
- Monitor personnel doses with passive personnel dosimeters according to local regulations, assuring that staff knows the appropriate position, such as above the protective apron at the chest level. Additional dosimeters may be required in case of institutions with a heavy workload, and/or equipment not-state-of-art.
- The effectiveness of the means applied to control patient and staff radiation burden has to be closely monitored in each medical facility and changes have to be carried out, if needed.

In conclusion, justification and optimization of the methods used for AAA treatment must commensurate with the medical purpose. Radiation dose and image quality strategies are important for ensuring a balance between cost and benefit. The optimum strategy has to be studied and justified in each medical facility, based on solid clinical and radiobiological evidence.

6. Acknowledgments

We gratefully acknowledge the staff of the Ioannina University Hospital Vascular Surgery unit (headed by assoc. professor M. Matsagas) and Prof L.K. Michalis of the Cardiology Department for their help with various clinical aspects of this study, as well as D. Dristiliaris of the Ioannina University Hospital Medical Physics Department and the post-graduate students S. Karavasilis and E. Katsarou on their contribution to aspects related with Medical Physics and Radiation Protection of this study. The author greatly appreciates I. Dostis and M. Eskinatzi for secretarial assistance.

7. References

Ainsbury, E.A.; Bouffler, S.D.; Dorr, W.; Graw, J.; Muirhead, C.R.; Edwards, A.A.; Cooper, J. (2009). Radiation cataractogenesis: a review of recent studies. *Radiat. Res.* Vol.172, pp.1-9

American Society for Gastrointestinal Endoscopy (2010). Minimizing occupational hazards in endoscopy: personal protective equipment, radiation safety and ergonomics. *Gastrointestinal Endocsopy*, Vol.72, pp.227-235

Badger, S.A.; Jones, C.; Boyd, C.S.; Soong, C.V. (2010). Determinants of radiation exposure during EVAR. *Eur. J. Vasc. Endovasc. Surg.* Vol.40, pp.320-325

Balter, S.; Hopewell, J.W.; Miller, D.L.; Wagner, L.K.; Zelefsky, M. (2010). Fluoroscopically guided procedures: a review of radiation effects on patient's skin and *hair. Radiology, Vol.*254, pp.326-341

Balter, S. and Mosses J. (2007) Managing patient dose in interventional cardiology. *Catheter/ Cardiovasc. Interv.* Vol.70, pp.244-249

Bannazadeh, M.; Altinel, O.; Kashyap. V.S.; Sun. Z.; Clair., D ; Sarac, T.P. (2009). Patterns of procedure-specific radiation exposure in endovascular era: impetus for further innovation. *J. Vasc. Surg.* Vol.49, pp.1520-1524

Best, P.J.M; Skelding, K; Mehran, R; Cheiffo, A; Kunandia, V; Madan M, et al. (2011). SCAI concesus document on occupational radiation exposure to the preganat cardiologist and technical presonnel. *Catheter. Cardiovasc. Inter.* Vol.77, pp.232-241

Blaszak, M.A.; Mayewska, N.; Juszkat, R.; Majewski, W (2009). Dose-area product to patients during stent-graft treatment of thoracic and abdominal aortic aneurysms. *Health Physics, Vol.*93, pp.206-211

Brent, R.L.; Lauriston S. (2007). Taylor lecture: fifty years of scientific research: the importance of scholarship and the influence of politics and controversy. *Health Phys.* Vol.93, pp.348-379.

Burris III, H.A; Hurtig, J. (2010). Radiation recall with anticancer agents. *The Oncologist,* Vol.15, pp.1227-1237

Camidge, R.; Price, A. (2001). Characterizing the phenomenon of radiation recall dermatitis. *Radioth. Oncol.* Vol.59, pp.237-245

Chambers, C.E.; Fetterly, K.A.; Holzer, R.; Paul Lin, P-J.; Blankenship, J.C.; Balter, S.; Laskey, W.K. (2011). Radiation safety program for the cardiac catheterization laboratory. *Catheter Cardiovasc. Interv.* Vol.77, pp.546-556

Challa, K.; Warren, S.G.; Danak, S.; Bates, M.C. (2009). Radundant protective barriers: minimizing operator occupational risk. *J. Interv. Cardiol.* Vol.22, pp.299-307

Chodick, G.; Bekiroglou. N.; Hauptmann, M.; Alexander, B.H.; Freedman, D.M.; Doody M.M.; Cheung, L.C., Simon, S.L.; et al. (2008). Risk of cataract after exposure to low doses of ionizing radiation: a 20-year prospective cohort study among US radiological technologist. *Am. J. Epidemiol.* Vol.168, pp.620-631

Christodoulou, E.G.; Goodsitt, M.M.; Larson, S.C.; Darner, K.L.; Satti, J.; Chan, H-P. (2003). Evaluation of the transmitted exposure through lead equivalent aprons used in a radiology department, including the contribution from backscatter. *Medical Physics,* Vol.30, pp.1033-1038

Ciraj-Bjelac, O.; Rehani, M.M.; Sim, K.; Liew, H.B.; Vano, E.; Kleiman, N.J. (2010). Risk for radiation-induced cataract for staff in interventional cardiology: is there reason for concern? *Catheter. Cardiovasc. Interv.* Vol.76, pp.826-834

Clairand, I., Bordy, J.M.; Daures, J.; Debroas, J., Deniziere, M.; Donadille L.; Ginjaume, M.; Itie, C.; et al. (2011). Active personal dosimeters in interventional radiology: tests in laboratory conditions and in hospitals. *Radiat. Prot. Dosim.* Vol.144, pp.453-458

Clark, J.M. (2003). Radiation protection program for declarred pregnany workers at Los Alamos National Laboratory. *Health Phys.* Vol.84(Suppl.2), pp.S66-S70.

Conference of Radiation Control Directors (CRCPD) (2010). Technical white paper: monitoring and tracking of fluoroscopic dose. CRCRD Publication E-10-7, CRCPD, Frankfort, Kentucky, Retrieved from www.crcpd.org

Damilakis, J.; Perisinakis, K.; Theocharopoulos, N.; Tzedakis, A.; Manios, E; Vardas, P.; Gourtzogiannis, N. (2005). Anticipation of radiation dose to the conceptus from occupational exposure of pregnant staff during fluoroscopically guided electrophysiological precedures. *J. Cardiovasc. Electrophysiol,* Vol.16, pp.773-780

Daniel, J. (1896). The X-rays. *Science, Vol.*3, pp.562

Dias, N.V.; Riva, L.; Ivancev. K.; Resch, T., Sonesson, B.; Malina, M. (2009). Is there a benefit of frequent CT follow-up after EVAR? *Eur. J. Va.c. Endovasc. Surg.* Vol.37, pp.425-430

Diehm, N.; Pena, C.; Benenati, J.F. Tsoukas; A.I.; Katzen, B.T. (2008). Adequacy of an early arterial phase low-volume contrast protocol in 64-detector computed tomography angiography for aortoiliac aneurysm, *J. Vasc. Surg.* Vol.47, pp.492-498

Dilmanian, F.; Morris, G,M.; Zhong, N.; Bacarian, T.; Hainfeld, .F.; Kalef-Ezra J.; Brewington, J.L.; Tammam, J.; Rosen, E. (2003). Murine EMT-6 carcinomas: High therapeutic efficacy of micro beam radiation therapy (MRT). *Radiation Research,* Vol.159, pp.632-641

Dilmanian, F.A.; Qu, Y.; Feinendegen, L.E.; Pena, L.A.; Bacarian, T.; Henn, F.A.; Kalef-Ezra J.; Liu, S.; Zhong, Z.; McDonald, J. W. (2007). Tissue-sparing effect of x-ray microplanar beams particular in CNS: is a bystander involved? *Experimental Hematology,* Vol.3, pp.69-77

Dimitriou, P.; Kalef-Ezra, J.; Pafilis, C.; Kamenopoulou, V. (2011). Educational and training activities in personal dosimetry in Greece. *Rad. Prot. Dosim.* Vol.144, pp.596-598

Domienick, J.; Brodecki, M.; Carinou, E.; Donadille, L.; Jankowski, J.; Koukourava, C.; et al. (2011) Extremity and eye lens doses in interventional radiology and cardiology procedures. First results of the ORAMED project. *Radiat. Prot. Dosim.* Vol.144, pp.442-447

Elkouri, S.; Panneton, J.M.; Andrews, J.C.; Lewism B.D.; McKusick, M.A.; Noel, AA.; Rowland, C.M.; Bower, T.C.; Cherry, K.J.; Cloviczki, P. (2004). Computed tomography and ultrasound in follow-up of patients after EVAR. *Ann. Vasc. Surg.* Vol.18, pp.271-279

European Commission (2000). Guidelines for education and training in radiation protection for medical exposures. Radiation Protection Report 116, E.C. Directorate-General Environment (http://ec.europa/energy/nuclear/radiation_protection/doc/publication/116.pdf)

Fadl, Y.Y.; Ellenbogen, K.A.; Grubb, R.L.; Khoo-Summers, L.; Lindsay, B.D. (2007). A review of spinal injuries in the invasive cardiologist II: prevention and treatment. *PACE*, Vol.30, pp.1149-1157

Farrar, A.V.; Mohan, I.V.; Steel, T.S.; Harris, J.P.; White, G.H.; Stephen, J.S. (2005). Radiation dose received by patient undergoing AAA repair. *ANZ. J. Surg.* Vol.75(Suppl), pp.A115 (abstract)

Feinendegen, L.E.; Brooks, A.L.; Morgan W.F. (2011). Final discussions, summary and recommendations. *Health Physics*, Vol:100, pp.342-34

Fellman, A. (2011). Fostering communication between physicians and patients. *Health Physics*, Vol.100, pp.S41-S43

Finnerty, M.; Brennan, P.C. (2005). Protective aprons in imaging departments: manufacturer stated lead equivalence values require validation. *Europ. Radiol.* Vol.15, pp.1477-1484

Foroozan, M.; Bracard, S.; Schmutz, JL. (2008). Alopecia after cerebral endovascular procedure. *JEADV*, Vol.23, pp.573-574

Forbes, T.L.; DeRose, G.; Lawlor, D.K.; Harris, K.A. (2007). The association between a surgeon's learning curve with endovascular aortic aneurysm repair and previous institutional experience. *Vasc. Endovasc. Surg.* Vol.41, pp.14- 18

Jacob, S.; Michel, M.; Spualding, C.; Boveda, S.; Bar, O.; Brezin, A.P.; et al. (2010). Occupational cataracts and lens opacities in interventional cardiology (O'CLOC study): are X-rays involved? *Radiation-induced cataracts and lens opacities. BMC Public Health*, Vol.10, pp.537-545

Johnson. D.R.; Kyriou, J.; Morton. E.J.; Clifton, A.; Fitzerald, M.; Macsweeney, E. (2001). Radiation protection in interventional radiology. *Clinical Radiology*, Vol.56, pp.99-106

Jones, C.; Badger, S.A.; Boyd, C.S.; Soong C.V. (2010). The impact of radiation dose exposure during endovascular aneurysm repair on patient safety. *J. Vasc. Surg.* Vol.52, pp.298-302

Johnson, O.N.; Sidawy, A.N.; Scalnon, J.M.; Walcott, R.; Arora, S.; Mascata, R.A.; Amdur, R.L.; Henderson, W.G. (2010). Impact of obesity on outcomes after surgical and endovascular abdominal aortic aneurysm repair. *J. Am. Coll. Surg.* Vol.210, pp.166-177

Hirshfeld, J.; Balter, S.; Brinker, J.; Kern, M.J.; Klein, L.W.; Lindsay, B.K.; Tommaso, C.L.; Tracy, C.M.; et al. (2005). ACCF/AHA/ HRS/SCI Clinical competence statement on physician knowledge to optimize patient safety and image quality in fluoroscopically guided invasive cardiovascular procedures. *Circulation*, Vol.111, pp.511-532

Ho, P.; Cheng, S.W.K.; Wu, P.M.; Ting, A.C.W.; Poon, J.T.C.; Cheng, C.K.M.; Mok, J.H.M.; Tsang, M.S. (2007). Ionizing radiation absorption of vascular surgeons during endovascular procedures. *J. Vasc. Surg.* Vol.46, pp.455-459

Hymes, S.R., Strom E.; Fife, C. (2006). Radiation dermatitis: clinical presentation, pathophysiology, and treatment. *J. Am. Acad. Dermatol.* Vol.54, pp.28-46

Geijer, H.; Larzon, T.; Popek, R.; Beckman, K.W. (2005). Radiation exposure in stent-grafting of abdominal aortic aneurysm. *Brit. J. Radiol.* Vol.78, pp.906-912

Germano, J.J.; Day, G.; Gregorious, D.; Natarajan, V.; Cohen, T. (2005). A novel radiation protection drape reduces radiation exposure during fluoroscopy-guided electrophysiological procedures. *J. Invas. Cardiol.* Vol.17, pp.469-472

Go, M.R.; Barbato, J.E.; Rhee, R.Y.; Makaroun, M.S. (2008). What is the clinical utility of a 6-month computed tomography in the follow-up of endovascular aneurysm repair patients? *J. Vasc. Surg.* Vol.47, pp.1181-1187

Iezzi, R.; Cotroneo, A.R.; Filippone, A.; DiFabio, F.; Quinto, F.; Colosimo, C.; Bonome, L. (2006). Multidetector CT in abdominal aortic aneurysm treated with endovascular repair: are unenhanced and delayed phase enhanced images effective for endoleak detection? *Radiology*, Vol.241, pp.915-921

Iezzi, R.; Cotroneo, A.R.; Giammarino, A.; Spigonardo, F.; Storto, M.L. (2009). Low dose multidetector-row CT-angiography of abdominal aortic aneurysm after endovascular repair. *Eur. J. Radiol.* doi.10.1016/j.ejrad.2009. 11.016

International Atomic Energy Agency (1998). *Diagnosis and treatment of radiation injuries.* STI/PUB/1040, IAEA, ISBN 92-0-100498, Vienna, Austria

International Atomic Energy Agency. (2002). *Follow-up of delayed health consequences of acute accidental radiation exposure.* IAEA-TECDOC-1300, IAEA, ISBN -92-0-133202-5, Vienna, Austria

International Atomic Energy Agency. (2004). *Personal protective equipment.* Practical radiation protection technical manual-5, IAEA, Vienna, Austria (www-pub.iaea.org/MTCD/publications/PDF/PRTM-5_web.pdf)

International Atomic Energy Agency (2010). *Patient dose optimization in fluoroscopy guided international procedures,* IAEA-TECDOC-1641, IAEA, IAEA, ISBN 978-92-0-100510-6, Vienna, Austria

International Commission on Radiological Protection. *Nonstochastic effects of ionizing radiation.* ICRP Peport 41, 1984, Pergamon Press, ISBN 0 08 032333-2, Oxford, UK.

International Commission on Radiological Protection. (1991). 1990 recommendations of the International Commission on Radiological Protection, ICRP publication 60, Pergamon Press, ISBN 0 08 041143 4, Oxford, *UK.*

International Commission Radiological Protection (1992). *The biological basis for dose limitation in the skin. ICRP* publication 59. Pergamon Press, ISBN 0 08 041143 6, Oxford, UK

International Commission on Radiological Protection. (2000) Avoidance of radiation injuries from medical interventional procedures. ICRP publication 85, *Annals of the ICRP,* Vol.30(2), pp.1-80

International Commission on Radiological Protection. (2000b) Pregnancy and medical radiation. ICRP publication 84 Annals of ICRP, Vol.30(1)

International Commission on Radiological Protection. (2003). Biological effects after prenatal irradiation (embryo and fetus). ICRP publication 90, *Annals of the ICRP,* Vol.33(1-2), pp.1-200

International Commission on Radiological Protection (2007) The 2007 recommendations of the ICRP, ICRP103 report. *Annals of the ICRP,* Vol.37(2-4), pp.1-332

International Commission on Radiological Protection. (2011). Education and training in radiological protection for diagnoistic and interventional procedures. ICRP publication 113, *Annals of the ICRP,* Vol.39(5), pp.1-68

International Electrochemical Commission (2000). Medical electric equipment-Dose area product meters, IEC publication 60580, 2nd edition, IEC, ISBN 2-8318-7178-6, Geneva

Kalef-Ezra, J.; Karava, K. (2008). Radiochromic film dosimetry: reflection vs transmission scanning. *Medical Physics*, Vol.35, pp.2308-2311

Kalef-Ezra, J.A.; Karavasilis, S.; Ziogas, D.; Dristiliaris, D.; Michalis, L.M.; Matsagas, M. (2009). Radiation burden of patients undergoing endovascular abdominal aneurysm repair. *Journal of Vascular Surgery*, Vol.49 pp.283-288

Kalef-Ezra, J.; Katsarou, E.; Karavasilis, S.; Matsagkas, M.; Michalis, L.K. (2010). Direct measurement of skin dose with radiochromic films in fluoroscopy guided vessel repairs. International Conference Radiation Protection in Medicine, Varna, Bulgaria, September 1-3, 2010 (abstract in Roentgenologia Radiologia Supp.10, p.51).

Kalef-Ezra, J.A ; Karavasilis, S.; Kouvelos, G.; Dristiliaris. D.; Michalis, L.K.; Matsagkas, M. Endovascular abdominal aneurysm repair: methods of radiological risk reduction. *J. Cardiovasc Surg.* (in press)

Kesley, C.A.; Mettler FA. (1990). Flexible protective gloves: the emperor's new clothes? *Radiology*, Vol.174, pp.275-276

Kim, S.H., Kin, S.R.; Lee, H.J.; Oh. H., Ryu, S.Y.; Lee, Y.S.; Kin, T.H., Jp, S.K. (2003). Apoptosis in growing hair follicles following gamma - irradiation and application for the evaluation of radioprotective agents. *In vivo,* Vol.17, pp.211-214

Kim, K.P.; Miller, D.L.; Balter, S.; Kleinerman, R.A.; Linet, M.S.; Kwon, D.; Simon, L. (2008). Occupationa; exposure doses to operators performing cardiac catherization procedures. *Health Physics,* Vol.94, pp.211-227

Kirby, J.M.; Jhaveri, K.S.; Kachura, J.R. (2007). Computed tomography angiography in abdominal aortic endoleaks: what is the optimal protocol? *Can. J. Assoc. Radiol.* Vol.58, pp.264-271

Klein, L.W.; Miller, D.L.; Balter, S.; Laskey, W.; Haines, D.; Norbash, A.; Mauro, M.A.; Goldstein J.A. (2009). Occupational health hazards in the interventional laboratory: time for a safer environment. *J. Vasc. Interv. Radiol.* Vol.20, pp.147-153

Koenig, T.R.; Wolff, D.; Mettler, F.A.; Wagner, L.K. (2001). Skin injuries from fluoroscopically guided procedures: Part 1, characteristics of radiation injury. *Am. J. Radiology,* Vol.177, pp.3-11

Kuhelj, D.; Zdesar, U.; Jevtic, V.; Skrk, D.; Omahen, G.; Zontar, D.; Surlan. M.; Glusics, M.; Popovic, P.; Kocijsncic, I.J.; Salapura, V. (2010). Risk of deterministic effects during endovascular aortic stent graft implanation. *Br. J. Radiol.* Vol.83, pp.958-963

Kuon, E.; Birkel. J.; Schmitt, M.; Dahm, J.B. (2003). Radiation exposure benefit of a lead cup in invasive cardiology. *Heart,* Vol.89, pp.1205-1210

Lambert, K.; McKeon, T. (2001). Inspection of lead aprons: criteria for rejection. *Health Physics,* Vol.80, pp.S67-S69

Lee, W.S.; Lee, S.W.; Lee, S.; Lee. J.W. (2004). Postoperative alopecia in five patients after treatment of aneurysm rapture with a Guglielmi detachable coil: pressure alopecia. Radiation induced, or both?. *J. Dermatol.* Vol.31, pp.848-851

Lie, O.O.; Paulsen, G.U., Wohni, T. (2008). Assessment of effective dose and dose to rhe lens of the eye fort he interventional cardiologist. *Radiat. Prot. Dosim.* Vol.132, pp.313-318

Lipsitz, E.C.; Veith, F.J.; Ohki, T.; Heller, S., Wain, R.A.; Suggs, W,D.; Lee, J,C.; Kwei, S.; Goldstein K.; Rabin J.; Chang, D.; Metha, M. (2005). Does the endovascular repair of aortoiliac aneurysms pose a radiation safety hazard to vascular surgeons? *J. Vasc. Surg.* Vol.32, pp.704-705

Macari, M.; Chandarana, H.; Schmidt, B.; Lee, J.; Lamparello, P.; Babb, J. (2006). Abdominal aneurysm: can the arterial phase at CT evaluation after endovascular repair be eliminated to reduce radiation dose? *Radiology*, Vol.241, pp.908-914

Manning, B.J.; O'Neill, S.M.; Haider, S.N.; Colgan, M.P.; Madhavan. P.; Moore, D.J. (2009). Duplex ultrasound in aneurysm surveillance following endovascular aneurysm repair: a comparison with computed tomography. *J. Vasc. Surg.* Vol.49, pp.60-65

Marti, N.; Lopez., V.; Pereda, C.; Nartin, J.M. (2008). Radiation-induced alopecia after embolization of cerebral aneurysm. *Dermatology Online Journal*, Vol.14, pp.19

Merriam, G.R.; Worgul B.V. (1983). Experimental radiation cataract – its clinical relevance, *Bull N.Y. Acad. Med.* Vol.59, pp.372-392

Muller, K.; Meineke, V. (2010). Advances in the management of localized radiation injuries. *Health Physics,* Vol.98, pp.843-850

Nakashima, E. (1994). Relationship of five anthropometric measurements at age 18 to radiation dose among atomic bomb survivors exposed in utero. *Radiation Res.,* Vol.140, pp.121-126

Nakashima, E.; Carter, R.L.; Naruushi, K.; Tanaka, S.; Funamoto, S. (1995). Height reduction among prenatally exposed atomic-bomb survivors: a longitudinal study of growth. *Health Physics,* Vol.68, pp.766-772.

Nakashima, E.; Neriishi, K.; Minamato, A. (2006). A reanalysis of atomic-bomb cataract data 2000-2002: a threshold analysis. *Health Physics,* Vol.90, pp154-160

Nakayama, Y.; Awai, K.; Funama. Y.; Liu. D.; Nakaura, T.; Tamura, Y.; Yamashita, Y. (2006). Lower tube voltage reduces contrast material on CT-MDCT aortography. *Am. J. Radiol.* Vol.187, pp.W490-W497

Nowakowski, R.S; Heyes N. (2008) Radiation, retardation and the developing brain: tome is the crucial variable. *Acta Paediatrica,* Vol.97, pp.527-531.

Osei, E.K; Kotre, C.J. (2001). Equivalent dose to fetus from occupational exposure of pregnant staff in diagnostic radiology. *Br. J. Radiol.,* Vol.74, pp.629-637

Otake, M.; Schull , W.J. (1984) In utero exposure to A-bomb radiation and mental retardation: a reassessment. *Br. J. Radiol.* Vol.57, pp.409-414.

Panuccio, G.; Greenberg, R.K.; Wunderle, K.; Mastracci, T.M.; Engelton, M.G.; Davros, W. (2011). Comparison of indirect radiation dose estimates with directly measured radiation dose for patients and operators during complex endovascular procedures. *J. Vasc. Surg.* Vol.53, pp.885-894

Peel, D.M.; Hopwell, J.W. (1984). Nonstochastic effects of different beta emitters on the pig skin. *Radiat Res*, Vol.99, pp.372-382

Rahimi, S.A.; Coyle, B.W.; Vogel, T.R.; Haser, P.B.; Graham A.M. (2011). Acute radiation syndrome after endovascular AAA repair. *Vasc Endovasc Surg*, Vol.45, pp.178-180

Rojas-Palma, C.; Liland, A.; Jersad, A.N.; Etherington, G.; Perez, M.R.; Rahola, T.; Smith, K. (2009). *Triange monitoring and treatment handbook*, Norwegian Radiation Protection Authority, ISBN 978-82-90362-27-5, Osteras, Norway

Schull, W.J; Otake M. (1999). Cognitive function and prenatal exposure to ionizing radiation. *Teratology*, Vol.59, p.222-226

Saether, H.K.; Davidson, T.M.; Winmark, A.; Wohni, T. (2005). Measurements of finger doses in X-ray guided surgery, nuclear medicine and research. *Radiat. Prot. Dosim.* Vol.113, pp.392-395

Schreiner-Karoussou, A. (2009). A preliminary study of issues and practices concerning pregnancy and ionising radiation. *Radiat. Prot. Dosim.*, Vol.135, pp.79-82

Shore, R.E.; Neriishi, K.; Nakashima, E. (2010). Epidemiological studies of cataract risk a low to moderate doses: (not) seeing is believing. *Radiat Res*, Vol.174, pp.889-894

Society of Interventional Radiology Device Forum. (2003). Imaging guidelines for abdominal repair with endovascular stent grafts. *J. Vasc. Interv. Radiol*, Vol.14, pp.262-264

Sommer, W.H.; Clevert, D.A.; Bamberg, F.; Helck, A.; Albrecht, E.; Reiser. M.F.; Becker, C.R.; Nikolaou, K. (2010). Time-resolved computed tomography imaging of the aorta: a feasibility study. *J. Thorac. Imaging*, Vol.25, pp.161-167

Stam, W.; Pillay, M. (2008). Inspection of lead aprons: a practical rejection model. *Health Physics*, Vol.95, pp.S133-S136

Sternbergh, W.C.; Greenberg, R.K; Chuter, T.A.M.; Tonnessen. B.H. (2008) Redefining postoperative surveillance after endovascular follow-up in the US Zenith multicenter trial. *J. Vasc. Surg.* Vol.48, pp.278-284

Tarbell, D.S.; Tarbell, A.T.; Hamilton J.H. (1981). An early report on the physiological effects of X-rays. *J. Chem. Edu.* Vol.58, p:275

Ten Bosch, J.A.; Rouwet, E.V.; Peters, C.T.; Jansen, L.; Verhagen, H.J.; Prins, M.H.; Teijink. J.A. (2010). Constrast-enhanced ultrasound versus computer tomographic angiography for surveillance of endovascular abdominal aortic aneurysm repair. *J. Vasc. Interv. Radiol.* Vol.21, pp.638-643

Thornton, R.H.; Dauer, L.T.; Altamirano, J.P.; Alvarado, K.J.; St Germain, J.; Solomon. S.M. (2010) Comparing strategies for operator eye protection in the interventional radiology suite. *J. Vasc. Interv. Radiol.* Vol.21, pp.1703-1707

Tomlison, J.; McNamara, J.; Matloubieg, J.; Singh, M.J., Davies, M.G.; Rhodes. J.M.; Illig, K.A. (2007) Intermediate follow-up after endovascular aneurysm repair- can we forgo CT scanning in certain patients? *Ann. Vasc. Surg.* Vol.21, pp.663-670

Tomlinson, J.; McNamara, J.; Matloubieh. J.; Hart, J.; Singh. M.J.; Davies, M.G.; Rhodes; J.M., Illing; Truijers, M.; Resch, T.; Van Den Berg, J.C.; Blankensteijn, J.D.; Lonn, L. (2009). Endovascular aneurysm repair: state-of art imaging techniques for preoperative planning and surveillance. *J. Cardiovasc. Surg.* Vol.50, pp.432-438

Truijers, M.; Resch, T.; van Den Berg J.C.; Blankensteijn J,D., Lonn, L. (2009). Endovascular aneurysm repair: state -of art imaging technique fro preoperative planning and surveillance. *J. Cardiovasc. Surg.* Vol.50, pp.423-438

US Department of Energy. (1999). Evaluation and control of radiation dose to the embryo / fetus guide for use with Title 10, Code of federal regulations, part 835, Occupational radiation protection, report DOE G 441.1-6, Assistant Sectretary for Environment, Safety and Health

Van de Aardeg, M.J.; Hopewell, J.W.; Simmons, R.H. (1988). Repair and recovery in the epithelial and vascular connective tissues of pig skin after irradiation. *Radiother. Oncol.* Vol.11, pp.73-82

Vano, E.; Gonzalez, L.; Fernandez, J.M.; Haskal, Z.J. (2008). Eye lens exposure to radiation in interventional suites: caution is warranted. *Radiology*, Vol.248, pp.945-953

Vano, E.; Kleiman, N.J.; Duran, A.; Rehani, M.M.; Echeverri, D.; Cabrera, M. (2010). Radiation cataract risk in interventional personnel. *Radiat. Res.* Vol.174, pp.490-495

Verhooven, E.L.; Oikonomou, K.; Ventin, F.C.; Lerut, P.; Fernandes, E.; Fernandes. R.; Mendes Pedro, L. (2011). Is it time to eliminate CT after EVAR as routine follow-up? *J. Cardiovasc. Surg.* Vol.52, pp.193-198

von Boetticher, H.; Lachmund, J.; Hoffmann, W. (2009). Cardiac chatheterization: impact of face and neck shielding on new estimates of effective dose. *Health Physics,* Vol.97, pp.622-627

Walsh, S.R., Cousins, C.; Tang, T.Y.; Gaunt, M.E.; Bolyle, J.R. (2008). Ionizing radiation in endovascular interventions. *J. Endovasc. Ther.* Vol.15, pp.680-687

Weerakkody, R.A.; Walsh, S.R.; Cousins. C.; Goldstone, K.E.; Tang, T.Y.; Gaunt, M.E. (2008). Radiation exposure during endovascular aneurysm repair. *Br. J. Surg.* Vol.95, pp.699-702

Weiss, D.J.; Pipinos, I.I.; Longo, G.M.; Rutar, F.J.; Johanning, J.M. (2008). Direct and indirect measurement of patient radiation exposure during endovascular aortic aneurysm repair. *Ann. Vasc. Surg.* Vol.22, pp.723-729

Wen, C,H.; Lin, S.M.; Chen, Y.; Chen, J-C.; Wang, Y-H.; Tseng. S-H. (2003). Radiation induced alopecia after embolization of cerebral arteriovenous malformations. *Clin. Neur. Neurosc.* Vol.105, pp.215-217

White, H.A., MacDonald, S. (2010). Estimating risk associated with radiation exposure during follow-up after endovascular repair. *J. Cardiovasc. Surg.* Vol.51, pp.95-104

Wintersprerger, B.; Jakobs, T.; Herzog, P.; Shaller, S.; Nikolaou, K.; Suess, S.; Weber, C.; Reiser, M.; Becker, C. (2005). Aorto-iliac multidetector-row angiography with low kV settings: improved vessel enhancement and simultaneous reduction of radiation dose. *Eur. J. Radiol.* Vol.15, pp.334-341

Wipper, A.; Katira, R.; Roberts, D.H. (2005). Interventional cardiology: it's a hairy business. *Heart,* Vol.91, pp.1428-1432

Worgul, B,V.; Kundiyev, Y,I.; Sergioyenko, N.M.; Chummak, V.V.; Vitte, P.M.; Medcedosky, C.; Bajhanova, E.V.; Junk, A.K.; et al. (2007). Cataracts among Chernobyl clean-up workers: implications regarding possible eye exposures. *Radiation Res.,*Vol.167, pp.233-243

Zhou, W. (2011). Radiation exposure of vascular surgery patients beyond endovascular procedures. *J. Vasc. Surg*. Vol.53, pp.39S-43S

Zuguchi, M.; Chida, K.; Taura, M.; Inaba, Y.; Ebata, A.; Yamada. S. (2008). Usefulness of non-lead aprons in radiation protection for physicians performing interventional procedures. *Radiat. Prot. Dosim*. Vol.131, pp.531-534

8

Ultrasound-Guided Peripheral Nerve Block in the Anesthetic Considerations for Vascular Surgery – An Alternative Choice for Neuroaxial Anesthesia Techniques

Yusuke Asakura[1] and Hideki Takagi[2]
[1]*Department of Anesthesiology,*
[2]*Department of Orthopedic Surgery,*
Nagoya Kyoritsu Hospital, Nagoya,
Japan

1. Introduction

Abdominal aortic aneurysm, with its incidence approaching approximately 8% in the population, accounts for more than 8,000 deaths annually in the United States. It is a multifactorial disease associated with atherosclerosis. Age, male gender, smoking, and the family history of abdominal aortic aneurysm are thought to be the risk factors for the disease (Ashton et al., 2002, Fleming et al., 2005). The natural history of abdominal aortic aneurysm is characterized by the progressive enlargement of the aneurysm, which ultimately leads to the rupture and the subsequent death of the patient.

The aorta wall consists of a thin intima, a thick tunica media, and an adventitia, composed of endothelium for a thin intima, smooth muscle layers for a thick tunica media, and a connective tissue including the vasa vasorum and nervi vascularis for the adventitia, respectively. The wall of aorta is particularly vulnerable to an injury owing to the continuous exposure to high pulsate blood pressure and shear stress. Once degenerated which most commonly occurs by atherosclerosis, cystic medial necrosis, a condition in which the collagen and elastic fibers in the tunica media of the aorta are degenerated and replaced by the mucoid connective tissues, will immediately take place. It will subsequently result in the circumferential weakness, dilatation, and as a consequence, the development of aneurysm. The other etiological conditions that lead to the development of aneurysm include some hereditary basis such as Marfan's and Ehlers-Dnlos syndromes, the infection including syphilis and tuberculosis, and vasculitis associated with autoimmune diseases such as Takayasu's arteritis and rheumatoid arthritis (White et al., 1993, Shah et al., 1997).

The prognosis of abdominal aortic aneurysm is strongly correlated with the size of aneurysm, and the risk of rupture is 1-2% for 5 years for an aneurysm less than 5cm in diameter, whereas it is more than 20-40% for those more than 5cm in diameter. Hence, an elective operation is indicated if the diameter of aneurysm is >5.5cm (Sakalihasan et al., 2005).

2. Treatment options for abdominal aortic aneurysm: Endovascular abdominal aortic aneurysm repair (EVAR)

Traditionally, abdominal aortic aneurysm had been treated with prophylactic open surgical repair, which usually had required the surgical procedure consisting of the cross-clamping of the aorta for more than 30 minutes. It exerted a profound impact on the peri-operative mortality of those with pre-existing impaired ventricular function and reduced coronary reserve through the increases in arterial blood pressure, systemic vascular resistance, and the reduction of cardiac output. In addition, ischemic complications may subsequently take place following a cross-clamping of aorta such as occlusive mesenteric ischemia, acute tubular necrosis of the kidneys, and paraplegia (Lloyd et al., 1996).

In 1991, Parodi and co-workers reported the first clinical application of endovascular surgery, namely endovascular aortic aneurysm repair (hereafter referred to as EVAR), for abdominal aortic aneurysm repair (Parodi et al., 1991). It has revolutionized the traditional approach for the treatment of abdominal aortic aneurysm. The prominent advantage of this approach is its less invasiveness as compared with the traditional open surgical abdominal aortic reconstruction, which is particularly suitable for those who are considered to unfit for open surgical abdominal aortic aneurysm reconstruction owing to their serious pre-existing comorbidities (EVAR trial participants, 2005). This approach has enabled to reconstruct abdominal aortic aneurysm surgically without the large incisions of abdominal walls and the prolonged aortic cross-clamp times, and with the significantly less blood loss and fluid shifts. The technique commonly is undertaken with the bilateral groin incisions to obtain an access to the common femoral arteries. Approximately two decades later since its first report in 1991, this approach has come to account for nearly a half of elective repairs of abdominal aortic aneurysm in the United States and in European countries (Shermerhorn et al., 2008).

Currently, two large randomized controlled trials evaluating the efficacy and the safety of EVAR in terms of 30-day peri-operative mortality as well as its long term durability as compared with the standard open surgical vascular reconstructions are undergoing in European countries (Prinssen et al, 2004, Greenhalgh et al., 2004). One is conducted in Netherland and Belgium, and the other is undergoing in the United Kingdom. Interestingly, the results of both trials were quite similar with each other. Although the 30-day peri-operative mortalities as well as the rate of complications were significantly lower in EVAR group than in the open surgical reconstruction group in both studies, the cumulative survival advantage of EVAR group over those with the open surgical reconstruction group had disappeared following 2 years after randomization (Blankensteijin et al., 2005, Greenhalgh et al., 2005). In addition, the rate of subsequent requirement of the secondary interventions was higher in EVAR group, and the quality of life as reported by the participants was also higher in the open repair group (Blankensteijin et al., 2005, Greenhalgh et al., 2005).

The other study is also now undergoing in the United Kingdom comparing the efficacy and the safety of EVAR as compared with no intervention on those who were especially considered to unfit for open repair and excluded for that reason, and it revealed no cumulative survival benefit of EVAR over no intervention group, presumably owing to the serious comorbidities of the participants (EVAR trial participants, 2005). However, the similar study now undergoing in the United States showed the more prominent lower peri-operative mortality in those who had undergone EVAR in highly comorbid participants, which suggests that EVAR, owing to its less invasive nature as compared with the standard open repair, is particularly suitable for those who were considered to unfit for open repair owing to their serious comorbidities (Timaran et al., 2007).

3. Anesthesia for endovascular aortic aneurysm repair

Shortly after the introduction of EVAR in the treatment of abdominal aortic aneurysm, general anesthesia was preferentially used for the anesthetic management of EVAR because of the following reasons;

1. The first generation device had required the induced hypotension technique during the deployment of the graft.
2. The procedure times were often long.
3. The considerable number of patients had required conversion to open repair during the EVAR procedure.

However, as the second-generation fully stented modular stent graft had come to be widely used, which, through the refinement of the first-generation brand, do not require the induced hypotension technique during the deployment of the graft, and as the physicians had gained the experiences with newer generation devices, which subsequently resulted in the shorter procedure times, a variety of regional anesthesia techniques has come to be used. These techniques include paravertebral peripheral nerve block, spinal anesthesia, continuous spinal anesthesia, epidural and combined spinal anesthesia, and regional anesthesia. Owing to the serious comorbidities of the patients who are undergoing EVAR procedure, the use of less invasive anesthetic techniques for the anesthetic management of EVAR, such as regional anesthesia techniques, has been shown to result in the lower peri-operative mortality, reduced ICU admission and stay, reduced hospital length of stay, and the reduced rate of early complications (Asakura et al. 2009b, Asakura, 2010a, Ruppert et al, 2006, Verhoeven et al., 2005).

The use of neuroaxial anesthesia including epidural and spinal anesthesia may have potentially beneficial effects on patients such as the suppression of the surgical stress, positive effect on post-operative nitrogen balance, and reduced blood loss, these advantages are often counterbalanced by the increased risk of developing subdural and epidural hematoma in patients undergoing EVAR who are frequently medicated with anticoagulants pre-operatively and with the use of heparin during the surgical procedure (Asakura et al. 2008a, Asakura, et al. 2009b, Asakura, 2010a, Park et al., 2001). The incidence of development of hematoma associated with the use of neuroaxial anesthesia is relatively low and is estimated to be approximately 1:150,000-1:200,000 in normal individuals (Horlocker et al., 2000). Although it is difficult to precisely ascertain the relative risk of the incidence of subsequent development of epidural/subdural hematoma in the population who is undergoing anticoagulant therapy, the consensus statement regarding the use of neuroaxial anesthesia and the concomitant use of anticoagulant drugs has been recently provided from the American Society of Regional Anesthesia, given the considerable number of case reports published thus far reporting the development of epidural hematoma in whom an anticoagulation therapy was administered (Horlocker et al., 2010).

Bleeding in the neuroaxial space which most commonly occurs in an epidural space due to the presence of prominent venous plexus, is a potentially catastrophic complication of neuroaxial anesthesia, and the only minor proportion of patients fully recovered neurologically after the prompt diagnosis and the immediate decompression laminectomy. Among 61 cases of spinal hematoma that had been previously reported in the review of literature, 25 of those had received intravenous or subcutaneous injection of heparin. Furthermore, 5 additional cases had undergone vascular surgery, which means that they were treated with heparin intra-operatively (Vandermeulen et al. 1994). Hence, nearly a half of reported cases were associated with the use of heparin. Although the use of neuroaxial anesthesia in patients who are going to receive heparin is not totally contraindicated, the consensus statement suggests that the careful cautions must be paid in patients receiving neuroaxial anesthesia who are treated with anticoagulant medications (Horlocker et al. 2010).

4. Peripheral nerve block; an alternative for neuroaxial anesthesia in the anesthetic management of EVAR

An alternative regional anesthesia technique that can be used is peripheral nerve blockade (PNB), which has been shown to provide an effective unilateral analgesia with a fewer serious neurological complications even with the use of heparin (Asakura, et al, 2008a, Gray, 2006). Historically, the technique of peripheral nerve block appeared in the early 20th century, but the needle advancement was guided by mostly the knowledge of anatomy. Hence, the rate of success was limited, and it was somewhat like an art of the skilled hands. However, as a result of the advance of ultrasound machine technology (Asakura, et al., 2008b), the anesthesiologists come to perform peripheral nerve block with more than 90% rate of success virtually without any complications. As such, ultrasound-guided peripheral nerve block has come to gain popularity recently worldwide (Marhofer et al. 2007).

4.1 Lumbar plexus block for the anesthetic management of EVAR

During the surgical procedure of EVAR, skin incisions are made in the groin areas to gain the access to the common iliac arteries. The nerve to the lower extremity and groin areas are supplied from the lumbar and sacral plexus (Fig.1). The plexus runs between the psoas major muscle and the quadrates lumborum muscle which is termed as the psoas compartment. The lumbar plexus is formed from ventral rami with L1-4 in addition to the various types of additional contribution from T12 and L5. The branches of lumbar plexus form iliohypogastric, ilioinguinal, genitofemoral, lateral femoral cutaneous, femoral, and obturator nerves. The first lumbar ventral ramus supplies iliohypogastric and ilioinguinal nerves. The genitofemoral and the lateral femoral cutaneous nerves originate from the second ramus. The femoral nerve is formed from the united ventral rami of L2-4. From the anterior division of L2-4, the obturator nerve is formed. The psoas compartment block is usually performed by advancing the needle into the space between the psoas major and the quadrates lumborum muscles, and the once the plexus is approached, a large volume of local anesthetics is injected which subsequently anesthetize the hip and anterolateral thigh.

For the standard lumbar plexus block, the patient is usually placed in the lateral decubitus position, with the hip fixated and the operative side uppermost. The block is conducted by the standard nerve stimulation method (Asakura, et al., 2008a). A 21-gauge 100-mm-long needle is advanced perpendicular to the skin until it contacts to the transverse process of the 5th lumbar spine. A nerve stimulator is set to deliver 0.5-1.0mA current impulse at 2Hz. By further advancing the needle, the localization of the lumbar plexus is confirmed by identifying the contraction of the quadriceps femoris (Asakura, et al., 2008a, Capdevila, et al., 2002).

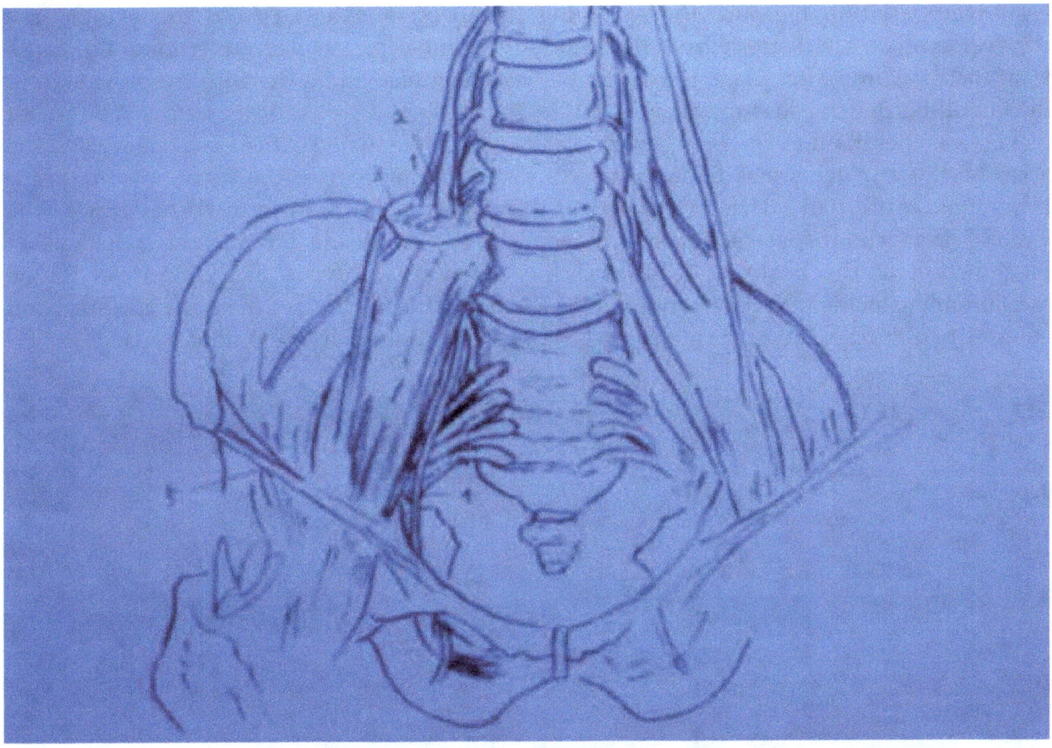

Fig. 1. A schematic presentation of the lumbar and the sacral plexus. 1) lateral femoral cutaneous nerve; 2) femoral nerve; 3) psoas major muscle; 4) obturator nerve; 5) inguinal ligament.

Following the confirmation of the negative aspiration of blood and the cerebrospinal fluids, a large volume of local anesthetics are usually injected. The procedure has been traditionally carried out by the nerve stimulation method under the confirmation of the landmarks of the body. After confirming the top of the iliac crest, a line is drawn to the spinous process of the 4th lumbar spine. Classically, a textbook describes to advance the needle 5cm lateral to the midline of the spine on this line. However, a considerable number of serious complications associated with the use of lumbar plexus block, such as intrathecal injection, epidural injection, inadvertent vascular puncture, and retroperitoneal bleeding (Aida et al., 1996, Aveline et al., 2004, Ludot, et al., 2008, Weller, et al., 2003) have been reported. These complications have, at least in part, resulted from the depth of the plexus inside the body, which also makes it difficult to perform ultrasound-guided lumbar plexus block partly owing to the presence of bony structures. In particular, the use of heparin during the surgical procedures of EVAR makes the retroperitoneal bleeding as the serious complication with the use of lumbar plexus block, although the complication is often self-limiting in contrast to the bleeding in neuroaxial space, which often results in the inreversible neurological damage. Hence, we analyzed the computed tomography of the consecutive patients in our facility that had undergone any elective surgery and characterized the precise localization of the lumbar plexus at the fourth lumbar spine level in the Japanese population.

In the study, axial transverse sections of computed tomography of the fourth lumbar spine level were used to measure the following distances; a distance from the skin to the transverse process, a distance from the skin to the lumbar plexus nervous trunks, a distance from the median sagital plane to the lumbar nerve trunks, and a distance from the skin to the lateral border of psoas major muscle (Fig.2). On the basis of cadaver study, the lumbar plexus was identified to run between the fleshy slip of the main part of psoas major and the accessory part of the psoas that constitutes the posterior part of the psoas major muscle (Kirchmair et al., 2001). These two parts of the muscle fuses to form the psoas major. The femoral nerve and the lateral femoral cutaneous nerve run inside a thin fascia at the level of the junction of the posterior third and the anterior two-thirds of the muscle. In the measurements made from the computed tomography, the junction of the posterior third and anterior two-third of the psoas major was used as the plane of the femoral nerve (Fig.3).

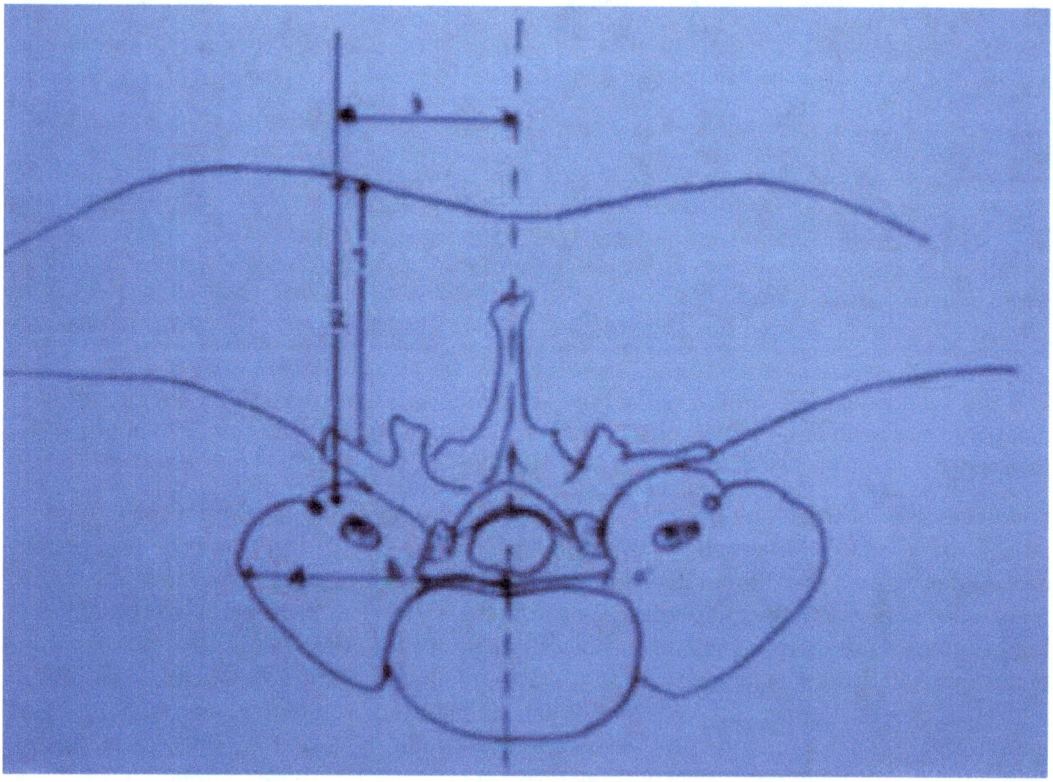

Fig. 2. The following variables were measured; 1)The distance from the skin to the transverse process, 2) The distance from the skin to the femoral nerve, 3) The distance from the median sagital line to the femoral nerve, 4) The distance from the median sagital line to the lateral border of the psoas major muscle.

4.2 Anatomical localization of the lumbar plexus in the Japanese population

Although several literatures have described the anatomical localization of lumbar plexus thus far, no similar information in the Japanese population is totally lacking (Farny et al., 1994, Kirchmair et al., 2001). The present study was undertaken in order to precisely identify the anatomical localization of the lumbar plexus in the Japanese population. The study included 100 Japanese adult patients (59 males and 41 females) who had undergone any elective surgical procedure in our facility. The measurements of the distance from the skin to the transverse process, the distance from the skin to the femoral nerve, the distance from the median sagital plane to the femoral nerve, and the distance from the median sagital plane to the lateral border of the psoas major muscle in the Japanese population are significantly smaller than those described previously in the Canadian population, which presumably had made the procedure to be complicated-prone one (Farny et al., 1994). In their report, the distance from the skin to the transverse process in the Canadian females was reported to be 70±13mm and the distance from the skin to the transverse process in the Canadian males was 75±22mm.

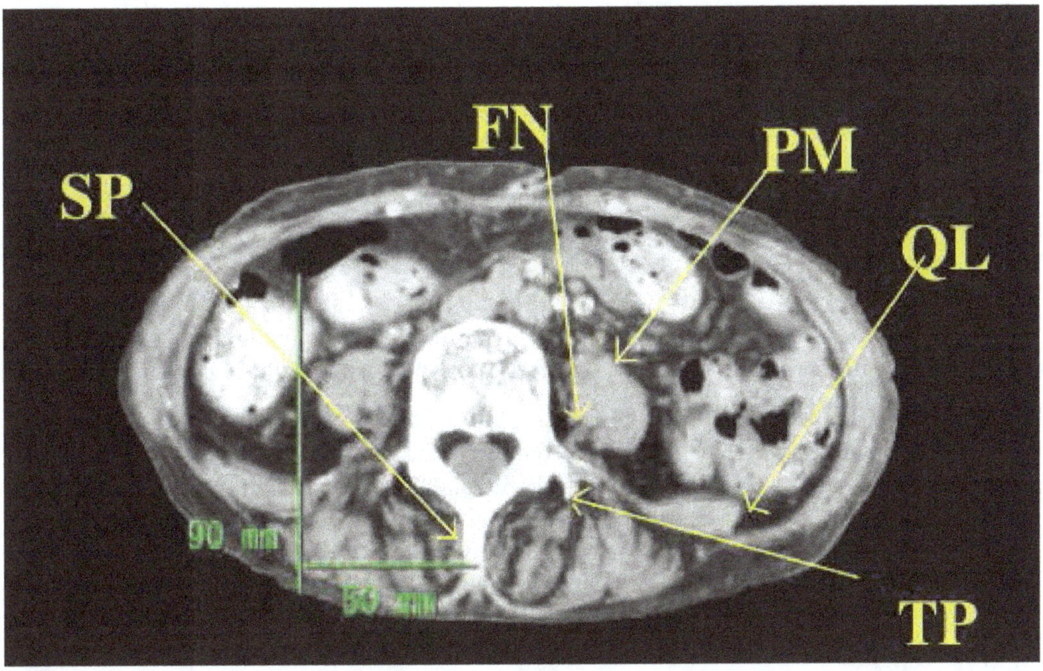

Fig. 3. Localization of the spinous process (SP), transverse process (TP), femoral nerve (FN), psoas major muscle (PM), and quadratus lumborum muscle (QL) on the computed tomography at the 4th lumbar spine level is shown.

By contrast, in our hands, the same distance that corresponds to the Japanese male was 49.32mm (median: 47, range: 30-72mm), and that corresponds to the Japanese female was 48.41mm (median: 47, range: 25-86mm) (Fig.4). Similarly, the average distance from the skin to the femoral nerve in the Canadian males and females were reported to be 99±21mm and 90±14mm, respectively, whereas that corresponds to the Japanese males was 66.6mm (median: 64, range: 64-90mm), and that to the Japanese female was 65.9mm (median: 66, range: 50-80mm) (Fig.5). The distance from the median sagital plane to the lateral border of the psoas muscle in the Canadian males and females were reported to be 72.7 ± 10mm and 60 ± 8mm, whereas those correspond to the Japanese males and females were 54.88mm (median: 55, range: 47-64), and 49.31mm (median: 50; range: 34-67mm) (Fig.6). In addition, although there was no description regarding the distance from the median sagital plane to the femoral nerve in the Canadian population, we measured those variables in the Japanese males and females. The distance from the median sagital plane to the femoral nerve in the Japanese male was 34.47mm (median: 35, range: 27-42mm), and that corresponds to the Japanese female was 32.63mm (median: 32, range 27-45mm) (Fig.7).

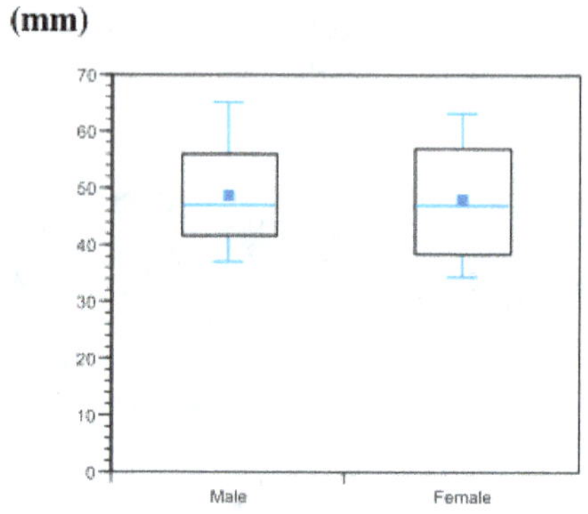

Fig. 4. The distance from the skin to the transverse process in the Japanese males (n=59) and the Japanese females (n=41). Results are expressed by the box-and-whisker plots.

In the standard textbook in the field of anesthesiology, the needle is suggested to advance at the point 3cm caudal to the line connecting the both iliac crest and 5cm lateral to the median sagital line (Wedel et al., 2005). However, the average distance from the median sagital line to the lateral border of the psoas major muscle in the Japanese female is 49.31mm, and there is a substantial risk of peritoneal puncture in approximately a half of this population if the needle is advanced at the point described in the textbook. In addition, although the needle is suggested to advance until it contacts to the transverse process of the fifth lumbar spine, there is some possibility that the needle will not contact to the transverse process if it is advanced at the point where the textbook recommends.

Moreover, the literature suggests that the nerve trunks are located approximately 90(female)-99(male) mm deep inside the body in the Canadian population (Farny et al., 1994). However, they are located far more superficial levels in the Japanese population (male; 66.6mm, female 65.9mm). Accordingly, there is a potential risk of peripheral nerve damage if the needle is advanced as suggested by the textbook.

In the Japanese population, the nerve trunks are located approximately 30mm lateral from the median sagital line (male; 34.47mm, female; 32.63mm). Literature suggests that the development of inadvertent epidural spread occurs in approximately 9-16% of the patients, and this adverse event is attributable to the retrograde diffusion of the local anesthetics to the epidural space (Enneking, et al., 2005). Given the nearer distance from the median sagital line to the femoral nerve in the Japanese population than in the Caucasion population, it must be always kept in mind that the Japanese patients carry more risks of inadvertent epidural spread than those described in the textbook previously.

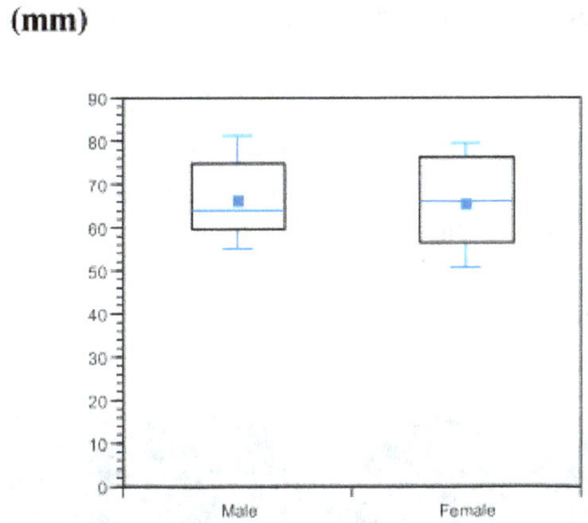

Fig. 5. The distance from the skin to the femoral nerve in the Japanese males (n=59) and females (n=41).

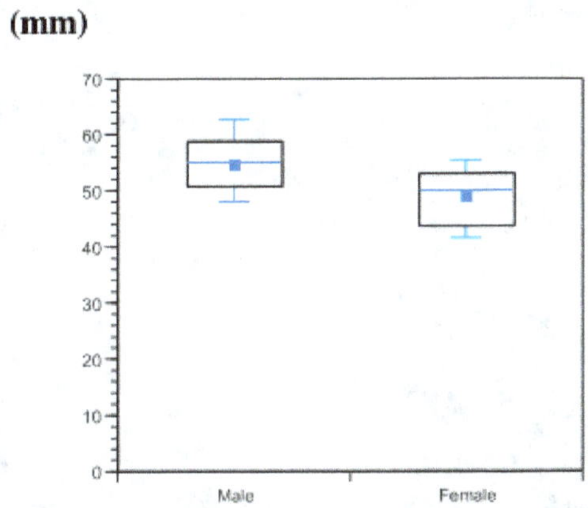

Fig. 6. The distance from the median sagital line to the lateral border of the psoas major muscle in the Japanese males (n=59) and females (n=41).

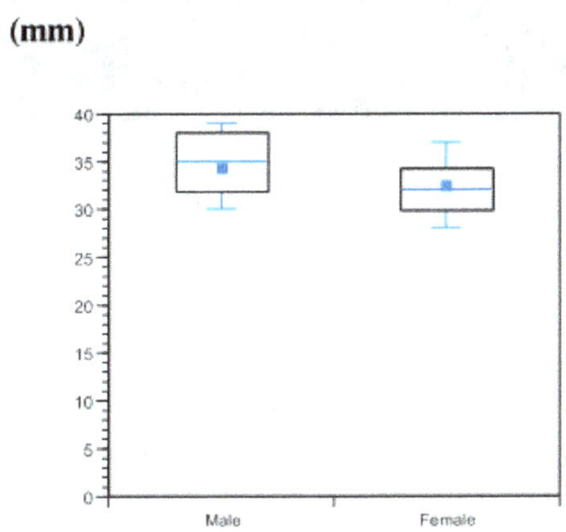

Fig. 7. The distance from the median sagital line to the femoral nerve in the Japanese males (n=59) and females (n=41).

4.3 Examples that would develop serious complications following lumbar plexus block

Followings are the typical examples of the Japanese patients who would develop serious complications if the needle would have advanced as suggested by the textbook. Figure 8 shows the computed tomography at the 4th lumbar supine level from the 70-year-old female. In this case, if the needle is advanced 5cm laterally from the median sagital line into the depth at 9cm level, the needle would puncture peritoneal cavity.

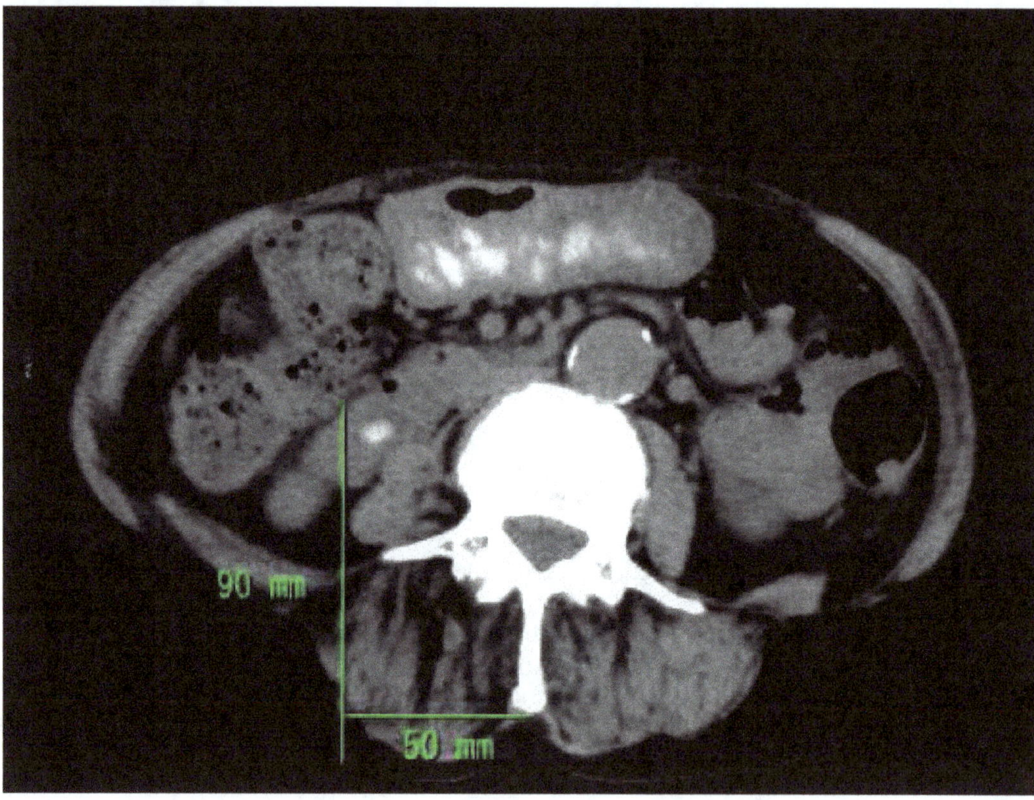

Fig. 8. The computed tomography of a 70-year-old female at the 4th lumbar spine level. Note that if the needle had advanced as suggested by the textbook, it would have punctured the peritoneal cavity.

Similarly, in cases which are shown in figure 9, 10, and 11, the inadvertent peritoneal puncture and possible colonic perforations would have developed if the needle had been advanced as suggested by the textbook.

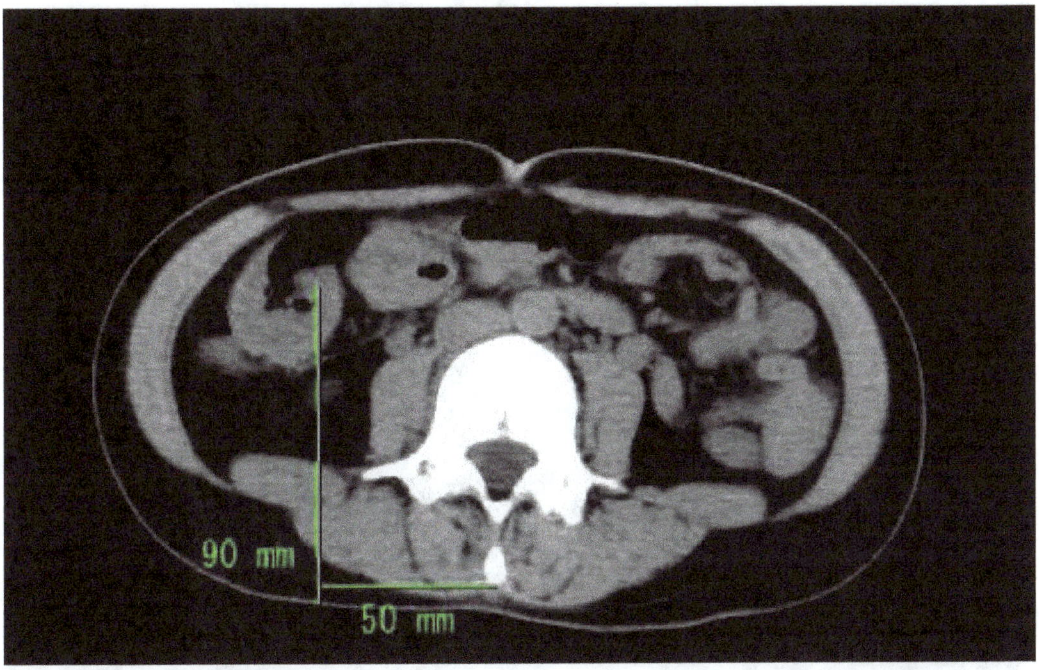

Fig. 9. Computed tomography of the 4th lumbar spine level from a 37-year-old female.

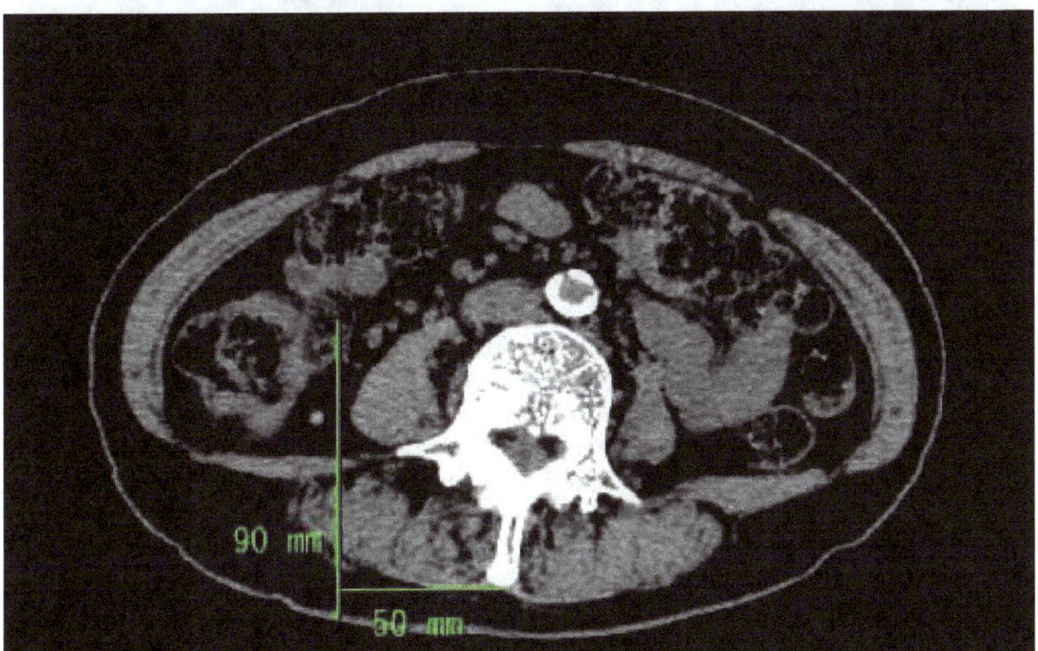

Fig. 10. Computed tomography of the 4th lumbar spine level from a 70-year-old female. Similarly, the needle would have penetrated the peritoneal cavity if the needle had been advanced as suggested by the textbook.

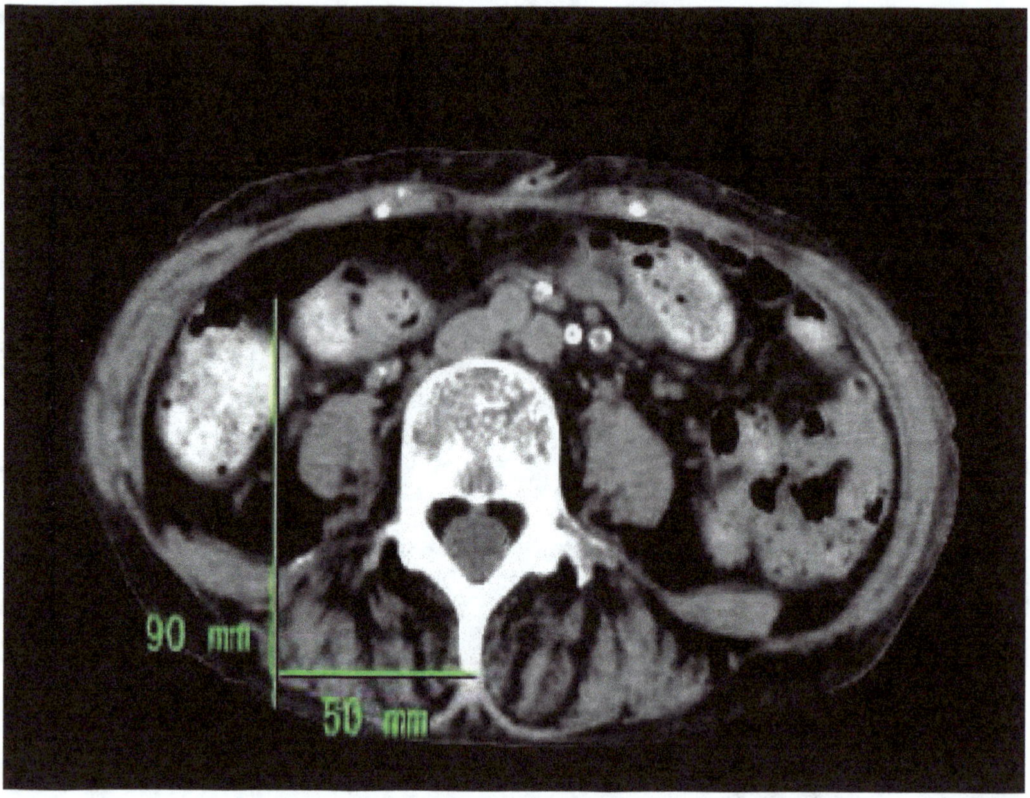

Fig. 11. The computed tomography at the 4th lumbar spine from a 74-year-old female.

In figure 12 and 13, the left kidney has descended as low as to the 4th lumbar supine level. In these cases, if the needle was advanced as suggested by the textbook, inadvertent renal puncture would have developed.

In figure 14 and 15, inferior vena cava is present 3cm laterally from the median sagital line at the depth of 9cm from the skin. Thus, if the needle would have advanced 3cm laterally from the median sagital line, there would be the risk of inadvertent inferior vena cava puncture, which may result in serious consequences such as retroperitoneal hematoma, and inadvertent vascular injection of local anesthetics.

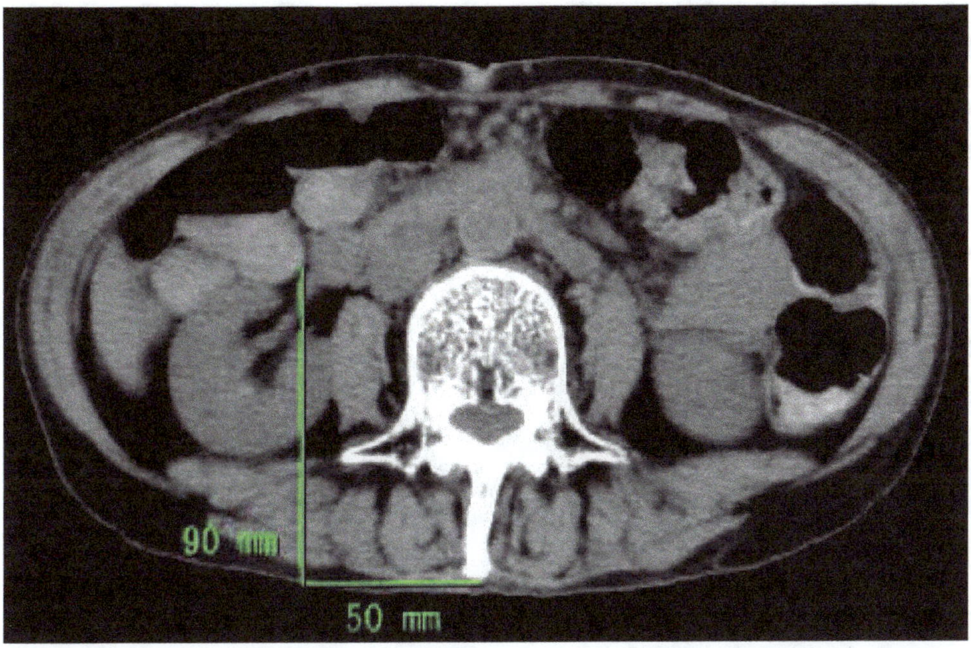

Fig. 12. Computed tomography of the 4th lumbar spine level from a 62-year-old female.

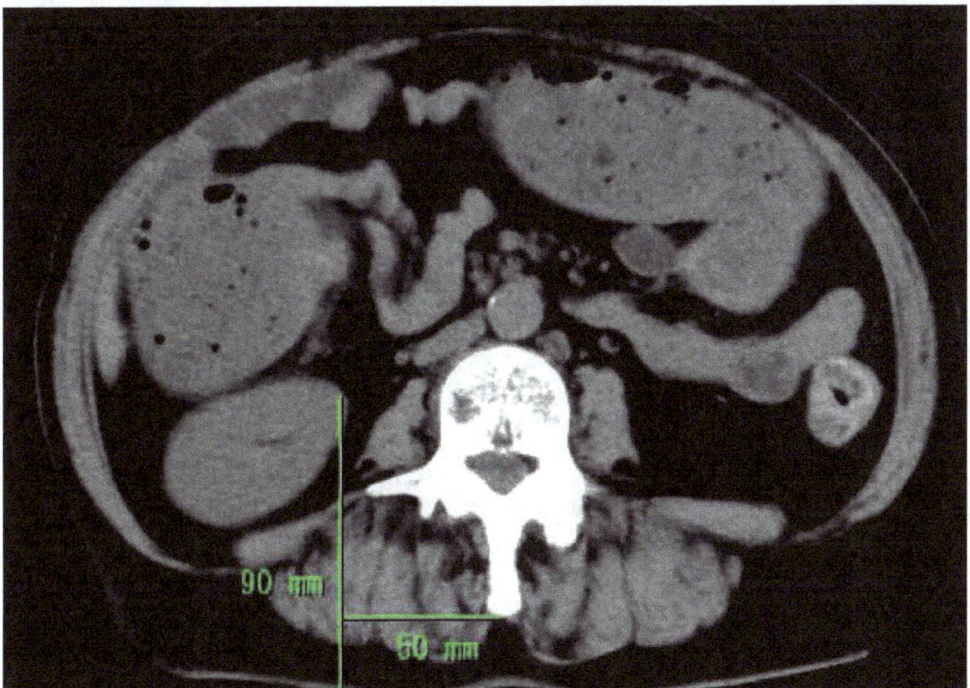

Fig. 13. Computed tomography of the 4th lumbar spine level from a 62-year-old female. In these two cases, if the needle had been advanced as suggested by the textbook, an inadvertent renal puncture would have developed.

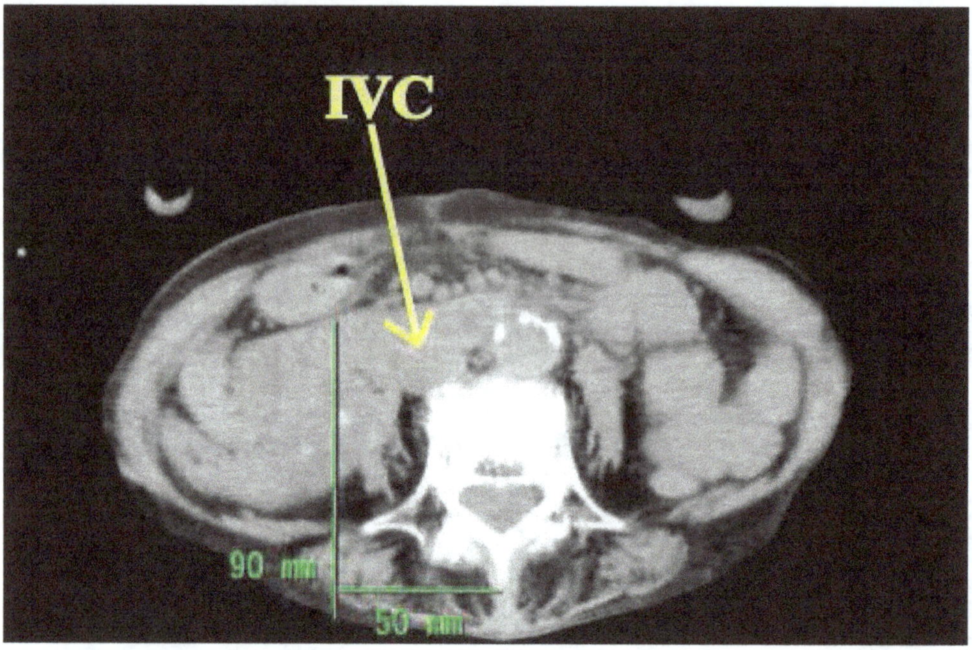

Fig. 14. The computed tomography at the 4th lumbar spine level from a 90-year-old female. Inferior vena cava is distended (indicated by the arrow), and there is a potential risk of inadvertent inferior vena cava puncture in this case.

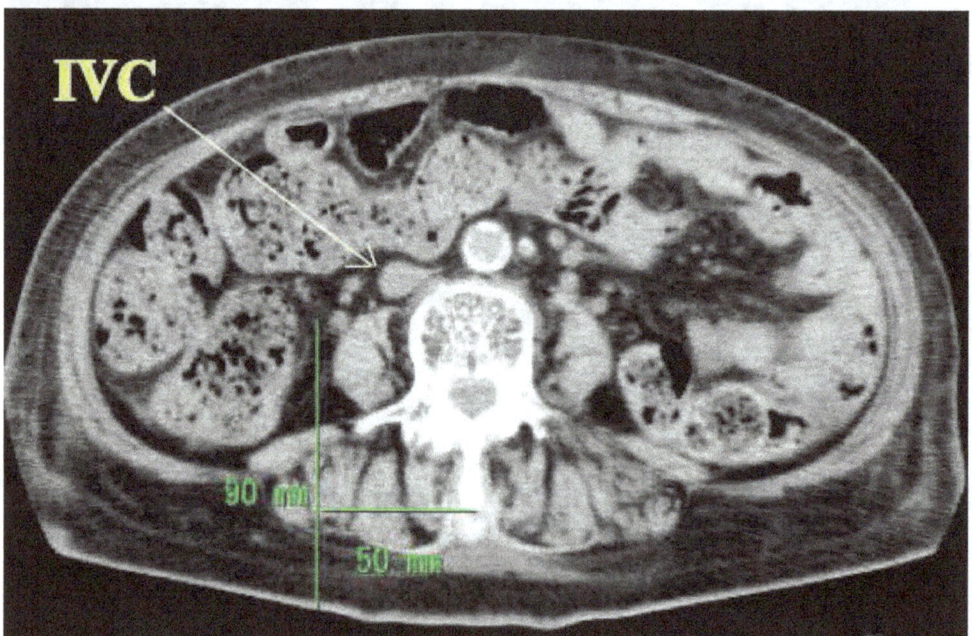

Fig. 15. The computed tomography at the 4th lumbar spine level from a 76-year-old female. In this case, inferior vena cava is laterally deviated (indicated by the arrow), and there is a potential risk of inadvertent inferior vena cava puncture.

From our observations, we suggest that the needle should be advanced 32 (female)-35 (male) mm laterally from the median sagital line in the Japanese population. If the needle puncture point is more than 5cm laterally from the median sagital line, there is a risk of inadvertent peritoneal puncture. In addition, the nerve trunks of lumbar plexus present at the depth of 64-66mm inside the body from the skin.

4.4 Ultrasound-guided lumbar plexus block

Lastly, the possibility of ultrasound-guidance for lumbar plexus block is going to be discussed. With the aid of ultrasound, it has come to be feasible to directly visualize the peripheral nerves, the needle, and the spread of local anesthetics. The ultrasound-guidance for peripheral nerve block has been shown to be efficacious in femoral nerve block, sciatic nerve block, brachial plexus block, and peripheral nerves of body trunks (Asakura, et al., 2010a, Asakura, et al., 2010b, Gray, 2006). However, bony structure has a high absorption coefficient of ultrasound, which makes the ultrasound-imaging of lumbar plexus limited in resolution, in addition to the location of nerve trunks deep inside the body. In general, the visualization of nerve structures by ultrasound requires the use of high frequency probes offering high-resolution images. However, the higher the frequency is, the smaller the penetration depth would be (Marhofer et al., 2007). In other words, for the blockade of nerves located deep inside the body, the ultrasound probes with lower frequency are required, which often are insufficient for offering high-resolution images required for identifying nerve structures. In the standard textbook in the field of anesthesiology, there are subtitles dealing with ultrasound-guided supraclavicular and interscalene brachial plexus block, infraclavicular block, axillary block, ilioinguinal block, femoral nerve block, and sciatic nerve block, but no single description of ultrasound-guided lumbar plexus block (Gray, 2005). The first attempt to identify the structures of lumbar plexus by ultrasound using a curved array transducer with a frequency at 4 MHz appeared in 2001 using the healthy volunteers (Kirchmair et al., 2001). They reported the successful identification of psoas muscle, erector spinae, and quadratus lumborum muscle by ultrasonography but not the nerve structures of lumbar plexus. Shortly thereafter, an attempt of ultrasound-guided lumbar plexus block using cadavers appeared from the same group, which confirmed the feasibility and accuracy of ultrasound guidance in advancing the needle to the psoas major muscle, but again without identifying the nerve structures (Kirchmair et al., 2002). Hence, the knowledge of anatomical localization of the nerve structures of the lumbar plexus would appear to be the prerequisite for performing the "ultrasound-assisted" lumbar plexus block. In 2004, however, the successful identification of the nerve trunks of lumbar plexus in the pediatric cases has been reported (Kirchmair et al., 2004). The successful identification of the lumbar plexs in these pediatric cases had resulted from the superficial localization of the nerve trunks, which allowed the researchers to utilize the higher frequency (5-8MHz) transducer ultrasound equipments. So far, the direct visualization of the nerve trunks of lumbar plexus in adult cases appears to be unsuccessful. However, by combining the nerve stimulation in addition to the ultrasound assistance, the identification of lumbar plexus becomes feasible even in adult cases (Asakura et al., 2008a). More importantly, the direct visualization of the adjacent structures such as the kidneys by ultrasound may prevent an inadvertent renal puncture or peritoneal puncture and hence may reduce the incidence of the development of complications associated with the lumbar plexus block.

5. Conclusion

Endovascular aortic aneurysm repair has provided a substantial improvement in the peri-operative patients' outcome including 30-day peri-operative mortality as compared with the traditional open surgical vascular reconstruction largely owing to its less invasive nature, especially in those whom serious comorbidities are present. In order to reduce the substantial risks associated with the anesthesia for EVAR in such seriously comorbid patients, various attempts have thus far been made. Particularly, the use of loco-regional anesthesia technique is a promising way to reduce the risks associated with the use of general anesthesia, such as the reduction in the incidence of development of respiratory complications. However, obstacles have also been met especially with the use of neuroaxial anesthesia because of the increased risks of developing subdural/epidural hematoma. Peripheral nerve block is the possible promising alternative for the use of neuroaxial anesthesia. During the surgical procedures of EVAR, skin incisions are made in the groin areas in order to gain the access to the femoral arteries. Anesthesia at the groin areas can be obtained by the posterior lumbar plexus block, which is traditionally approached by the nerve stimulation method. In comparison with the Caucasian population, the nerve trunks of lumbar plexus are located far more superficial and far more close to the median sagital plane in the Japanese and possibly in Asian populations. In order to prevent the potential risks of inadvertent renal and peritoneal puncture as well as inadvertent epidural spread, the lumbar plexus block should be carried out with the assistance of ultrasound-guidance.

6. References

Asakura, Y.; Kandatsu, N.; Hashimoto, A.; Kamiya, M.; Akashi, M.; & Komatsu, T. (2009a) Ultrasound-guided neuroaxial anesthesia: accurate diagnosis of spina bifida occulta by ultrasonography. *Journal of Anesthesia,* Vol.23, 2009, 312-3

Asakura, Y.; Ishibashi, H.; Ishiguchi, T.; Kandatsu, N.; Akashi, M.; & Komatsu, T. (2009b) General versus locoregional anesthesia for endovascular aortic aneurysm repair: influences of the type of anesthesia on its outcome. *Journal of Anesthesia,* Vol. 23, 2009, 158-61

Asakura, Y. (2010a) In reply: The anesthetic technique of choice for better outcomes in high-risk elderly patients undergoing endovascular repair of aortic aneurysm. *Journal of Anesthesia,* Vol.24, 2010, 500-501

Asakura, Y.; Kandatsu, N.; Kato, N.; Sato, Y.; Fujiwara, Y.; & Komatsu T. (2008a) Ultrasound guided sciatic nerve block combined with lumbar plexus block for infra-inguinal artery bypass graft surgery. *Acta Anaesthesiologica Scandinavica* Vol.52, 2008, 721-2

Asakura, Y.; Mizuno, T.; Kato, N.; Sato, Y.; Fujiwara, Y.; & Komatsu T. (2008b) Respiratory status that facilitates subclavian venous catheterization. *Acta Anaesthesiologica Scandinavica* Vol. 52, 2008, 867-9

Asakura, Y.; Tsuchiya, H.; Nieda, Y.; Yano, T.; Kato, T.; & Takagi H. (2010b) Deep vein thrombosis: how long will it remain? *Journal of Anesthesia* Vol.24, 2010, 490-1

Asakura, Y.; Yano, T.; Takagi, H.; Tsuchiya, H.; & Kato T. (2010c) The incidence of development of motor blockade by ropivacaine is concentration dependent, and most studies regarding the continuous FNB after total knee arthroplasty used 0.2% to 0.3% ropivacaine. *Journal of Arthroplasty* Vol.25, 2010, 837-8

Ashton, H.A.; Buxton, M.J.; Day, N.E.; Kim, L.G.; Marteau, T.M.; Scott, R.A.; Thompson, S.G.; Walker, N.M.; Multicenter Aneurysm Screening Study (MASS) Group. The multicenter aneurysm screening study (MASS) into the effect of abdominal aortic aneurysm screening on mortality in men: a randomized controlled trial. *Lancet* Vol.360, 2002, 1531-9

Aveline, C.; & Bonnet, F. Delayed retroperitoneal hematoma after failed lumbar plexus block. *British Journal of Anaesthesia* Vol.93, 2004, 589-91

Capdevila, X.; Macaire, P.; Dadure, C.; Choquet, O.; Biboulet, P.; Ryckwaert, Y.; & D'Athis F. Continuous psoas compartment block for post-operative analgesia after total hip arthroplasty. New landmarks, technical guidelines, and clinical evaluation. *Anesthesia and Analgesia* Vol.94, 2002,1606-13.

Ennecking, F.K.; Chan, V.; Greger, J.; Hadzic, A.; Lang, S.A.; & Horlocker, T.T. Lower extremity peripheral nerve blocks: Essentials of our current understanding. *Regional Anesthesia and Pain Medicine* Vol.30, 2005, 4-35.

EVAR trial participants. Endovascular aneurysm repair and outcome in patients unfit for open repair of abdominal aortic aneurysm (EVAR trial 2): randomized controlled trial. *Lancet* Vol.365, 2005, 2187-92

Farny, J.; Drolet, P.; & Girald, M. Anatomy of the posterior approach to the lumbar plexus block. *Canadian Journal of Anaesthesia*, Vol.41, 1994, 480-5

Fleming, C.; Whitlock, E.P.; Beil, T.L.; & Lederle, F.A. Screening for abdominal aortic aneurysm: a best-evidence systematic review for the U.S. preventive service task force. *Annals of Internal Medicine* Vol.142, 2005, 203-11

Gray, A.T. (2005) Ultrasound-guidance for regional anesthesia. In: *Miller's Anesthesia, 7th edition,* Miller R.D. (Eds.), 1675-1704, Elsevier, Churchill Livingstone, ISBN: 978-0-8089-2413-5.

Gray, A.T. Ultrasound-guided regional anesthesia: current state of the art. *Anesthesiology* Vol.104, 2006, 368-73.

Greenhalgh, R.M.; Brown, L.C.; Kwong, G.P.; Powell, J.T.; & Thompson, S.G.; EVAR trial participants. Comparison of endovascular aneurysm repair with open repair in patients with abdominal aortic aneurysm (EVAR trial 1), 30-day operative mortality results: randomized controlled trial. *Lancet* Vol.364, 843-8.

Horlocker, T.T.; & Wedel, D.J. Neurologic complications of spinal and epidural anesthesia. *Regional Anesthesia and Pain Medicine* Vol.25, 2000, 83-98

Horlocker, T.T.; Wedel, D.J.; Rowlingson, J.C.; Enneking, F.K.; Kopp, S.L.; Benzon, H.T.; Brown, D.L.; Heit, J.A.; Mulroy, M.F.; Rosenquist, R.W.; Tryba, M.; & Yuan, C.S. Regional anesthesia in the patient receiving antithrombotic or thrombolytic therapy. *Regional Anesthesia and Pain Medine* Vol.35, 2010, 64-101.

Kirchmair, L.; Entner, T.; Wissel, J.; Moriggl, B.; Kapral, S.; & Mitterschiffthaler, G. A study of the paravertebral anatomy for ultrasound-guided posterior lumbar plexus block. *Anesthesia and Analgesia* Vol.93, 2001, 477-81

Kirchmair, L.; Entner, T.; Kapral, S.; & Mitterschiffthaler, G. Ultrasound guifance for the psoas compartment block: an imaging study. *Anesthesia and Analgesia* Vol.94, 2002, 706-10

Kirchmair, L.; Enna, B.; Mitterschiffthaler, G.; Moriggl, B.; Greher, M.; Marhofer, P.; Kapral, S.; & Gassner I. Lumbar plexus in children. A sonographic study and its relevance to pediatric regional anesthesia. *Anesthesiology* Vol.101, 2004, 445-50

Lloyd, W.E.; Paty, P.S.; Darling, R.C. 3rd; Chang, B.B.; Fitzgerald, K.M.; Leather, R.P.; & Shah, D.M. Results of 1000 consecutive elective abdominal aortic aneurysm repairs. *Cardiovascular Surgery* Vol.4, 1996, 724-26.

Ludot, H.; Thari, J.Y.; Belouadah, M.; Mazoit, J.X.; & Malinovsky, J.M. Successful resuscitation after ropivacaine and lidocaine-induced ventricular arrhythmia following posterior lumbar plexus block in a child. *Anesthesia & Analgesia* Vol.106, 2008,1572-4

Marhofer, P.; & Chan, V.W. Ultrasound-guided regional anesthesia: Current concepts and future trends. *Anesthesia and Analgesia* Vol.104, 2007, 1265-9

Park, W.Y.; Thompson, J.S.; & Lee, K.K. Effect of epidural anesthesia and analgesia on periperative outcome. A randomized controlled veterans affairs cooperative study. *Annals of Surgery* Vol.234, 2001, 560-571

Parodi, J.C.; Palmaz, J.C.; & Barone, H.D. Transfemoral intraluminal graft implantation for abdominal aortic aneurysm. *Annals of Vascular Surgery* Vol.5, 1991, 491-499

Ruppert, V.; Leurs, L.J.; Steckmeier, B.; Buth, J.; & Umscheid, T. Influence of anesthesia type on outcome after endovascular aortic aneurysm repair: an analysis based on EUROSTAR data. *Journal of Vascular Surgery* Vol.44, 2006,16-21

Shah, P.K. Inflammation, metalloproteinases, and increased proteolysis: an emerging pathophysiological paradigm in aortic aneurysm. *Circulation* Vol.96, 1997, 2115-17

Schermerhorn, M.L.; O'Malley, A.J.; Jhaveri, A.; Cotterill, P.; Pomposelli, F.; & Landon, B.E. Endovascular versus open repair of abdominal aortic aneurysms in the Medicare population. *New England Journal of Medicine* Vol.358, 2008, 464-74

Sakalihasan, N.; Limet, R.; & Defawe, O.D. Abdominal aortic aneurysm. *Lancet* Vol.365, 2005, 1577-89

Timaran, C.H.; Veith, F.J.; Rosero, E.B.; Modrall, J.G.; Arko, F.R.; Clagett, G.P.; & Valentine, R.J. Endovascular aortic aneurysm repair in patients with the highest risk and in-hospital mortality in the United States. *Archives of Surgery* Vol.142, 2007, 520-524

Vandermeulen, E.P.; Van Ake, H.; & Vermylen, J. Anticoagulants and spinal-epidural anesthesia. *Anesthesia and Analgesia* Vol.79, 1994, 1165-77

Verhoeven, E.L.; Cina, C.S.; Tielliu, I.F.; Zeebregts, C.J.; Prins, T.R.; Eindhoeven, G.B.; Span, M.M.; Kapma, M.R.; & van den Dungen, J.J. Local anesthesia for endovascular abdominal aortic aneurysm repair. *Journal of Vascular Surgery* Vol.42, 2005, 402-9.

Wedel, D.J.; & Horlocker, T. (2005) Nerve blocks. In: *Miller's Anesthesia, 7th edition,* Miller R.D. (Eds.), 1639-74, Elsevier, Churchill Livingstone, ISBN: 978-0-8089-2413-5.

Weller, R.S.; Gerancher, J.C.; Crews, J.C.; & Wade, KL. Extensive retroperitoneal hematoma without neurologic deficit in two patients who underwent lumbar plexus block and were later anticoagulated. *Anesthesiology,* Vol.98, 2003, 581-5.

Part 4

Molecular Management in Aortic Disease

9

Nutrition and the Aorto-Iliac Atherosclerotic Disease

Sergio Santana Porbén
Nutritional Support Group, "Hermanos Ameijeiras" Clinical surgical Hospital,
La Habana,
Cuba

1. Introduction

ESRV Elective Surgical Revascularization is the ultimate intervention in atherosclerotic aorto-iliac disease which has progressed up to the arterial insufficiency state [**1**]. Surgical solution of extreme forms of aorto-iliac atherosclerotic disease (such as aortic aneurysm) implies removal of the stenotic/dilated arterial segment, creation of an arterial derivation, and/or placement of a vascular prosthesis [**2**]. Surgical act entails a metabolic aggression whose cost might override the patient's homeostatic mechanisms, resulting in complications and death [**3-4**]. Consequently, the medical team should care for the safe completion of the surgical procedure through identification and proactive modification of factors existing in the patient that might place him/her at risk of complication and death.

Patient's nutritional status can determine the result of surgical activity. An increased risk of surgical failures has been reported as patient's nutritional status deteriorates [**5-7**]. However, relationship between the response to the surgical act and nutritional status might not be that straightforward, and could be modified by fuzzy variables such as age and presence of co-morbidities [**8-9**].

The present essay gives the opportunity for assessing the relationship between nutritional status of the patient and surgical activity from a different, entirely new, perspective. That is: it would be interesting to examine if body weight excess can also modify the results of surgical activity non-related to tumor-reduction, as would be the case of ESRV. This study model of systemic response to surgical aggression could be more appealing in view of the fact that abnormalities of the great abdominal vessels intended to be surgically corrected represent different stations in the progression of atherosclerotic disease, and this, in turn, is associated with Obesity. Thus, it could be anticipated that surgical failures rate to increase as patient's body fat does.

2. Atherosclerosis and nutrition

Any discussion on the possible links between atherosclerotic aorto-iliac disease and nutrition should take into account the influence of subject's food habits upon onset and history (in absence of intervention) of this illness, the nutritional status of the patient prior to ESRV, and nutritional influence upon the response to the surgical act.

Atherosclerosis is intimately related with disorders of blood lipids homeostasis [**10-11**]. Although fat strip has been described as the originary atherosclerotic lesion in the aorta of

newborn babies, its conversion into an atheroma, with subsequent calcification, rupture and thrombosis, or weakening of the arterial wall, are all associated with chronic states of hypercholesterolemia **[11-12]**. However, it should be noticed that causes of hypercholesterolemia can be multiple and chaotic in their presentation and influences **[13]**.
Obesity, established from the disproportionate participation, and anomalous distribution, of body fat in the subject's body composition, and the repercussion that specified topographical locations of adipose tissue have upon endocrine activity of human economy as well as cell and tissue metabolism, is an important factor in the progression of atherosclerotic damage **[14-15]**. Obesity results from the incapacity of the organism to correctly use food energy quantities incongruent with subject's physical activity, in particular if present in his/her regular diet as refined sugars and energetically dense foods. Coincidently, elevated food fats intakes, with an important participation of saturated fats and *trans* fatty acids, have been described in obese subjects **[15-18]**. Hypercholesterolemia could also be the result of unbalanced intakes of long-chain, poly-unsaturated fatty acids, and poor representation of ω3 fatty acids in the diet **[13,19]**. All these food influences converge to configure the so-called Metabolic syndrome, which eventually leads to hyperuricemia, blood lipids disorders, and disruption of the peripheral utilization of carbohydrates, that might evolve towards hyperglycemia and insulin resistance; molecular events all that accelerate the progression of atherosclerotic disease **[20-21]**.

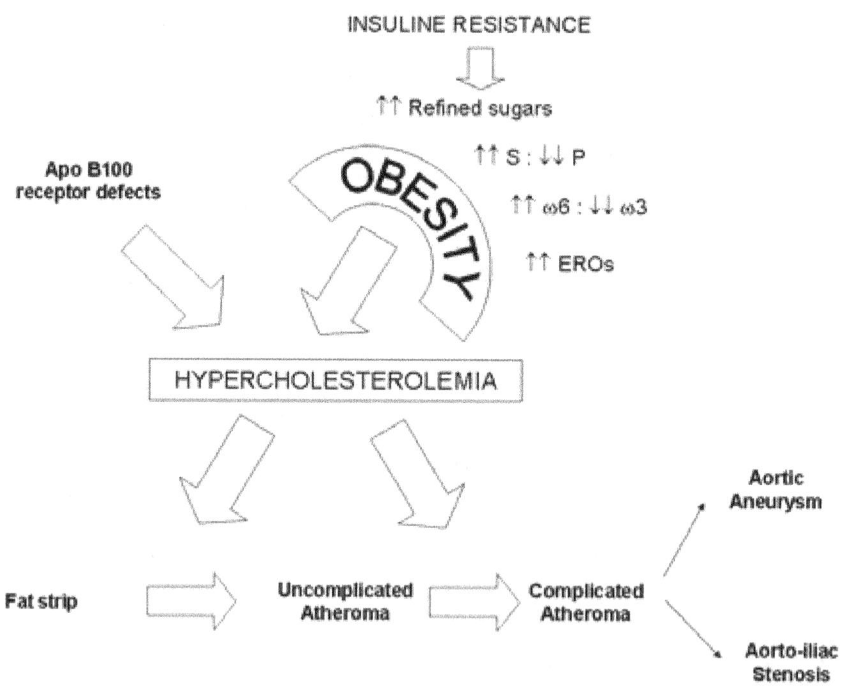

Legends: S: Saturated fats. P: Poly-unsaturated fats. ORSs: Oxygen-reactive species

Fig. 1. Some influences in the progression of the originary atherosclerotic lesion. The figure intends to call the attention upon factors involved in atherosclerosis dependant on Obesity as well as molecular defects in LDL-Cholesterol clearance. The presentation does not exhaust the events related with atherosclerosis, nor the relationships they sustain among them. For further details: See pertinent references at the end of the essay.

3. Nutritional phenotypes in atherosclerotic aorto-iliac disease

Corresponding with what has been said previously, it should not come as a surprise to see that a significant proportion of aorto-sclerosis patients considered for ESRV show a body weight higher that the one expected regarding the height of their peers, as seen in Figure 2. Regarding BMI Body Mass Index, 69 patients assisted between 2000 - 2007 due to aorto-iliac atherosclerosis (more than half presenting with aortic aneurysm) at a Angiology and Vascular surgery of a referral, tertiary hospital of the city of Havana (Cuba) were distributed as follows: Malnourished: < 18.5 $Kg.m^{-2}$: 4.3%; Non-Malnourished: Between 18.5 - 24.9 $Kg.m^{-2}$: 41.4%; and Body weight excess: > 24.9 $Kg.m^{-2}$: 54.3%; respectively. Fourteen point 2 percent of the patients was obese on admission to the Service.

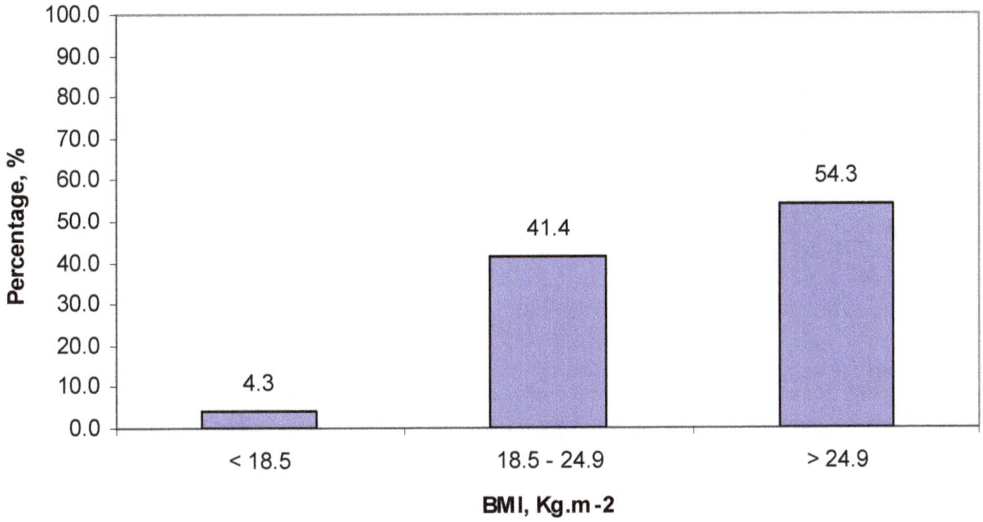

Legend: BMI: Body Mass Index.
Source: Records of the Nutritional Support Group. Clinical surgical Hospital "Hermanos Ameijeiras". La Habana. Cuba.
Records closed on: Monday, October 10th, 2010.

Fig. 2. Distribution of different nutritional phenotypes among patients awaiting elective surgical revascularization in a referral, tertiary, Angiology service. More than half of patients presented with aortic aneurysm.

Having reached this point in the essay, a relevant question is pertinent: Can body weight excess (in either of its two forms: overweight or obesity) affect the response to ESRV? In other words: does the risk of complications after ESRV increase because of size/distribution of body fat? If this is to be the case, patient's response to ESRV could be improved, and in the process, a higher-quality medical-surgical care offered, by means of the conduction of proactive measures oriented to modify the size as well as topographical distribution of body fat.

The relevance of these considerations is not to be ignored. ESRV includes technically-demanding procedures, such as aorto-femoral derivation, and placement of vascular prostheses. Complications that might occur after completion of such procedures can encompass from sepsis to derivation/prosthesis failure, with subsequent amputation of the vascular compromised limb [**3-4,22**]. Interestingly, considerations about the association between surgical activity and nutritional status have been dominated by the discussion on how weight loss affects the result of surgical tumor-reduction [**5-8**]. On the contrary, documented evidences on the influence of body weight excess upon the response of the patient to surgical activity non-related with oncology practice are scarce. However, it has been hypothesized that the relationship between risk of complication after a surgical act and nutritional status of the patient might adopt a "U" or "J" shape, as shown in Figure 3 [**23-24**]. The shape of this relationship is striking, because it stresses that polar nutritional phenotypes can be equivalent in their influences upon the response of the patient to the surgical activity[1].

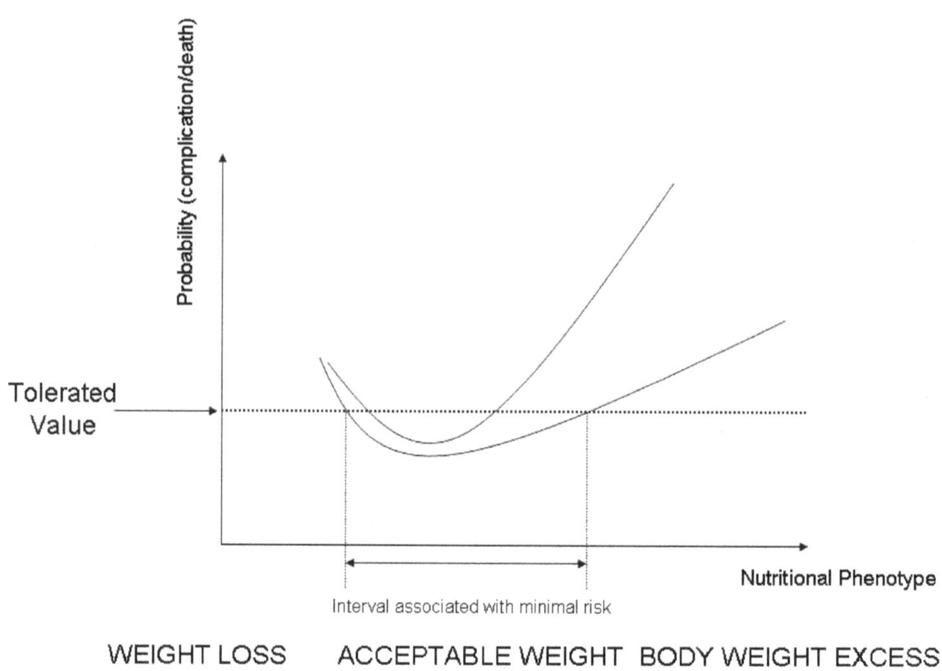

Drawn with data taken from: References [23-24].

Fig. 3. Influence of nutritional phenotype upon response to the surgical act.

4. Why polar nutritional phenotypes are equally deleterious for the response to ESRV?

ENM Energy Nutrient Malnutrition is that disorder of body composition resulting from depletion of Potassium-rich, metabolic-active, lean tissues [**26**]. Reduction of body lean mass beyond a critical size is associated with an increased risk of complications after ESRV, not to

[1] Unfortunately, the author has not been able to validate this hypothesis. After research completed in a Angiology and Vascular Surgery referral, tertiary Service, it was concluded that post-surgical complications were independent from nutritional phenotype, affecting two-thirds of non-malnourished patients, and half plus one of those with body weight excess [**25**].

mention death[2]. ENM deeply affects all the orders of subject's economy, and profoundly alters inner milieu homeostasis. Malnutrition usually associates with impaired liver protein synthesis and tissue repair and healing processes, and defective collagen deposition, thus difficulting the formation of an effective scar callous [**24, 27**]. Malnutrition also brings about disruption of the natural barriers for restraining invading pathogen bacteria, antigen-presentation mechanisms, production and release of cytokines, immunoglobulins and cell mobilization factors, and the proliferation and differentiation of cells involved in immune response [**28**]. Far from exhausting the topic, malnutrition can affect ventilatory function, making the subject prone to failure in weaning from a mechanical ventilator and pneumonia [**29**]; as well as kidney function, thus altering depuration of toxins and other by-products of tissue metabolism [**30**].

By comparison, influence of body weight excess upon response to surgical activity has been little explored, above all in settings non-related with tumor-reduction. Excess of subcutaneous adipose tissue can result in an increased rate of surgical wound sepsis due to failure in obliterating the incision line, and subsequent appearance of dead spaces. Poor vascularity of subcutaneous adipose tissue can also contribute to an insufficient irrigation of surgically lacerated tissues, and thus, inflammation, bacterial colonization, and surgical wound sepsis. Suture dehiscence, incisional hernias and eventrations could then become the most visible face of the influence of body weight excess upon surgical activity.

But body weight excess can also exert remote influences through altered states of peripheral utilization of carbohydrates. Indeed, hyperglycemia has been described as a post-surgical sepsis risk factor [**31**]. It is to be kept in mind that cells involved in immune response are important consumers of energy as glucose [**32**]. Hyperglycemia can result from disorders in the peripheral utilization of carbohydrates as well as hyper-insulinism states. Insulin action target-cell can express a reduced number of hormone-specific receptors, or uncouple the receptor from post-receptor cascade of events, inhibiting in one way or the other stimulation by insulin, a phenomenon recognized as "down-regulation". Incapacity of using glucose as the energy substrate of choice forces the cell to turn to alternative energy fuels, which in the end, worsens hypertrigliceridemia resulting from improper cell utilization of metabolic energy.

Body weight excess can be also associated with chronic states of inflammation. Depending on the topographical location, the adipocyte is able to produce cytokines (αTNF Tissue Necrosis Factor among them), and other inflammation-promoting molecules [**33**]. These blood products also contribute to insulin resistance, hyperglycemia and hypertrigliceridemia. Hence, and given what has been said before, body weight excess can become a powerful negative predictor of complications after ESRV.

5. Can age independently influence upon response to ESRV?

Relationship between probability of complication after ESRV and nutritional phenotype has been documented in subjects younger than 60 years of age [**23, 24**]. However, such dependence relationship has not been established in older subjects. As a matter of fact, it has come to the attention of researchers that body weight excess is associated with a lesser risk of complications after completion of surgical acts non-related with tumor-reduction in

[2] There is also depletion of adipose tissue in ENM, but this phenomenon is secondary to the reduction of the size of body lean mass. As a matter of fact, post-surgical complications can occur in a patient with a nearly constant adipose tissue.

elderly subjects [**34**]. In a recently concluded research at a referral, terminal Angiology Service, it was observed that age was an independent predictor of after-ESRV failures when higher complications rates concentrated among younger subjects notwithstanding nutritional phenotype [**25**]. Hence, it is only attractive to explore why age transit can cause such a profound transformation of the relationship discussed throughout this essay.

Significant changes occur in subject's body composition with aging. These changes could result from "turning off" molecular signals responsible for tissue accretion (explaining, at least in part, the phenomenon of "sarcopenia"); redistribution of body compartments, with preponderance of adipose tissue deposition at the scapular waist, and concomitant reduction of the circumference of body segments and/or substitution of body lean mass with adipose tissue [**35**]. These changes could, in turn, modify subject's hormonal status, reducing insulin resistance, and thus, altered states of peripheral utilization of carbohydrates [**36**]. The morpho-functional substrate such as the one early described might then explain why Obesity, understood as an increase in body fat size, can act as a protecting factor in the third age of life. Hence, others events/circumstances aside, a subject with +60 years of age could tolerate ESRV better if he/she presents to the surgical act with body weight excess, when compared with younger peers.

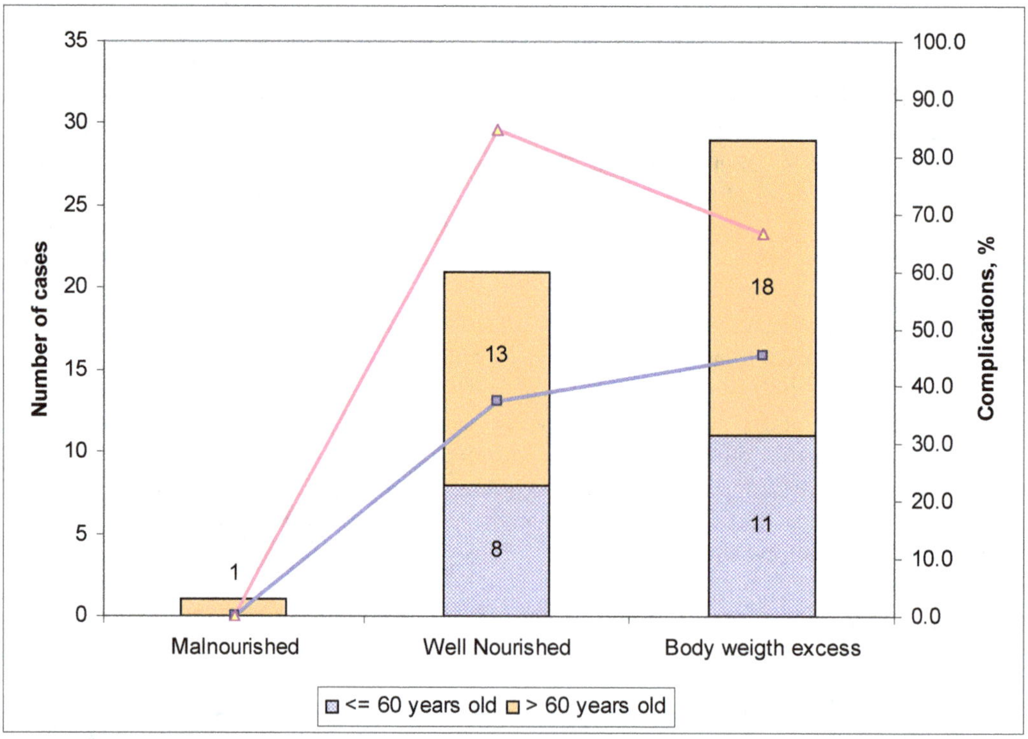

Reproduced from: Reference [25] with the authorization of the Editorial board of ANGIOLOGIA, bimonthly journal of the Spanish Society of Angiology and Vascular Surgery.

Fig. 4. Complications observed after completion of ESRV in a referral, terminal Angiology Service. Cases are distributed according with nutritional status and age. Blue solid line: Complications observed in subjects younger than 60 years. Pink solid line: Complications observed in elder subjects. More than half of patients presented with aortic aneurysm.

6. On perioperatory nutritional intervention in ESRV

Having discussed the aforementioned issues, it is time to dwell about interventions oriented to secure the success of ESRV by supplying the patient with selected nutrients incorporating intrinsic pharmacological actions, such as ω3 fatty acids and dietetic fiber.

Pharmacological actions of ω3 fatty acids have been intensively studied in recent years. ω3 fatty acids, brought by oily seeds and deep waters fishes, might act as precursors of 3- and

Nutrient	Recommended intake	Foods	Enteral Nutrients	Parenteral Nutrients
ω3 fatty acids • DHA	200 mg.24 h-1	Flaxseed oil Deep water fishes: herring, cod	SUPPORTAN ω3 (Fresenius-Kabi, Germany) NUTRICOMP IMMUN (BBRAUN, Germany) NUTRICOMP Diabetes (BBRAUN, Germany)	LIPOPLUS (BBRAUN, Germany) STRUCTOLIPIDS (Fresenius-Kabi, Germany)
ω3 fatty acids • DPA	Not established	Flaxseed oil Deep water fishes: herring, cod	SUPPORTAN ω3 (Fresenius-Kabi, Germany) NUTRICOMP IMMUN (BBRAUN, Germany) NUTRICOMP Diabetes (BBRAUN, Germany)	LIPOPLUS (BBRAUN, Germany) STRUCTOLIPIDS (Fresenius-Kabi, Germany)
ω3 fatty acids • EPA	200 mg.24 h-1	Flaxseed oil Deep water fishes: herring, cod	SUPPORTAN ω3 (Fresenius-Kabi, Germany) NUTRICOMP IMMUN (BBRAUN, Germany) NUTRICOMP Diabetes (BBRAUN, Germany)	LIPOPLUS (BBRAUN, Germany) STRUCTOLIPIDS (Fresenius-Kabi, Germany)
Dietetic fiber • Soluble	10-15 g/day	Fruits, beans, selected vegetables	NUTRICOMP Diabetes (BBRAUN, Germany)	Non available
Dietetic fiber • Non-soluble	10-15 g/day	Non-digested parts of fruits, beans, vegetables	NUTRICOMP Standard w/ Fibre (BBRAUN, Germany): 7.5 g/500 mL	Non available
Glycerol	Not established	Lards, butter, margarines	Non available	LIPOFUNDIN LCT/MCT (BBRAUN, Germany): 25 g/1000 mL LIPOPLUS (BBRAUN, Germany): 25 g/1000 mL ProcalAmine (BBRAUN, Germany): 25 g/1000 mL

Legend: DHA: Docosahexanoic acid. DPA: Docosapentanoic acid. EP: Eicosapentanoic acid.
Note: Soluble, dietetic fiber refers to mucins and pectins. Insoluble, dietetic fiber refers to cellulose and hemi-cellulose.

Table 1. Nutrients known for their effect upon insulin resistance and peripheral utilization of sugars. It is not intended to be a comprehensive list of presented items.

5-series prostanoids, with documented anti-inflammatory, anti-clotting, and smooth muscle-relaxing properties [**37**]. Supply of such fatty acids, be either as foods or chemically defined preparations, could then become an intervention resulting in a lesser systemic inflammatory activity, and thus, a better utilization of cell as well as tissue energy substrates [**38**]. Use of ω3 fatty acids as part of nutritional intervention in ESRV might also result in stabilization of the atherosclerotic plaque, thus facilitating the work of angiologist surgeon [**39**]. Morever, it has been reported that use of parenteral lipids solutions incorporating fish oil as a source of ω3 fatty acids shortened hospital length of stay of patients electively subjected to abdominal aortic aneurysm surgery [**40**]. However, is should be remembered that prolonged use of ω3 fatty acids might modify shape, size, distribution and lipid composition of HDL High density Lipoproteins that have been linked to a reduced risk of atherosclerotic damage [**41**].
Dietetic fiber could be another nutrient capable to influence upon response to ESRV. Low dietetic fiber intakes have been described after surveys completed in obese subjects [**42-43**]. Low dietetic fiber intakes have been associated with occurrence of blood lipid disorders and increased peripheral resistance to insulin action [**44**]. Supply of dietetic fiber might improve cell/tissue response to insulin's stimulatory action, and hence, altered states of carbohydrates peripheral utilization [**45**]. Likewise, dietetic fiber might also modify features and distribution of plasma lipoproteins in charge of Cholesterol and triglycerides transportation [**46**].
Finally, being hyperglycemia the first complication associated with/derived from body weight excess upon which to intervene after ESRV, alternative sugars solutions to Glucose should be made available to the angiologist surgeon for energy supply to the patient. Several alternative sugars have been proposed, such as xylitol, glucitol and sorbitol [**47**]. Glycerol: the poly-alcohol supplying the carbon backbone sustaining triglycerides's structure, has also been proposed as an alternative substrate to Glucose in post-surgical settings where insulin resistance, hyperglycemia, and hypertrygliceridemia are to be expected [**48**].

7. Clinical case: Ischemia-reperfusion syndrome - Influence upon nutritional status and response to ESRV

Complicated atherosclerosis is associated with a reduced blood irrigation of regions distal to atherosclerotic lesion, and hence, chronic tissue ischemia. When blood supply is restored after ESRV, molecular signals generated by until-that-moment ischemic tissues enter the blood stream. Systemic influence of such molecular signals might simulate the shock picture firstly described in people trapped in collapses [**49**]. Ischemia-reperfusion syndrome thus configured might affect nutritional status of patient subjected to ESRV, and complicate the implementation of designed nutritional support scheme.
Case presentation: The case is presented of a 55 years-old, white female, being admitted to a referral, terminal Angiology and Vascular Surgery Service for surgical correction of a mesenteric-aorto-iliac atheromatosis. The list with health problems identified in this patient is displayed in Table 2. During the surgical act, an aorto-iliac derivation was made, along with reopening of the superior mesenteric artery and placement of a bypass. Post-surgical evolution was torpid, marked by a Multiple Organs Dysfunction event, local as well as systematic sepsis, and a SIRS Systemic Inflammatory Response System. Health problems presented during post-operatory follow-up were all medically treated. Eventually the patient overcome these problems and was discharged from the Service.

Pr 1. Chronic tobacco use.
Pr 2. Complicated mesenteric-aorto-iliac Atherosclerosis.
Pr 3. Moderate Energy Nutrient Malnutrition of the Marasmatic type.
  sPr 3.1 Sixteen Kg weight loss during the last 6 months.
  - Volitional enteral Nutrition: Generic, fiberless, polimeric diet: 400 Kcal.24 h-1

H1: Mesenteric insufficiency.
  - Jejunum biopsy: No villous atrophy is observed. Mild congestion of lymph and blood vessels.

Pr 4. Peripheral arterial insufficiency.
  sPr 4.1 Intermittent claudication.
  - Oriented pharmacological treatment.
  - Laparotomy.
  - Aortic endarteriectomy.
  - Placement of an end-to-end aortic prosthesis.
  - Aorto-iliac bypass.
  - Superior mesenteric-aortic bypass.

Pr 5. Complicated Endarteriectomy Post-operatory Status.
  sPr 5.1 Systemic sepsis: Bacterial bronchopneumonia.
  - ATB: Cefotaxime+Gentamicine

  sPr 5.2 Local sepsis: Moniliasic glosytis
  - Nistatine mouth washes.

Pr 6. Multiple Organ Disfunction
  sPr 6.1 Small bowel dysfunction: Diarrheas.
  - Nils per Oris
  - Central Parenteral Nutrition: Dextrose 10%: 800 Kcal.24 h-1 + Aminoacids 10%: 50 g.24 h-1

  sPr 6.2 Lung dysfunction: Lung congestion.
  sPr 6.3 Liver dysfunction: Prolonged coagulogram.
  - K Vitamin administration.

  sPr 6.4 Heart dysfunction: Acute heart insufficiency.
  - Treatment w/ Digitalics.
  - Heart function support w/ Amines

  sPr 6.5 Bone marrow dysfunction: Anemia
  - Blood transfusion: Two 500 mL-bags of blood.

Pr 7. SIRS Systemic Inflammatory Response Syndrome.
  sPr 7.1 Hydroelectrolitic disorders.
  sPr 7.2 Upper digestive bleeding.
  H2: Stress ulcers
  - Nils per Oris
  - Interruption of Central Parenteral Nutrition scheme.

Table 2. Patient's health problems listing.

Table 3 shows the evolution of selected nutritional as well as welfare markers collected during the patient's treatment window. Weight loss accentuated during post-operatory evolution, as expression of existing tissue catabolism. Haemoglobin values never went beyond the 120 $g.L^{-1}$ limit. Observed anemia might compound several causes, among them, insufficient supply of nutrients. A marked lymphopenia was observed, as expression of the immune suppression accompanying SIRS installed during post-operatory evolution. Serum Cholesterol values were lower than 3.5 mmol.L^{-1}, confirming inflammatory status present in the patient as response to the ischemia-reperfusion syndrome. Interestingly, depletion of serum Albumin values was not observed, pointing to a liver function preserved enough to sustain nitrogen anabolism. This circumstance might explain the patient's favorable evolution, in spite of recorded events. There was also constancy of serum Creatinine values, indicating a conserved depurative kidney function for securing inner milieu homeostasis.

Day of Evolution	Weight, Kg	MAC, Cm	Hb, g.L-1	TLC, cél.mm3	S-Cre, umol.L-1	S-Alb, g.L-1	S-Chol, mmol.L-1
-58	36.0		102	2478	59.7	40.0	
-26	35.0						
-15			117		61.0	44.0	3.9
-12	33.0	20.3					
-3	35.0	20.0					
-1			105				
0			90				
+2			111		67.6		
+3	37.0	21.0	141	1782			
+4			157	1496	53.0	32.5	
+9	40.0						
+11			75		46.6		
+12	40.0	20.0					
+13			75	1188			
+14					41.0		
+17			92	888	67.0		
+19			99		52.0		3.1
+22			54	459			
+24			105				
+30				1320	56.0		
+37	32.0	17.0	116				
+44			109	3960	67.6	38.0	4.7
+132	41.0						
+151			108		91.3		4.5

Legend: MAC: Mid-arm-circumference. Hb: Hemoglobin. TLC: Total Lympochytes Count. S-Cre: Serum Creatinine. S-Alb: Serum Albumin. S-Chol: Serum Cholesterol.

Table 3. Behavior of selected nutritional as well as welfare markers of the patient discussed in the "Clinical case presentation" section. Shaded boxes indicate abnormal values of the corresponding marker. See text for further details.

Hemodynamic instability situation experienced by the patient during post-operatory course prevented the installment of coherent nutritional support schemes. This can be better appreciated in Figure 5. Important discontinuities in the use of the oral route for sustaining nutritional status were observed during the 20 days following the surgical act. Bowel insufficiency warned against the use of enteral nutrients during this stage as a substitute for oral feedings. In spite of all these events, the hospital NST Nutritional Support Team always stood for timely rehabilitation of the oral route, and prescribed the supply of energy as low-density Dextrose solutions. A hyperglycemia event (serum Glucose: 22.1 mmol.L^{-1}) was identified on day +13 of post-surgical evolution, forcing to momentarily interrupt the infusion of Dextrose solutions. Eventually, once hemodynamic stability was achieved, organic function recovered, and sepsis foci controlled, oral route was used for satisfying patient's nutrients needs. This action, along with parenteral aminoacids supplementation, might have been determinant in patient's response to ESRV.

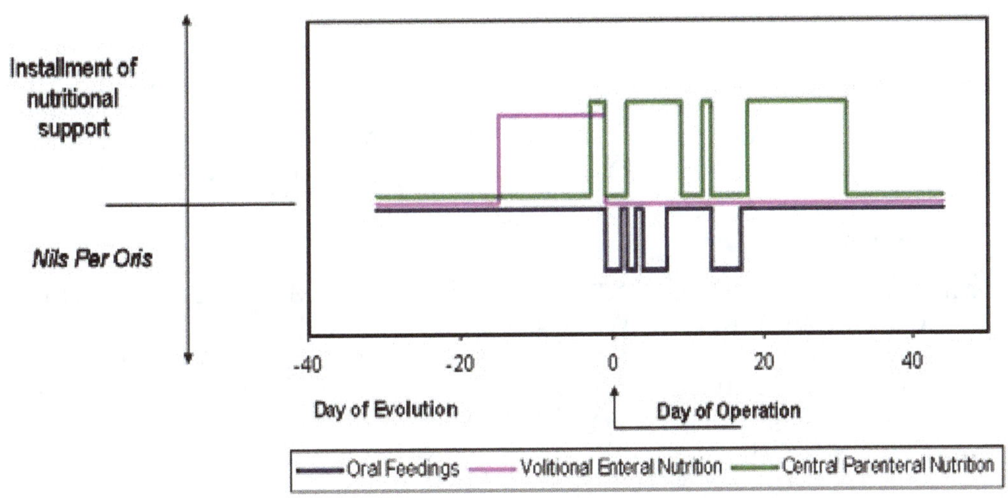

Fig. 5. Behavior of nutritional support during follow-up of the patient discussed in "Clinical case presentation" section. Discontinuities in the use of oral route are represented as falls of the solid blue line. Conduction of artificial nutritional schemes is symbolized as surges arising from the corresponding baseline. See text for further details.

8. Conclusions

The results of a study model of metabolic response to stress conveyed by ESRV have been presented in this work. Body weight excess might become a predictor of post-surgical complications. This hypothesis will be reformulated in future works in order to explore if occurrence of complications after ESRV can be traced back to the different facets of Insulin resistance Syndrome associated to body weight excess, such as arterial hypertension, hyperglycemia, blood lipid disorders, and hyperuricemia, among others. It is expected that complications risk to be minimal among obese patients presenting with few stigmas of insulin resistance, but maximal in those exhibiting a critical number of such stigmas.

9. Final notice

The preceding discussion has focused on the link between nutrition and aortic aneurysm as an extreme form of aorto-iliac atherosclerotic disease, given the involvement of the author with the practice of a referral, tertiary Angiology Service. However, aortic aneurysm might result from other, atherosclerosis-independent causes. The case is presented of a teen-ager suffering from an aortic aneurysm of probable mycological origin being assisted at a medical surgical clinic in Havana City [**50**]. Size of aneurysm prevented oral feeding, thus causing a significant nutritional derangement. Central Parenteral nutrition using premixed, all-in-one admixtures (NutriFlex Lipid Peri, B | BRAUN, Melsungen, Germany) was started in order to sustain patient's nutritional status, and improve metabolic response to surgical trauma.

10. Acknowledgements

Dr. Fernando Vaquero Morillo, Director of ANGIOLOGIA, bimonthly journal of the Spanish Society of Angiology and Vascular Surgery, for his support and cooperation.

11. References

Hirsch AT, Haskal ZJ, Hertzer NR, Bakal CW, Creager MA, Halperin JL, Hiratzka LF, Murphy WR, Olin JW, Puschett JB, Rosenfield KA, Sacks D, Stanley JC, Taylor LM Jr, White CJ, White J, White RA, Antman EM, Smith SC Jr, Adams CD, Anderson JL, Faxon DP, Fuster V, Gibbons RJ, Hunt SA, Jacobs AK, Nishimura R, Ornato JP, Page RL, Riegel B; American Association for Vascular Surgery; Society for Vascular Surgery; Society for Cardiovascular Angiography and Interventions; Society for Vascular Medicine and Biology; Society of Interventional Radiology; ACC/AHA Task Force on Practice Guidelines Writing Committee to Develop Guidelines for the Management of Patients With Peripheral Arterial Disease; American Association of Cardiovascular and Pulmonary Rehabilitation; National Heart, Lung, and Blood Institute; Society for Vascular Nursing; TransAtlantic Inter-Society Consensus; Vascular Disease Foundation. ACC/AHA 2005 Practice Guidelines for the management of patients with peripheral arterial disease (lower extremity, renal, mesenteric, and abdominal aortic): a collaborative report from the American Association for Vascular Surgery/Society for Vascular Surgery, Society for

Cardiovascular Angiography and Interventions, Society for Vascular Medicine and Biology, Society of Interventional Radiology, and the ACC/AHA Task Force on Practice Guidelines (Writing Committee to Develop Guidelines for the Management of Patients With Peripheral Arterial Disease): endorsed by the American Association of Cardiovascular and Pulmonary Rehabilitation; National Heart, Lung, and Blood Institute; Society for Vascular Nursing; TransAtlantic Inter- Society Consensus; and Vascular Disease Foundation. Circulation 2006;113:e463- e654.

Mariné ML, Valdés EF, Mertens MR, Krämer SchA, Bergoeing RM, Rivera DD, Vergara GJ, Carvajal NC. Open and endovascular surgery for the treatment of abdominal aortic aneurysm. Review of the available evidence. Rev Med Chil 2009;137:1081-8.

Jaakkola P, Hippeläinen M, Oksala I. Infrarenal aortofemoral bypass surgery: risk factors and mortality in 330 patients with abdominal aortic aneurysm or aortoiliac occlusive disease. Ann Chir Gynaecol 1996;85(1):28-35.

Fontaine R, Kolh P, Creemers E, Gerard P, Kerstenne MA, Van Damme H, Limet R. Open surgery for abdominal aortic aneurysm or aorto-iliac occlusive disease--clinical and ultrasonographic long-term results. Acta Chir Belg. 2008 Jul-Aug;108(4):393-9.

Mullen JL, Gertner MH, Buzby GP, Goodhart GL, Rosato EF. Implication of malnutrition in the surgical patient. Arch Surg 1979;114:121-5.

Windsor JA, Hill GL. Protein depletion and surgical risk. Aust NZ J Surg 1988;58:711-5.

Sungurtekin H, Sungurtekin U, Balci C, Zencir M, Erdem E. The influence of nutritional status on complications after major intraabdominal surgery. J Am Coll Nutr 2004;23:227-32.

Ortiz Reyes S, Aguilar Martínez F, Llanes Díaz G, González Díaz ME, González Villalonga JA, Santana Porbén S, Barreto Penie J. Valor predictivo de la encuesta subjetiva global en la conducta quirúrgica y la evolución posoperatoria del cancer colorrectal Revista Mexicana de Coloproctología 2005;11:114-22.

Pacelli F, Bossola M, Rosa F, Tortorelli AP, Papa V, Doglietto GB. Is malnutrition still a risk factor of postoperative complications in gastric cancer surgery? Clin Nutr 2008;27:398-407.

Anónimo. Etiology of atherosclerosis- special reference to humoral and neurogenic factors. Nippon Rinsho 2011;69:39-44.

Hermus L, Lefrandt JD, Tio RA, Breek JC, Zeebregts CJ. Carotid plaque formation and serum biomarkers. Atherosclerosis 2010;213:21-9.

Weingärtner O, Lütjohann D, Böhm M, Laufs U. Cholesterol homeostasis and cardiovascular risk. Dtsch Med Wochenschr 2011;136:34-8.

Motoyama A, Saito R, Fujibayashi K, Aoki H, Kajinami K.Disorder in lipid metabolism. Nippon Rinsho 2010;68(Suppl 8):364-9.

Ashburn DD, Reed MJ. Endocrine system and obesity. Crit Care Clin 2010;26:633-6.

Gilardini L, Pasqualinotto L, Di Matteo S, Caffetto K, Croci M, Girola A, Invitti C. Factors associated with early atherosclerosis and arterial calcifications in young subjects with a benign phenotype of obesity. Obesity (Silver Spring). 27 de Enero del 2011. Epub ahead of print.

García Lorda P. Role of lipid intake in obesity. Nutr Hosp 2002;17(Suppl 1):67-72. Astrup A. The role of dietary fat in obesity. Semin Vasc Med 2005;5:40-7.

Gaesser GA. Carbohydrate quantity and quality in relation to body mass index. J Am Diet Assoc 2007;107:1768-80.

Siri-Tarino PW, Sun Q, Hu FB, Krauss RM. Saturated fatty acids and risk of coronary heart disease: modulation by replacement nutrients. Curr Atheroscler Rep 2010;12:384-90.

Glinsberg HN. Insulin resistance and its relation to coronary artery disease. J Clin Invest 2000;106:453-8.

Tomkin GH. Atherosclerosis, diabetes and lipoproteins. Expert Rev Cardiovasc Ther 2010;8:1015-29.

Wójkowska-Mach J, Bulanda M, Cencora A, Jawień A, Szczypta A, Rózańska A y cols. Surgical site infections following vascular surgery. Przegl Epidemiol 2007;61: 683-91.

Dempsey DT, Mullen JL, Buzby GP. The link between nutritional status and clinical outcome: can nutritional intervention modify it? Am J Clin Nutr 1988;47: 352-6.

Kavalukas SL, Barbul A. Nutrition and wound healing: an update. Plast Reconstr Surg 2011;127 (Suppl 1):38S-43S.

García Lizame ML, Eliseo Mussenden O, Peguero Brínguez Y, Díaz Hernández O, Santana Porbén S. Influencia del estado nutricional en los resultados de la cirugía revascularizadora del sector aortoilíaco. Angiología [España] 2009;61:315-24.

Kotler DP, Tierney AR, Wang J, Pierson RN Jr. Magnitude of body-cell-mass depletion and the timing of death from wasting in AIDS. Am J Clin Nutr 1989;50:444-7.

Harris CL, Fraser C. Malnutrition in the institutionalized elderly: the effects on wound healing. Ostomy Wound Manage 2004;50:54-63.

Esposito S. Immune system and surgical site infection. J Chemother 2001;13 Spec No 1: 12-6.

Barchfeld T, Schönhofer B. Difficult weaning. Pneumologie 2006;60:616-28.

Stratton RJ, Marinos E. Who benefits from nutritional support: what is the evidence? Eur J Gastroenterol Hepatol 2007;19:353-8.

Mowery NT, May AK, Collier BC, Dossett LA, Gunter OL, Dortch MJ, Diaz JJ Jr. Glucose metabolism, not obesity, predicts mortality in critically ill surgical patients. Am Surg 2010;76:1377-83.

Santana Porbén S, Barreto Penié J. Metabolismo de los sustratos. En: Manual de Nutrición Enteral y Parenteral (Editores: Arenas Márquez H, Anaya Prado R). Editorial Interamericana McGraw-Hill. Ciudad México: 2007. pp 23

Rosen ED, Spiegelman BM. Adipocytes as regulators of energy balance and glucose homeostasis. Nature 2006;444:847-53.

Mullen JT, Moorman DW, Davenport DL. The obesity paradox: body mass index and outcomes in patients undergoing nonbariatric general surgery. Ann Surg 2009;250:166-72.

Kuk JL, Saunders TJ, Davidson LE, Ross R. Age-related changes in total and regional fat distribution. Ageing Res Rev 2009;8:339-48.

Lerman Garber I, Rosales Calderón M. Changes in glucose tolerance in elderly. Rev Invest Clin 2010;62:312-7.

Chapkin RS, Kim W, Lupton JR, McMurray DN. Dietary docosahexaenoic and eicosapentaenoic acid: emerging mediators of inflammation. Prostaglandins Leukot Essent Fatty Acids 2009;81:187-91.

Saremi A, Arora R. The utility of omega-3 fatty acids in cardiovascular disease. Am J Ther 2009;16:421-36.

Cawood AL, Ding R, Napper FL, Young RH, Williams JA, Ward MJ, Gudmundsen O, Vige R, Payne SP, Ye S, Shearman CP, Gallagher PJ, Grimble RF, Calder PC. Eicosapentaenoic acid (EPA) from highly concentrated n-3 fatty acid ethyl esters is incorporated into advanced atherosclerotic plaques and higher plaque EPA is associated with decreased plaque inflammation and increased stability. Atherosclerosis 2010;212:252-9.

Berger MM, Tappy L, Revelly JP, Koletzko BV, Gepert J, Corpataux JM, Cayeux MC, Chiolero RL. Fish oil after abdominal aorta aneurysm surgery. Eur J Clin Nutr 2008 ;62 :1116-22.

Balk EM, Lichtenstein AH, Chung M, Kupelnick B, Chew P, Lau J. Effects of omega-3 fatty acids on serum markers of cardiovascular disease risk: a systematic review. Atherosclerosis 2006;189:19-30.

Gaesser GA. Carbohydrate quantity and quality in relation to body mass index. J Am Diet Assoc 2007;107:1768-80.

Linde JA, Utter J, Jeffery RW, Sherwood NE, Pronk NP, Boyle RG. Specific food intake, fat and fiber intake, and behavioral correlates of BMI among overweight and obese members of a managed care organization. Int J Behav Nutr Phys Act 2006;3:42.

Liese AD, Roach AK, Sparks KC, Marquart L, D'Agostino RB Jr, Mayer-Davis EJ. Whole-grain intake and insulin sensitivity: the Insulin Resistance Atherosclerosis Study. Am J Clin Nutr 2003;78:965-71.

Li SC, Liu YH, Liu JF, Chang WH, Chen CM, Chen CY. Almond consumption improved glycemic control and lipid profiles in patients with type 2 diabetes mellitus. Metabolism 2011;60:474-9.

Estruch R, Martínez-González MA, Corella D, Basora-Gallisá J, Ruiz-Gutiérrez V, Covas MI, Fiol M, Gómez-Gracia E, López-Sabater MC, Escoda R, Pena MA, Diez-Espino J, Lahoz C, Lapetra J, Sáez G, Ros E; PREDIMED Study Investigators. Effects of dietary fibre intake on risk factors for cardiovascular disease in subjects at high risk. J Epidemiol Community Health 2009; 63:582-8.

Georgieff M, Moldawer LL, Bistrian BR, Blackburn GL. Xylitol, an energy source for intravenous nutrition after trauma. JPEN J Parenter Enter Nutr 1985;9:199-209.

Sun LC, Shih YL, Lu CY, Chen FM, Hsieh JS, Chuang JF, Wang JY. Randomized controlled study of glycerol versus dextrose in postoperative hypocaloric peripheral parenteral nutrition. J Invest Surg 2006;19:381-5.

Haglund U. The splanchnic organs as the sources of toxic mediators in shock. Prog Clin Biol Res 1988;264:135-45.

Alvarez Rodríguez A. Soporte Nutricional en un caso de aneurisma aorto-abdominal. Uso de los lípidos parenterales. RCAN Rev Cubana Aliment Nutr 2010;20:S17-S20. Available at: http://www.revicubalimentanut.sld.cu/Vol_20_1/SimposioLipidosNutricionArtif icial.pdf. Last visited on: Wednesday, June 01, 2011.

10

Role of Cathepsin K, L and S in Blood Vessel Remodeling

Andriy O. Samokhin and Dieter Brömme
University of British Columbia, Vancouver, Canada

1. Introduction

The development of cardiovascular diseases is characterized by the loss of structural integrity of blood vessels that requires extensive remodeling of the extra-cellular matrix (Michel et al., 2011; Garcia-Touchard et al., 2005). The entire aorta and some medium-sized arteries have elastic properties and mechanical strength allowing these vessels to withstand a surge of blood ejected from the heart. Such properties of blood vessels are contributed mostly by two major components of the extracellular matrix: elastin and collagen (Barbour et al., 2007; Wagenseil & Mecham, 2009; Sawabe, 2010). Elastin fibers are responsible for the elastic properties and collagen fibers provide mechanical strength to the arterial wall (Arteaga-Solis et al., 2000). These two proteins have a fibrillar structure and in their mature forms are very resistant to proteolysis. Thus elastin has a half-life around 50 years (Wagenseil & Mecham, 2009). However in some pathological conditions, excessive proteolytic activity results in extracellular matrix breakdown that is a key factor of arterial wall damage and the development of potential rupture. Sites of atherosclerotic and aneurysmatic lesions are characterized by increased elasto- and collagenolytic activity (Diehm et al., 2007; Shimizu et al., 2006; Barbour et al., 2007; Sukhova et al., 1998). The dominant histological feature of aneurysmatic lesions is a chronic medial and adventitial inflammation resulting in medial degeneration and smooth muscle cell apoptosis. One of the most important contributors to aneurysmatic degeneration is an excessive loss of extracellular matrix. Fragmentation of elastin and collagen fibers is a characteristic feature of aneurysm formation and their loss is the ultimate cause of aneurysmatic rupture as well as rupture of atherosclerotic plaques (Shimizu et al., 2006; Sakalihasan et al., 2005; Diehm et al., 2007). Recently it has been shown that together with some matrix metalloproteinases, cathepsin K, L and S are the primary proteolytic culprits responsible for the breakdown of extracellular matrix proteins in blood vessels (Abdul-Hussien et al., 2010; Rizas et al., 2009; Sukhova & Shi, 2006). Cysteine proteinases cathepsin K, L and S belong to the most potent elasto- and/or collagenolytic proteinases with potent abilities to degrade extracellular matrix. These enzymes attracted attention due to their upregulation within the aortic wall under different pathological conditions (Lutgens et al., 2007; Lafarge et al., 2010; Liu et al., 2004). Their expression was revealed in macrophages, smooth muscle cells and endothelial cells in atherosclerotic and aneurismal lesions in humans. These results instigated a series of studies on the involvement of cathepsin K, L and S in the development of cardiovascular diseases based on animal models of atherosclerosis and abdominal aortic aneurysm formation (Lutgens et al., 2007; Lafarge et al., 2010; Liu et al., 2004). The lack of these proteases resulted in a plaque size reduction and delay of plaque progression as well as in reduced level of medial elastin degradation and smooth muscle cell transmigration from the media to the intima (Lutgens et al., 2006a; Rodgers et al., 2006; Samokhin et al., 2008; Sukhova et al., 2003). These results were corroborated by in vitro experiments that revealed the differences in collageno- and elastolytic activities of smooth muscle cells and macrophages from mice expressing and lacking these cathepsins.

The availability of specific cathepsin inhibitors allowed the conduction of *in vitro* and *in vivo* experiments that confirmed the involvement of cathepsins in aortic extracellular matrix destruction and atherosclerosis progression (Samokhin et al., 2010b) Immunostaining for cathepsin K revealed its high level of expression in multinucleated giant cells in human specimens from carotid arteries and abdominal aortic aneurysm as well as in mouse atherosclerotic plaques (Samokhin et al., 2010c; Chapman et al., 1997). High level of cathepsin K expression is a marker of active osteoclasts; in these giant cells cathepsin K is a major enzyme responsible for bone resorption (Bromme et al., 1996). Similarly, cathepsin K-expressing giant cells were found close to damaged elastin laminae in aorta, suggesting an important role for this enzyme in the development of cardiovascular diseases (Samokhin et al., 2010c; Chapman et al., 1997).

2. Extracellular matrix of the aortic wall

Elastin and fibrillar collagen are the main components of the arterial wall responsible for its mechanical properties (Wagenseil & Mecham, 2009; Arteaga-Solis et al., 2000; Sawabe, 2010). Elastin is the major protein that confers elastic properties to the arterial wall. It is produced by smooth muscle cells of the tunica media in form of the soluble precursor tropoelastin and after polymerization by lysyl oxidase, forms interconnecting concentric rings around the arterial lumen. A high number of cross-links (15-20 per tropoelastin unit) is responsible for elastin insolubility, long half-life and resistance to proteolysis (Wagenseil & Mecham, 2009; Arteaga-Solis et al., 2000; Sawabe, 2010). Elastin fibers are formed by elastin and associated microfibrils. Microfibrils form a scaffold for elastin polymerization and they are mainly composed of fibrillin and a collagen type IV (Sawabe, 2010; Pasquali-Ronchetti & Baccarani-Contri, 1997). This three-dimensional network of interconnecting elastin fibers is designed to transfer stress throughout the arterial walls and is responsible for their dilation and recoil (Wagenseil & Mecham, 2009; Shadwick, 1999). The aortic wall is characterized by the abundant presence of elastic fibers associated with smooth muscle cells in the medial area (Barbour et al., 2007, Sakalihasan et al., 2005). Elastic fibers are also interconnected with collagen bundles (Wagenseil & Mecham, 2009).

Collagen is made up of a triple helix of three polypeptide chains. Types I, II and III collagens belong to "fibrillar" collagens that are the most abundant (van der Rest & Garrone, 1991). Types I and III collagens provide tensile strength and maintain the structural integrity of the blood vessels. In aorta these two types of collagens are mostly found in media and adventitia (Wagenseil & Mecham, 2009; Barbour et al., 2007; Sakalihasan et al., 2005). Types IV, V, and VI are nonfibrillar collagens highly present in the basement membrane. Fibrillar collagens type I and III are highly resistant towards proteolysis. They can be degraded only by specific collagenases that are able to cleave within the triple helix of native fibrillar collagen (Abdul-Hussien et al., 2007).

Medial elastin and collagens types I and II in the media and adventitia determine much of the structural integrity and stability of arteries (Shimizu et al., 2006; Arteaga-Solis et al.,

2000). The increased turnover of elastin and collagen results in aortic dilation and possible rupture (Shimizu et al., 2006). The fragmentation and loss of collagen and elastin fibers is one of the most important and consistent histological features of aneurismal changes in aorta (Dobrin & Mrkvicka, 1994; Barbour et al., 2007).

Because of the long half-life of collagen fibers and the extremely long half-life of elastin, loss of these two extracellular matrix proteins almost certainly results from increased degradation rather than decreased synthesis. Indeed, the predominant role of increased proteolysis is well described for the pathogenesis of aneurysm formation (Barbour et al., 2007; Sakalihasan et al., 2005; Michel et al., 2011). Traditionally, matrix metalloproteinases were considered the main culprits in blood vessel extracellular matrix cleavage (Kadoglou & Liapis, 2004; Newby, 2008), whereas some recent data point out to the important role of cathepsin K, L and S in this pathological process (Chapman et al., 1997; Shimizu et al., 2006; Abisi et al., 2007).

3. Cathepsin K, L and S are strong extracellular matrix-degrading enzymes

Cathepsin K, L and S are lysosomal cysteine proteases of the papain family. These enzymes share many common features but also have significant differences in distribution, activity and corresponding physiological functions. Cathepsin K has the highest level of expression in osteoclasts and plays a major role in collagen turnover in bones (Bromme et al., 1996). This protease is also expressed at lower levels in macrophages, epithelial cells, fibroblasts, smooth muscle cells which can be elevated under pathological conditions (Chapman et al., 1997). Thus, high cathepsin K concentration was found in rheumatoid arthritic joints, in epithelioid and multinucleated giant cells in lungs, and in thyroid glands (Buhling et al., 2004; Samokhin et al., 2010a; Tepel et al., 2000). Cathepsin K is not detectable in normal blood vessels, but is highly expressed in macrophages, smooth muscle cells, endothelial and multinucleated giant cells in atherosclerotic lesions and in giant cell aortitis (Sukhova et al., 1998; Platt et al., 2007; Chapman et al., 1997; Samokhin et al., 2010c). Cathepsin K is the most efficient elastinolytic enzyme (Bromme et al., 1996) and, in contrast to other cathepsins, has the ability to cleave triple-helical collagens both outside and inside the helical regions (Lecaille et al., 2008; Garnero et al., 1998). This unique feature enables cathepsin K to perform complete cleavage of collagens, a process that usually requires a cooperative action of several extracellular matrix-degrading enzymes.

Cathepsin S is predominantly expressed in spleen and antigen-presenting cells, including B cells, macrophages, dendritic and epithelial cells (Chapman et al., 1997; Gupta et al., 2008). In these cells, cathepsin S plays an important role in the proteolytic degradation of the invariant chain, thus regulating antigen presentation to $CD4^+$ T-cells by MHC II molecules (Honey & Rudensky, 2003; Hsing & Rudensky, 2005). In addition to its role in the immune response, cathepsin S can be secreted by such cells as macrophages, smooth muscle cells, endothelial cells and some tumor cells (Gupta et al., 2008) and plays an important role in extracellular matrix remodeling. Similarly to cathepsin K, cathepsin S shows strong collagenolytic and elastolytic activities and in contrast to cathepsin K and L, this protease is more stable and retains activity at neutral pH (Chapman et al., 1997; Taleb & Clement, 2007). Under pathological conditions, cathepsin S is upregulated in lung and blood vessel tissues and its stability at neutral pH may significantly contribute to the degradation of the extracellular matrix (Deschamps et al., 2010; Samokhin et al., 2011; Hirakawa et al., 2007; Williams et al., 2009).

Cathepsin L is ubiquitously expressed and similarly to cathepsin S, plays an important role in the immune system by degrading the invariant chain in MHC class II processing (Honey & Rudensky, 2003; Hsing & Rudensky, 2005). Mice lacking cathepsin L have epidermal hyperplasia with periodic hair loss, older animals develop dilative cardiomyopathy (Lankelma et al., 2010; Reinheckel et al., 2005). This enzyme is also involved in the development of kidney diseases in mice and humans and is upregulated in a variety of cancers (Reiser et al., 2010). Cathepsin L is a potent elastase (equivalent to cathepsin S) and collagenase (similar to cathepsin K) (Chapman et al., 1997). The physiological role of mouse cathepsins L is most likely replaced by cathepsin V in human tissues (Tolosa et al., 2003).

A common feature of these cathepsins is their strong ability to degrade elastin and collagen fibers. Cathepsins have attracted attention as extracellular matrix-degrading enzymes only recently. Previously it was assumed that they are inactive outside of cells due to their instability at neutral pH. However under pathological conditions, the acidification of the pericellular environment creates optimal conditions for lysosomal cathepsins. Thus, the destruction of elastin-rich arteries is associated with the accumulation of macrophages. In inflammatory conditions, macrophages secrete cathepsin K, L and S and at the same time increase expression of vacuolar-type H^+-ATPase (Punturieri et al., 2000; Reddy et al., 1995). H^+-ATPase acidifies the local environment and creates optimal conditions for cathepsin activities. Such increased expression of H^+-ATPase has been revealed by immunohistochemical analysis in AAA in infiltrating monocytes and to a lesser extend in SMCs (Abdul-Hussien et al., 2010).

In addition to their direct destructive role in blood vessel remodeling, cathepsins may promote the development of cardiovascular diseases by degrading lipoproteins and through their involvement in the regulation of apoptosis (Linke et al., 2006; Conus & Simon, 2008; Repnik & Turk, 2010).

4. Increased expression of cathepsin K, L and S under pathological conditions in blood vessels

4.1 Atherosclerosis

Increased expression of cathepsin K and S in human atherosclerotic lesions was first described in 1998 (Sukhova et al., 1998). Until that time cathepsin K, L and S were already known as strong collagenases and elastases and researchers found a correlation between increased immunostaining for cathepsin K and S and increased elastase-degrading activity in atheromatous tissues extracts. The use of cathepsin and MMP inhibitors revealed that cathepsins had significantly greater contribution to elastolytic activity of atherosclerotic lesions extracts. Cathepsin K and S immunoreactivities were mostly localized in the fibrous cap region that suggested their important role in plaque destabilization (Sukhova et al., 1998; Rodgers et al., 2006). In addition, smooth muscle cells cultured with IFN-γ or interleukin-1β secreted active cathepsin S and showed significantly increased ability to degrade elastin. This elastolytic activity was abrogated by a selective cathepsin S inhibitor (Sukhova et al., 1998). In a similar experiment, a selective cathepsin S inhibitor or endogenous cathepsin inhibitor cystatin C significantly decreased SMC migration across an elastin gel (Cheng et al., 2006). In human atherosclerotic plaques cathepsins were localized in macrophages, SMCs and endothelial cells (Platt et al., 2007; Sukhova et al., 1998). The destructive role of cathepsin K in macrophage foam cells was confirmed by immunohistochemical analysis that revealed accumulation of collagen type I degradation products close to cathepsin K immunoreactivity. These results were supported by an *in vitro* experiment where incubation of human macrophage foam cells on a collagen matrix resulted in the accumulation of collagen degradation products (Barascuk et al., 2010). Cathepsin K expression in endothelial cells in human atherosclerotic plaques also correlated with internal elastic lamina destruction (Platt et al., 2007).

Similarly to cathepsin K and S, cathepsin L shows weak or no immunostaining in normal human arteries but its immunoreactivity increases significantly in atherosclerotic lesions and localizes in the fibrous cap and tunica media (Liu et al., 2006). Double immunostaining revealed that cathepsin L is mostly expressed in macrophages of the plaque shoulder regions, endothelial and smooth muscle cells. Serum cathepsin L level correlated with the development of atherosclerotic lesions (Liu et al., 2006). Furthermore, expression of cathepsin L correlated with apoptosis, formation of the necrotic core, decrease in collagen content and rupture of the fibrous cap (Li et al., 2009; Liu et al., 2006).

4.2 Aortic aneurysm

Increased expression of cathepsin K, L and S was found in abdominal aortic aneurysm and in popliteal artery aneurysm (Sukhova and Shi, 2006; Abdul-Hussien et al., 2010). Similarly to atherosclerosis, these enzymes were identified as major proteolytic culprits in abdominal aortic aneurysm and their expresion correlated with excessive collagen degradation (Abdul-Hussien et al., 2007). The activities of cathepsin S and L were increased in abdominal aortic aneurysms and ruptured abdominal aortic aneurysms, whereas cathepsin K activity was not elevated despite a significant increase in the level of activated cathepsin K protein in aortic extracts (Abdul-Hussien et al., 2007; Abisi et al., 2007). Increased expression of cathepsin L in abdominal aortic aneurysm was localized in SMCs, Ecs and macrophages (Li et al., 2009).

5. Studies of cathepsin K, L and S in mouse models of cardiovascular diseases

5.1 Atherosclerosis

The results of human studies prompted *in vivo* studies of the involvement of cathepsins in cardiovascular diseases using murine disease models. Apolipoprotein E- and low density lipoprotein receptor-deficient mice are widely used as animal models of atherosclerosis. These mice develop severe hypercholesterolemia and atherosclerosis similar to human atherosclerosis and atherosclerotic lesions progression can be accelerated by high fat diet. Firstly, the high expression of cathepsin L and S was shown in aorta of apolipoprotein E-deficient mice. Immunohistochemical analysis showed positive staining for cathepsins L and S in the intima and within fibrous caps and cathepsin S was also detected in the medial area (Jormsjo et al., 2002). Soon after that, the effect of cathepsin S deficiency on atherosclerosis development was reported in experiments with low density lipoprotein receptor-deficient mice (Sukhova et al., 2003). Low density lipoprotein receptor-deficient mice lacking cathepsin S showed significant reduction of plaque size and area, preserved integrity of elastic lamina and reduced smooth muscle cell and collagen contents in the intima when compared to mice expressing cathepsin S. Absence of cathepsin S also resulted in decreased macrophage and leukocyte accumulation in atherosclerotic plaques (Sukhova et al., 2003). The atheroprotective effect of cathepsin S deficiency was also confirmed by experiments with apolipoprotein E-deficient mice lacking this protease. (Rodgers et al., 2006). Atherosclerotic lesions in brachiocephalic arteries of apolipoprotein E-deficient and cathepsin S double deficient mice were significantly smaller and had fewer acute plaque ruptures. These mice also had a lower number of buried fibrous caps, which are believed to be a marker of unstable atherosclerotic plaques. The fibrous caps in plaques of double knockout mice were also thicker compared to cathepsin S-expressing mice that most likely rendered higher stability to those plaques (Rodgers et al., 2006). Recently, the role of cathepsin S in atherosclerosis was investigated in chimeric low density lipoprotein receptor-deficient mice lacking this protease in leukocytes (de Nooijer et al., 2009). The absence of cathepsin S in leukocytes did not change the lesion size but reduced the necrotic core and changed plaque morphology. Chimeric mice contained more macrophages and less intimal smooth muscle cells and collagen. The lower number of intimal smooth muscle cells correlated with the marked decrease in the number of elastin lamina ruptures providing evidence for an important role of leukocyte-derived cathepsin S in elastin lamina disruption in atherosclerosis (de Nooijer et al., 2009).

The role of cathepsin K in atherosclerotic lesions development was investigated in apolipoprotein E-deficient mice (Lutgens et al., 2006b; Samokhin et al., 2008; Lutgens et al., 2006a). Cathepsin K deficiency reduced the total plaque area in the aortic arch of mice receiving normal diet (Lutgens et al., 2006a) as well as the plaque size in the brachiocephalic artery after 16 weeks of high fat diet (Samokhin et al., 2008). In both experiments mice lacking cathepsin K had a smaller number of elastin lamina ruptures and increased collagen content compared to cathepsin K-expressing mice. Cathepsin K-deficient mice on normal diet had a borderline significant decrease in plaque macrophage content but the individual size of macrophages was increased and showed increased lipid uptake (Lutgens et al., 2006b). Atherosclerotic plaques in the brachiocephalic artery of mice on high fat diet had a significant decrease in their macrophage content and an increase in collagen content after 8 weeks of high fat diet. Smooth muscle cell loss in medial area was significantly lower in cathepsin K-deficient mice after 16 weeks of high fat diet that correlated well with the decreased number of elastin lamina breaks (Samokhin et al., 2008). Atherosclerotic plaques in brachiocephalic arteries had thicker fibrous caps and a smaller number of buried fibrous caps in cathepsin K-deficient mice. Similarly to cathepsin S, the effect of cathepsin K deficiency in leukocytes was studied in chimeric low density lipoprotein receptor-deficient mice (Guo et al., 2009). Leukocytes cathepsin K deficiency did not affect the plaque size but decreased elastin lamina fragmentation as well as collagen content and increased plaque macrophage content and the necrotic area. The effect of cathepsin L deficiency was studied on low density lipoprotein receptor-deficient mice (Kitamoto et al., 2007). Double knockout mice developed reduced atherosclerotic lesions with smaller lipid core compared to cathepsin L-expressing mice. They also had a lower number of elastin lamina ruptures and a decreased amount of plaque macrophages, $CD4^+$ T-cells, smooth muscle cells and collagen. In *in vitro* experiments, cathepsin L-deficient smooth muscle cells showed delayed transmigration through an elastin layer, whereas cathepsin L-deficient monocytes and lymphocytes demonstrated reduced ability to migrate through collagen type I and IV coated transwell membranes. Based on these results, authors suggested that cathepsin L plays a significant role in medial smooth muscle cells and blood-borne leukocytes migration during development of atherosclerotic lesions (Kitamoto et al., 2007).

5.2 Aortic aneurysm

Increased expression of cathepsin K, L and S in blood vessels have been shown in several animal models of aneurysm induction. Cathepsin K and S were upregulated in a porcine model of abdominal aortic aneurysm (Sadek et al., 2008) and cathepsin L showed increased expression in a rabbit model of elastase-induced saccular aneurysm (Kadirvel et al., 2004).

The role of cathepsin K in aneurysm formation was investigated in a mouse model of aneurysm induction (Bai et al., 2010). Surprisingly, cathepsin K deficiency did not prevent aneurysm formation after angiotensin II infusion. Cathepsin K-lacking mice had the same aneurysm size and severity. The absence of cathepsin K did not prevent elastin degradation, whereas the collagen content was significantly increased in the aneurysm area in cathepsin K-lacking mice (Bai et al., 2010).

6. Cathepsin inhibitors in the prevention of pathological aortic remodeling

The highly destructive potential of cysteine cathepsins requires their tight regulation and one of such restrictive mechanisms is a presence of cathepsin inhibitors. Cystatin C is the most important inhibitor of cysteine cathepsins. It is a small protein expressed in virtually all organs and found in high concentration in biological fluids including blood (Shi et al., 1999). Cystatin C is present in normal blood vessels but its concentration significantly decreases in atherosclerotic and aneurismal lesions (Lindholt et al., 2001). Serum cystatin C level inversely correlated with abdominal aortic diameter in patients with abdominal aortic aneurysm (Shi et al., 1999). Animal experiments have shown that lack of cystatin C expression in apolipoprotein E-deficient mice results in more advanced atherosclerotic lesions with increased elastin lamina degradation and higher macrophage content (Bengtsson et al., 2005; Sukhova et al., 2005). In an angiotensin II-induced model of abdominal aortic aneurysm such mice showed aggravated destruction of elastin, increased cathepsin activity, fewer number of smooth muscle cells in tunica media and increased macrophage content and number of $CD4^{+}$ T cells (Schulte et al., 2010). Recently cathepsin K, L and S attracted a lot of attention as a potential therapeutic target in cardiovascular, bone and cartilage diseases (Turk, 2006; Bromme & Lecaille, 2009). The atheroprotective effect of a potent and selective cathepsin S inhibitor was tested in apolipoprotein E-deficient mice (Samokhin et al., 2010b). Animals receiving high fat diet containing the cathepsin S inhibitor developed significantly smaller plaques in brachiocephalic arteries, had smaller number of elastin ruptures, and lower levels of macrophages in plaques. Mice treated with cathepsin S inhibitor also showed a reduced number of buried fibrous caps providing evidence of more stable plaques. In this study, the cathepsin S inhibitor was also tested in peritoneal macrophages where cells showed reduced elastolytic activity (Samokhin et al., 2010b). This study also revealed some gender-related differences in atherosclerotic lesions development in response to inhibitor treatment. Female mice showed an almost 2-fold greater reduction in plaque sizes compared to the male group. The effectiveness of the cathepsin S inhibitor was verified by the build-up of intermediate invariant chain breakdown products in spleen. Cathepsin S plays an important role in MHC class II-associated antigen presentation by participating in proteolytic processing of invariant chain and its inhibition results in accumulation of invariant chain breakdown products (Honey & Rudensky, 2003). The inhibition of cathepsin S reflected most of the phenotype observed in experiments with cathepsin S-deficient mice (Sukhova, 2003; Rodgers, 2006) suggesting the high specificity of the inhibitor and the potential feasibility of the treatment of atherosclerosis with cathepsin inhibitors.

7. Cathepsin K is highly expressed in multinucleated giant cells in aortic wall

The presence of multinucleated giant cells within the aortic wall is described in giant cell arteritis and atherosclerosis. In these two diseases, multinucleated giant cells are formed by the fusion of macrophages in inflammatory infiltrates of the arterial wall (Weyand et al., 2005; Eberhardt & Dhadly, 2007; Soilleux et al., 2002). It was shown by immunohistochemical analysis and *in situ* hybridization that multinucleated giant cells from different organs and from patients with different pathological conditions have strong cathepsin K expression (Buhling et al., 2001; Chapman et al., 1997).

7.1 Multinucleated giant cells in human atherosclerotic plaques show strong staining for cathepsin K

The analysis of atherosclerotic plaques from carotid arteries and lesions from patients with abdominal aortic aneurisms revealed the presence of multinucleated giant cells (Fig. 1). Similarly to giant cells arteritis, they were mostly localized in the media-intima junction (Samokhin, 2010c). The lesions contained Langhans-type multinucleated giant cells recognizable by their circular arrangement of nuclei and foreign body-type giant cells with random arrangement of nuclei.

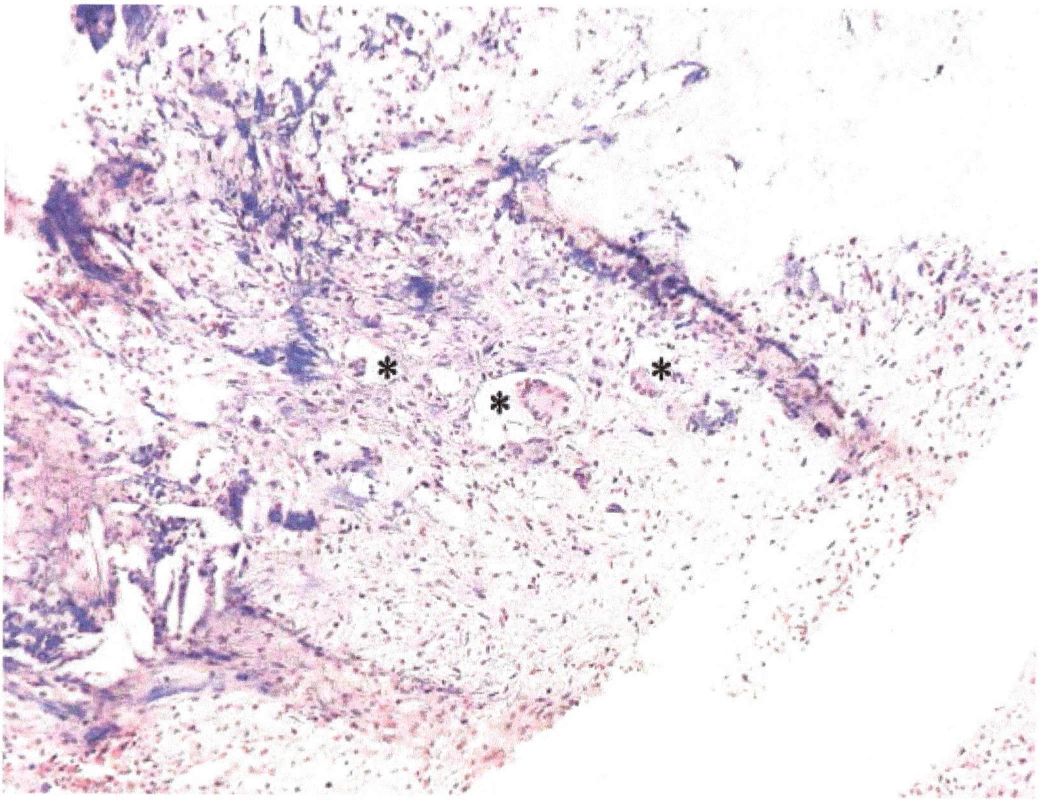

Fig. 1. Multinucleated giant cells in atherosclerotic lesions from carotid artery (trichrome staining, x10, asterisks show multinucleated giant cells).

Immunohistochemical analysis revealed strong expression of cathepsin K in multinucleated giant cells (Fig. 2). These results suggest an important role of cathepsin K from multinucleated giant cells in aortic wall damage in atherosclerosis and abdominal aortic aneurisms.

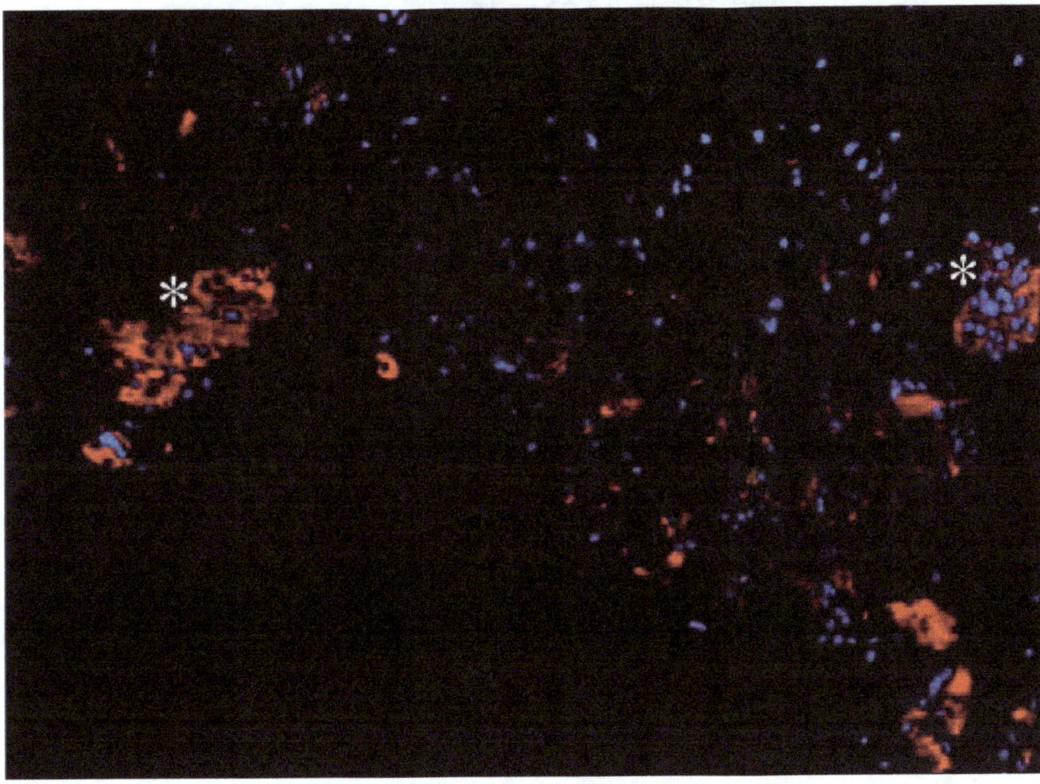

Fig. 2. Cathepsin K-positive multinucleated giant cells in atherosclerotic lesions from carotid artery (red - cathepsin K, blue - nuclei, x20, asterisks show multinucleated giant cells).

7.2 Multinucleated giant cells in mouse atherosclerotic plaques

Apolipoprotein E-deficient mice on cholate-containing high fat diet developed atherosclerotic lesions containing multinucleated giant cells (Fig. 3). These giant cells were observed in atherosclerotic plaques within the brachiocephalic artery and the aortic root and were easily detectable by intensive cathepsin K immunostaining (Samokhin et al., 2010c). They were mostly localized in the fibrous cap region and close to the elastin laminae. The presence of multinucleated giant cells correlated with the disruption of elastin fibers (Fig. 4) and the absence of smooth muscle cells within the tunica media. Similarly, in giant cell arteritis, multinucleated giant cells have been implicated in internal elastic laminae damage and their presence strongly correlated with smooth muscle cell migration (Kaiser et al., 1999; Penn & Dasgupta, 2003; Nordborg & Nordborg, 2003).

Cathepsin K plays a major role in the destructive potential of osteoclasts and is suggested as a marker of macrophage differentiation (Brömme et al., 1996; Buhling et al., 2001). In contrast to macrophages, multinucleated giant cells in atherosclerotic lesions of apolipoprotein E-deficient mice do not show strong immunostaining for cathepsin L and S (Samokhin; 2010c). These results suggest that cathepsin K plays a crucial role in the destructive potential of multinucleated giant cells in the aortic wall.

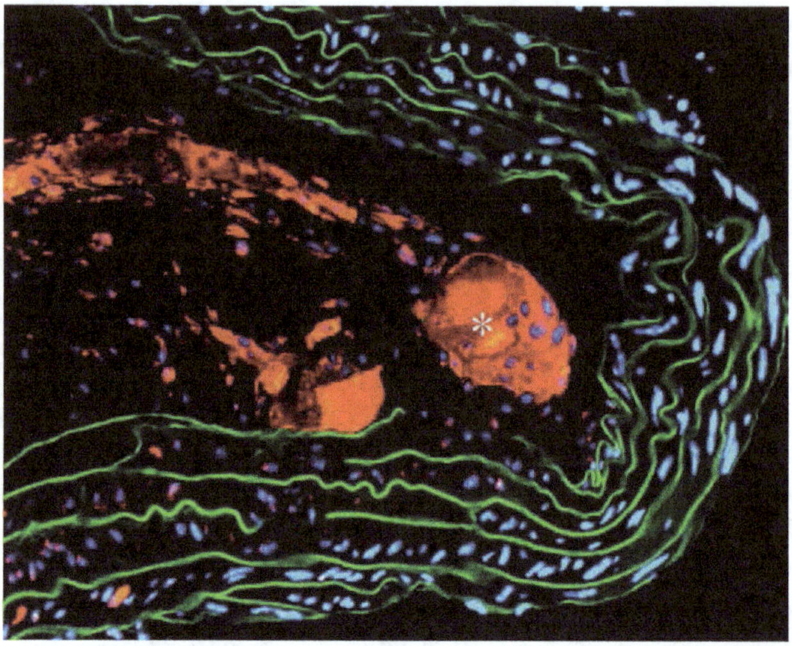

Fig. 3. Cathepsin K immunostaining of atherosclerotic lesions in brachiocephalic artery of ApoE-/- mice (red- cathepsin K, green - elastin fibers autofluorescence, blue - nuclei, x20, asterisk shows multinucleated giant cell).

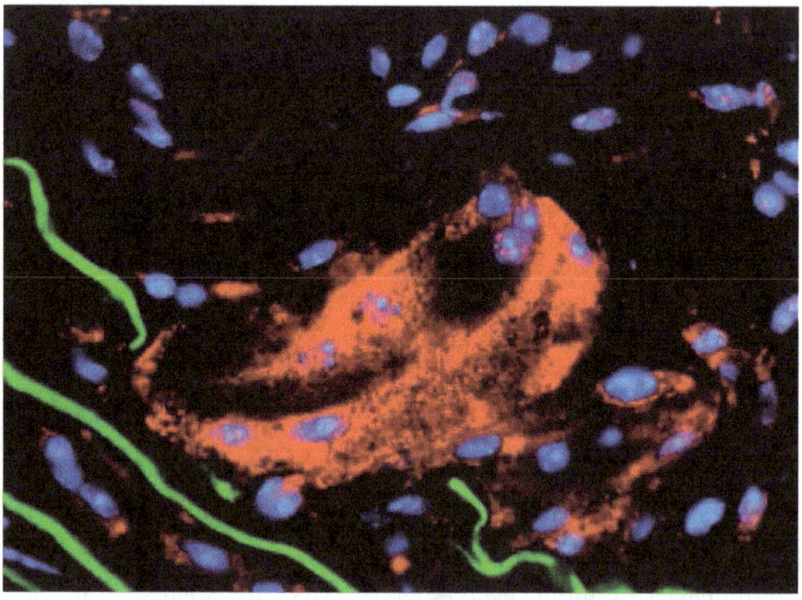

Fig. 4. Cathepsin K-positive multinucleated giant cell at the site of an elastin fiber break (red- cathepsin K, green - elastin fibers autofluorescence, blue- nuclei, x63).

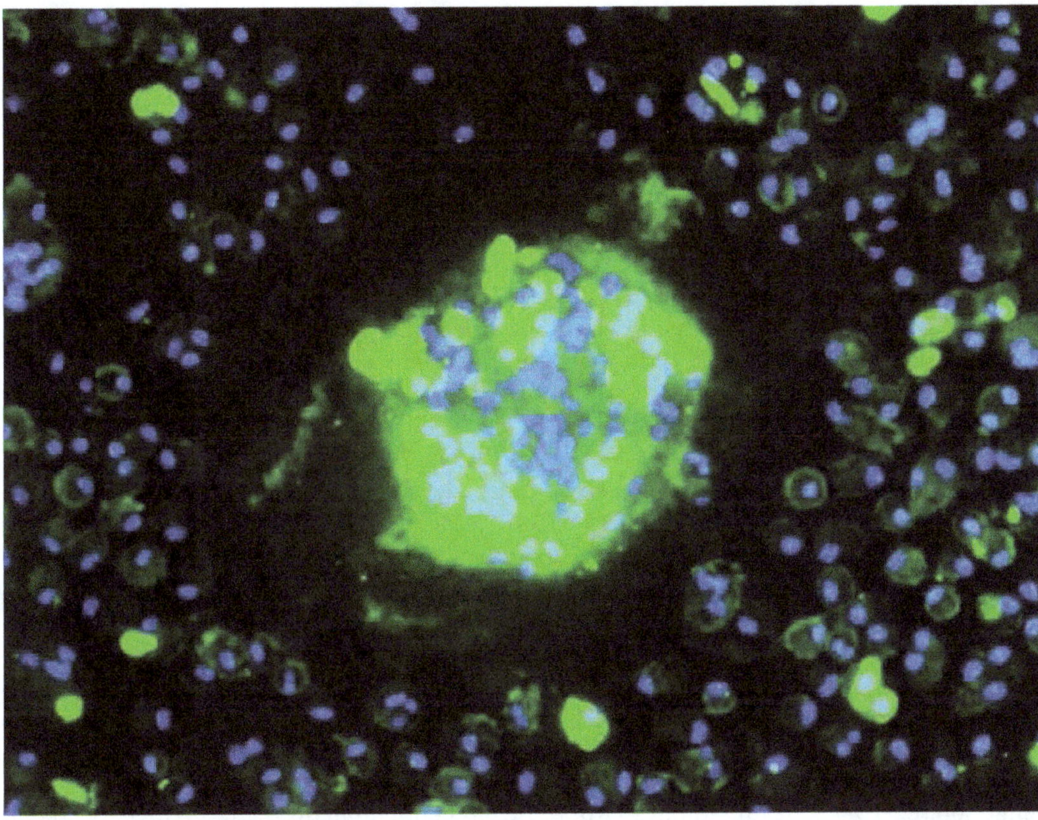

Fig. 5. Predominant accumulation of elastin-FITC complexes on/inside of multinucleated giant cell (olive green - phalloidin-FITC, neon green - elastin-FITC, blue nuclei, x20).

The involvement of cathepsin K in the increased elastolytic potential of multinucleated giant cells was further supported by an in vitro experiment where peritoneal macrophages were incubated with IL-4 to induce fusion and multinucleated giant cell formation. The fusion of macrophages resulted in dramatic increase in their elastolytic activity as was revealed by the cleavage of FITC-labeled elastin. On the third day of macrophage fusion, cells from cathepsin K-deficient mice showed a 30% reduction in their elastolytic activity compared to cells derived from cathepsin K-expressing animals (Samokhin, 2010c). Notably, most of the elastin fibers were attached to or engulfed by MGCs (Fig. 5) demonstrating that the observed increase in elastolytic activity was due to the process of giant cell formation.

8. Conclusion

The results of recent studies in humans and animal models provide evidences for the pivotal roles of cathepsin K, L and S in aortic extracellular matrix remodeling during pathological conditions. Their elasto- and/or collagenolytic activities render them into main culprits of matrix destruction observed in cardiovascular diseases and make these proteases attractive pharmaceutical targets for therapeutic interventions.

9. References

Abdul-Hussien, H., Hanemaaijer, R., Kleemann, R., Verhaaren, B.F., van Bockel, J.H. & Lindeman, J.H. (2010). The pathophysiology of abdominal aortic aneurysm growth: corresponding and discordant inflammatory and proteolytic processes in abdominal aortic and popliteal artery aneurysms. *J Vasc Surg,* Vol. 51, No. 6, pp. 1479-87.

Abdul-Hussien, H., Soekhoe, R.G., Weber, E., von der Thusen, J.H., Kleemann, R., Mulder, A., van Bockel, J.H., Hanemaaijer, R. & Lindeman, J.H. (2007). Collagen degradation in the abdominal aneurysm: a conspiracy of matrix metalloproteinase and cysteine collagenases. *Am J Pathol,* Vol. 170, No. 3, pp. 809-17.

Abisi, S., Burnand, K.G., Waltham, M., Humphries, J., Taylor, P.R. & Smith, A. (2007). Cysteine protease activity in the wall of abdominal aortic aneurysms. *J Vasc Surg,* Vol. 46, No. 6, pp. 1260-6.

Arteaga-Solis, E., Gayraud, B. & Ramirez, F. (2000). Elastic and collagenous networks in vascular diseases. *Cell Struct Funct,* Vol. 25, No. 2, pp. 69-72.

Bai, L., Beckers, L., Wijnands, E., Lutgens, S.P., Herias, M.V., Saftig, P., Daemen, M.J., Cleutjens, K., Lutgens, E., Biessen, E.A. & Heeneman, S. (2010). Cathepsin K gene disruption does not affect murine aneurysm formation. *Atherosclerosis,* Vol. 209, No. 1, pp. 96-103.

Barascuk, N., Skjot-Arkil, H., Register, T.C., Larsen, L., Byrjalsen, I., Christiansen, C. & Karsdal, M.A. (2010). Human macrophage foam cells degrade atherosclerotic plaques through cathepsin K mediated processes. *BMC Cardiovasc Disord,* Vol. 10, pp. 19.

Barbour, J.R., Spinale, F.G. & Ikonomidis, J.S. (2007). Proteinase systems and thoracic aortic aneurysm progression. *J Surg Res,* Vol. 139, No. 2, pp. 292-307.

Bengtsson, E., To, F., Hakansson, K., Grubb, A., Branen, L., Nilsson, J. & Jovinge, S. (2005). Lack of the cysteine protease inhibitor cystatin C promotes atherosclerosis in apolipoprotein E-deficient mice. *Arterioscler Thromb Vasc Biol,* Vol. 25, No. 10, pp. 2151-6.

Bromme, D. & Lecaille, F. (2009). Cathepsin K inhibitors for osteoporosis and potential off-target effects. *Expert Opin Investig Drugs,* Vol. 18, No. 5, pp. 585-600.

Bromme, D., Okamoto, K., Wang, B.B. & Biroc, S. (1996). Human cathepsin O2, a matrix protein-degrading cysteine protease expressed in osteoclasts. Functional expression of human cathepsin O2 in Spodoptera frugiperda and characterization of the enzyme. *J Biol Chem,* Vol. 271, No. 4, pp. 2126-32.

Buhling, F., Reisenauer, A., Gerber, A., Kruger, S., Weber, E., Bromme, D., Roessner, A., Ansorge, S., Welte, T. & Rocken, C. (2001). Cathepsin K--a marker of macrophage differentiation? *J Pathol,* Vol. 195, No. 3, pp. 375-82.

Buhling, F., Rocken, C., Brasch, F., Hartig, R., Yasuda, Y., Saftig, P., Bromme, D. & Welte, T. (2004). Pivotal role of cathepsin K in lung fibrosis. *Am J Pathol,* Vol. 164, No. 6, pp. 2203-16.

Chapman, H.A., Riese, R.J. & Shi, G.P. (1997). Emerging roles for cysteine proteases in human biology. *Annu Rev Physiol,* Vol. 59, pp. 63-88.

Cheng, X.W., Kuzuya, M., Nakamura, K., Di, Q., Liu, Z., Sasaki, T., Kanda, S., Jin, H., Shi, G.P., Murohara, T., Yokota, M. & Iguchi, A. (2006). Localization of cysteine protease, cathepsin S, to the surface of vascular smooth muscle cells by association with integrin alphanubeta3. *Am J Pathol,* Vol. 168, No. 2, pp. 685-94.

Conus, S. & Simon, H.U. (2008). Cathepsins: key modulators of cell death and inflammatory responses. *Biochem Pharmacol,* Vol. 76, No. 11, pp. 1374-82.

de Nooijer, R., Bot, I., von der Thusen, J.H., Leeuwenburgh, M.A., Overkleeft, H.S., Kraaijeveld, A.O., Dorland, R., van Santbrink, P.J., van Heiningen, S.H., Westra, M.M., Kovanen, P.T., Jukema, J.W., van der Wall, E.E., van Berkel, T.J., Shi, G.P. & Biessen, E.A. (2009). Leukocyte cathepsin S is a potent regulator of both cell and matrix turnover in advanced atherosclerosis. *Arterioscler Thromb Vasc Biol,* Vol. 29, No. 2, pp. 188-94.

Deschamps, K., Cromlish, W., Weicker, S., Lamontagne, S., Huszar, S.L., Gauthier, J.Y., Mudgett, J.S., Guimond, A., Romand, R., Frossard, N., Percival, M.D., Slipetz, D. & Tan, C.M. (2010). Genetic and Pharmacological Evaluation of Cathepsin S in a Mouse Model of Asthma. *Am J Respir Cell Mol Biol.*

Diehm, N., Dick, F., Schaffner, T., Schmidli, J., Kalka, C., Di Santo, S., Voelzmann, J. & Baumgartner, I. (2007). Novel insight into the pathobiology of abdominal aortic aneurysm and potential future treatment concepts. *Prog Cardiovasc Dis,* Vol. 50, No. 3, pp. 209-17.

Dobrin, P.B. & Mrkvicka, R. (1994). Failure of elastin or collagen as possible critical connective tissue alterations underlying aneurysmal dilatation. *Cardiovasc Surg,* Vol. 2, No. 4, pp. 484-8.

Duca, L., Floquet, N., Alix, A.J., Haye, B. & Debelle, L. (2004). Elastin as a matrikine. *Crit Rev Oncol Hematol,* Vol. 49, No. 3, pp. 235-44.

Eberhardt, R.T. & Dhadly, M. (2007). Giant cell arteritis: diagnosis, management, and cardiovascular implications. *Cardiol Rev,* Vol. 15, No. 2, pp. 55-61.

Garcia-Touchard, A., Henry, T.D., Sangiorgi, G., Spagnoli, L.G., Mauriello, A., Conover, C. & Schwartz, R.S. (2005). Extracellular proteases in atherosclerosis and restenosis. *Arterioscler Thromb Vasc Biol,* Vol. 25, No. 6, pp. 1119-27.

Garnero, P., Borel, O., Byrjalsen, I., Ferreras, M., Drake, F.H., McQueney, M.S., Foged, N.T., Delmas, P.D. & Delaisse, J.M. (1998). The collagenolytic activity of cathepsin K is unique among mammalian proteinases. *J Biol Chem,* Vol. 273, No. 48, pp. 32347-52.

Guo, J., Bot, I., de Nooijer, R., Hoffman, S.J., Stroup, G.B., Biessen, E.A., Benson, G.M., Groot, P.H., Van Eck, M. & Van Berkel, T.J. (2009). Leucocyte cathepsin K affects atherosclerotic lesion composition and bone mineral density in low-density lipoprotein receptor deficient mice. *Cardiovasc Res,* Vol. 81, No. 2, pp. 278-85.

Gupta, S., Singh, R.K., Dastidar, S. & Ray, A. (2008). Cysteine cathepsin S as an immunomodulatory target: present and future trends. *Expert Opin Ther Targets,* Vol. 12, No. 3, pp. 291-9.

Hirakawa, H., Pierce, R.A., Bingol-Karakoc, G., Karaaslan, C., Weng, M., Shi, G.P., Saad, A., Weber, E., Mariani, T.J., Starcher, B., Shapiro, S.D. & Cataltepe, S. (2007). Cathepsin S deficiency confers protection from neonatal hyperoxia-induced lung injury. *Am J Respir Crit Care Med,* Vol. 176, No. 8, pp. 778-85.

Honey, K. & Rudensky, A.Y. (2003). Lysosomal cysteine proteases regulate antigen presentation. *Nat Rev Immunol,* Vol. 3, No. 6, pp. 472-82.

Hsing, L.C. & Rudensky, A.Y. (2005). The lysosomal cysteine proteases in MHC class II antigen presentation. *Immunol Rev,* Vol. 207, pp. 229-41.

Jormsjo, S., Wuttge, D.M., Sirsjo, A., Whatling, C., Hamsten, A., Stemme, S. & Eriksson, P. (2002). Differential expression of cysteine and aspartic proteases during progression of atherosclerosis in apolipoprotein E-deficient mice. *Am J Pathol,* Vol. 161, No. 3, pp. 939-45.

Kadirvel, R., Ding, Y.H., Dai, D., Lewis, D.A. & Kallmes, D.F. (2004). Differential expression of genes in elastase-induced saccular aneurysms with high and low aspect ratios. *Neurosurgery,* Vol. 66, No. 3, pp. 578-84; discussion 584.

Kadoglou, N.P. & Liapis, C.D. Matrix metalloproteinases: contribution to pathogenesis, diagnosis, surveillance and treatment of abdominal aortic aneurysms. *Curr Med Res Opin,* Vol. 20, No. 4, pp. 419-32.

Kaiser, M., Younge, B., Bjornsson, J., Goronzy, J.J. & Weyand, C.M. (1999). Formation of new vasa vasorum in vasculitis. Production of angiogenic cytokines by multinucleated giant cells. *Am J Pathol,* Vol. 155, No. 3, pp. 765-74.

Kitamoto, S., Sukhova, G.K., Sun, J., Yang, M., Libby, P., Love, V., Duramad, P., Sun, C., Zhang, Y., Yang, X., Peters, C. & Shi, G.P. (2007). Cathepsin L deficiency reduces diet-induced atherosclerosis in low-density lipoprotein receptor-knockout mice. *Circulation,* Vol. 115, No. 15, pp. 2065-75.

Lafarge, J.C., Naour, N., Clement, K. & Guerre-Millo, M. (2010). Cathepsins and cystatin C in atherosclerosis and obesity. *Biochimie,* Vol. 92, No. 11, pp. 1580-6.

Lankelma, J.M., Voorend, D.M., Barwari, T., Koetsveld, J., Van der Spek, A.H., De Porto, A.P., Van Rooijen, G. & Van Noorden, C.J. (2010). Cathepsin L, target in cancer treatment? *Life Sci,* Vol. 86, No. 7-8, pp. 225-33.

Lecaille, F., Bromme, D. & Lalmanach, G. (2008). Biochemical properties and regulation of cathepsin K activity. *Biochimie,* Vol. 90, No. 2, pp. 208-26.

Li, W., Kornmark, L., Jonasson, L., Forssell, C. & Yuan, X.M. (2009). Cathepsin L is significantly associated with apoptosis and plaque destabilization in human atherosclerosis. *Atherosclerosis,* Vol. 202, No. 1, pp. 92-102.

Lindholt, J.S., Erlandsen, E.J. & Henneberg, E.W. (2001). Cystatin C deficiency is associated with the progression of small abdominal aortic aneurysms. *Br J Surg,* Vol. 88, No. 11, pp. 1472-5.

Linke, M., Gordon, R.E., Brillard, M., Lecaille, F., Lalmanach, G. & Bromme, D. (2006). Degradation of apolipoprotein B-100 by lysosomal cysteine cathepsins. *Biol Chem,* Vol. 387, No. 9, pp. 1295-303.

Liu, J., Sukhova, G.K., Sun, J.S., Xu, W.H., Libby, P. & Shi, G.P. (2004). Lysosomal cysteine proteases in atherosclerosis. *Arterioscler Thromb Vasc Biol,* Vol. 24, No. 8, pp. 1359-66.

Liu, J., Sukhova, G.K., Yang, J.T., Sun, J., Ma, L., Ren, A., Xu, W.H., Fu, H., Dolganov, G.M., Hu, C., Libby, P. & Shi, G.P. (2006). Cathepsin L expression and regulation in human abdominal aortic aneurysm, atherosclerosis, and vascular cells. *Atherosclerosis,* Vol. 184, No. 2, pp. 302-11.

Lutgens, E., Lutgens, S.P., Faber, B.C., Heeneman, S., Gijbels, M.M., de Winther, M.P., Frederik, P., van der Made, I., Daugherty, A., Sijbers, A.M., Fisher, A., Long, C.J., Saftig, P., Black, D., Daemen, M.J. & Cleutjens, K.B. (2006a). Disruption of the cathepsin K gene reduces atherosclerosis progression and induces plaque fibrosis but accelerates macrophage foam cell formation. *Circulation,* Vol. 113, No. 1, pp. 98-107.

Lutgens, S.P., Cleutjens, K.B., Daemen, M.J. & Heeneman, S. (2007). Cathepsin cysteine proteases in cardiovascular disease. *FASEB J*, Vol. 21, No. 12, pp. 3029-41.

Lutgens, S.P., Kisters, N., Lutgens, E., van Haaften, R.I., Evelo, C.T., de Winther, M.P., Saftig, P., Daemen, M.J., Heeneman, S. & Cleutjens, K.B. (2006b). Gene profiling of cathepsin K deficiency in atherogenesis: profibrotic but lipogenic. *J Pathol*, Vol. 210, No. 3, pp. 334-43.

Michel, J.B., Martin-Ventura, J.L., Egido, J., Sakalihasan, N., Treska, V., Lindholt, J., Allaire, E., Thorsteinsdottir, U., Cockerill, G. & Swedenborg, J. (2011). Novel aspects of the pathogenesis of aneurysms of the abdominal aorta in humans. *Cardiovasc Res*, Vol. 90, No. 1, pp. 18-27.

Newby, A.C. (2008). Metalloproteinase expression in monocytes and macrophages and its relationship to atherosclerotic plaque instability. *Arterioscler Thromb Vasc Biol*, Vol. 28, No. 12, pp. 2108-14.

Nordborg, E. & Nordborg, C. (2003). Giant cell arteritis: epidemiological clues to its pathogenesis and an update on its treatment. *Rheumatology (Oxford)*, Vol. 42, No. 3, pp. 413-21.

Pasquali-Ronchetti, I. & Baccarani-Contri, M. (1997). Elastic fiber during development and aging. *Microsc Res Tech*, Vol. 38, No. 4, pp. 428-35.

Penn, H. & Dasgupta, B. (2003). Giant cell arteritis. *Autoimmun Rev*, Vol. 2, No. 4, pp. 199-203.

Platt, M.O., Ankeny, R.F., Shi, G.P., Weiss, D., Vega, J.D., Taylor, W.R. & Jo, H. (2007). Expression of cathepsin K is regulated by shear stress in cultured endothelial cells and is increased in endothelium in human atherosclerosis. *Am J Physiol Heart Circ Physiol*, Vol. 292, No. 3, pp. H1479-86.

Punturieri, A., Filippov, S., Allen, E., Caras, I., Murray, R., Reddy, V. & Weiss, S.J. (2000). Regulation of elastinolytic cysteine proteinase activity in normal and cathepsin K-deficient human macrophages. *J Exp Med*, Vol. 192, No. 6, pp. 789-99.

Reddy, V.Y., Zhang, Q.Y. & Weiss, S.J. (1995). Pericellular mobilization of the tissue-destructive cysteine proteinases, cathepsins B, L, and S, by human monocyte-derived macrophages. *Proc Natl Acad Sci U S A*, Vol. 92, No. 9, pp. 3849-53.

Reinheckel, T., Hagemann, S., Dollwet-Mack, S., Martinez, E., Lohmuller, T., Zlatkovic, G., Tobin, D.J., Maas-Szabowski, N. & Peters, C. (2005). The lysosomal cysteine protease cathepsin L regulates keratinocyte proliferation by control of growth factor recycling. *J Cell Sci*, Vol. 118, No. Pt 15, pp. 3387-95.

Reiser, J., Adair, B. & Reinheckel, T. Specialized roles for cysteine cathepsins in health and disease. (2010).*J Clin Invest*, Vol. 120, No. 10, pp. 3421-31.

Repnik, U. & Turk, B. Lysosomal-mitochondrial cross-talk during cell death. *Mitochondrion*, Vol. 10, No. 6, pp. 662-9.

Rizas, K.D., Ippagunta, N. & Tilson, M.D., 3rd (2009). Immune cells and molecular mediators in the pathogenesis of the abdominal aortic aneurysm. *Cardiol Rev*, Vol. 17, No. 5, pp. 201-10.

Rodgers, K.J., Watkins, D.J., Miller, A.L., Chan, P.Y., Karanam, S., Brissette, W.H., Long, C.J. & Jackson, C.L. (2006). Destabilizing role of cathepsin S in murine atherosclerotic plaques. *Arterioscler Thromb Vasc Biol*, Vol. 26, No. 4, pp. 851-6.

Sadek, M., Hynecek, R.L., Goldenberg, S., Kent, K.C., Marin, M.L. & Faries, P.L. (2008). Gene expression analysis of a porcine native abdominal aortic aneurysm model. *Surgery,* Vol. 144, No. 2, pp. 252-8.

Sakalihasan, N., Limet, R. & Defawe, O.D. (2005). Abdominal aortic aneurysm. *Lancet,* Vol. 365, No. 9470, pp. 1577-89.

Samokhin, A.O., Buhling, F., Theissig, F. & Bromme, D. (2010a). ApoE-deficient mice on cholate-containing high-fat diet reveal a pathology similar to lung sarcoidosis. *Am J Pathol,* Vol. 176, No. 3, pp. 1148-56.

Samokhin, A.O., Gauthier, J.Y., Percival, M.D. & Bromme, D. Lack of cathepsin activities alter or prevent the development of lung granulomas in a mouse model of sarcoidosis. (2011). *Respir Res,* Vol. 12, pp. 13.

Samokhin, A.O., Lythgo, P.A., Gauthier, J.Y., Percival, M.D. & Bromme, D. (2010b). Pharmacological inhibition of cathepsin S decreases atherosclerotic lesions in Apoe-/- mice. *J Cardiovasc Pharmacol,* Vol. 56, No. 1, pp. 98-105.

Samokhin, A.O., Wilson, S., Nho, B., Lizame, M.L., Musenden, O.E. & Bromme, D. (2010c). Cholate-containing high-fat diet induces the formation of multinucleated giant cells in atherosclerotic plaques of apolipoprotein E-/- mice. *Arterioscler Thromb Vasc Biol,* Vol. 30, No. 6, pp. 1166-73.

Samokhin, A.O., Wong, A., Saftig, P. & Bromme, D. (2008). Role of cathepsin K in structural changes in brachiocephalic artery during progression of atherosclerosis in apoE-deficient mice. *Atherosclerosis,* Vol. 200, No. 1, pp. 58-68.

Sawabe, M. (2010) Vascular aging: from molecular mechanism to clinical significance. *Geriatr Gerontol Int,* Vol. 10 Suppl 1, pp. S213-20.

Schulte, S., Sun, J., Libby, P., Macfarlane, L., Sun, C., Lopez-Ilasaca, M., Shi, G.P. & Sukhova, G.K. (2010). Cystatin C deficiency promotes inflammation in angiotensin II-induced abdominal aortic aneurisms in atherosclerotic mice. *Am J Pathol,* Vol. 177, No. 1, pp. 456-63.

Senior, R.M., Griffin, G.L., Mecham, R.P., Wrenn, D.S., Prasad, K.U. & Urry, D.W. (1984). Val-Gly-Val-Ala-Pro-Gly, a repeating peptide in elastin, is chemotactic for fibroblasts and monocytes. *J Cell Biol,* Vol. 99, No. 3, pp. 870-4.

Shadwick, R.E. (1999). Mechanical design in arteries. *J Exp Biol,* Vol. 202, No. Pt 23, pp. 3305-13.

Shi, G.P., Sukhova, G.K., Grubb, A., Ducharme, A., Rhode, L.H., Lee, R.T., Ridker, P.M., Libby, P. & Chapman, H.A. (1999). Cystatin C deficiency in human atherosclerosis and aortic aneurysms. *J Clin Invest,* Vol. 104, No. 9, pp. 1191-7.

Shimizu, K., Mitchell, R.N. & Libby, P. (2006). Inflammation and cellular immune responses in abdominal aortic aneurysms. *Arterioscler Thromb Vasc Biol,* Vol. 26, No. 5, pp. 987-94.

Soilleux, E.J., Morris, L.S., Trowsdale, J., Coleman, N. & Boyle, J.J. (2002). Human atherosclerotic plaques express DC-SIGN, a novel protein found on dendritic cells and macrophages. *J Pathol,* Vol. 198, No. 4, pp. 511-6.

Sukhova, G.K. & Shi, G.P. (2006). Do cathepsins play a role in abdominal aortic aneurysm pathogenesis? *Ann N Y Acad Sci,* Vol. 1085, pp. 161-9.

Sukhova, G.K., Shi, G.P., Simon, D.I., Chapman, H.A. & Libby, P. (1998). Expression of the elastolytic cathepsins S and K in human atheroma and regulation of their production in smooth muscle cells. *J Clin Invest,* Vol. 102, No. 3, pp. 576-83.

Sukhova, G.K., Wang, B., Libby, P., Pan, J.H., Zhang, Y., Grubb, A., Fang, K., Chapman, H.A. & Shi, G.P. (2005). Cystatin C deficiency increases elastic lamina degradation and aortic dilatation in apolipoprotein E-null mice. *Circ Res,* Vol. 96, No. 3, pp. 368-75.

Sukhova, G.K., Zhang, Y., Pan, J.H., Wada, Y., Yamamoto, T., Naito, M., Kodama, T., Tsimikas, S., Witztum, J.L., Lu, M.L., Sakara, Y., Chin, M.T., Libby, P. & Shi, G.P. (2003). Deficiency of cathepsin S reduces atherosclerosis in LDL receptor-deficient mice. *J Clin Invest,* Vol. 111, No. 6, pp. 897-906.

Taleb, S. & Clement, K. (2007). Emerging role of cathepsin S in obesity and its associated diseases. *Clin Chem Lab Med,* Vol. 45, No. 3, pp. 328-32.

Tepel, C., Bromme, D., Herzog, V. & Brix, K. (2000). Cathepsin K in thyroid epithelial cells: sequence, localization and possible function in extracellular proteolysis of thyroglobulin. *J Cell Sci,* Vol. 113 Pt 24, pp. 4487-98.

Tolosa, E., Li, W., Yasuda, Y., Wienhold, W., Denzin , L.K., Lautwein, A., Driessen, C., Schnorrer, P., Weber, E., Stevanovic, S., Kurek, R., Meims, A. & Bromme, D. (2003). Cathepsin V is involved in the degradation of invariant chain in human thymus and is overexpressed in myasthenia gravis. *J Clin Invest,* Vol. 112, No. 4, pp. 517-526.

Turk, B. (2006). Targeting proteases: successes, failures and future prospects. *Nat Rev Drug Discov,* Vol. 5, No. 9, pp. 785-99.

van der Rest, M. & Garrone, R. (1991). Collagen family of proteins. *FASEB J,* Vol. 5, No. 13, pp. 2814-23.

Wagenseil, J.E. & Mecham, R.P. (2009). Vascular extracellular matrix and arterial mechanics. *Physiol Rev,* Vol. 89, No. 3, pp. 957-89.

Weyand, C.M., Ma-Krupa, W. & Goronzy, J.J. (2004). Immunopathways in giant cell arteritis and polymyalgia rheumatica. *Autoimmun Rev,* Vol. 3, No. 1, pp. 46-53.

Weyand, C.M., Ma-Krupa, W., Pryshchep, O., Groschel, S., Bernardino, R. & Goronzy, J. J. (2005). Vascular dendritic cells in giant cell arteritis. *Ann N Y Acad Sci,* Vol. 1062, pp. 195-208.

Williams, A.S., Eynott, P.R., Leung, S.Y., Nath, P., Jupp, R., De Sanctis, G.T., Resnick, R., Adcock, I.M. & Chung, K.F. (2009). Role of cathepsin S in ozone-induced airway hyperresponsiveness and inflammation. *Pulm Pharmacol Ther,* Vol. 22, No. 1, pp. 27-32.

Permissions

All chapters in this book were first published by InTech Open; hereby published with permission under the Creative Commons Attribution License or equivalent. Every chapter published in this book has been scrutinized by our experts. Their significance has been extensively debated. The topics covered herein carry significant findings which will fuel the growth of the discipline. They may even be implemented as practical applications or may be referred to as a beginning point for another development.

The contributors of this book come from diverse backgrounds, making this book a truly international effort. This book will bring forth new frontiers with its revolutionizing research information and detailed analysis of the nascent developments around the world.

We would like to thank all the contributing authors for lending their expertise to make the book truly unique. They have played a crucial role in the development of this book. Without their invaluable contributions this book wouldn't have been possible. They have made vital efforts to compile up to date information on the varied aspects of this subject to make this book a valuable addition to the collection of many professionals and students.

This book was conceptualized with the vision of imparting up-to-date information and advanced data in this field. To ensure the same, a matchless editorial board was set up. Every individual on the board went through rigorous rounds of assessment to prove their worth. After which they invested a large part of their time researching and compiling the most relevant data for our readers.

The editorial board has been involved in producing this book since its inception. They have spent rigorous hours researching and exploring the diverse topics which have resulted in the successful publishing of this book. They have passed on their knowledge of decades through this book. To expedite this challenging task, the publisher supported the team at every step. A small team of assistant editors was also appointed to further simplify the editing procedure and attain best results for the readers.

Apart from the editorial board, the designing team has also invested a significant amount of their time in understanding the subject and creating the most relevant covers. They scrutinized every image to scout for the most suitable representation of the subject and create an appropriate cover for the book.

The publishing team has been an ardent support to the editorial, designing and production team. Their endless efforts to recruit the best for this project, has resulted in the accomplishment of this book. They are a veteran in the field of academics and their pool of knowledge is as vast as their experience in printing. Their expertise and guidance has proved useful at every step. Their uncompromising quality standards have made this book an exceptional effort. Their encouragement from time to time has been an inspiration for everyone.

The publisher and the editorial board hope that this book will prove to be a valuable piece of knowledge for researchers, students, practitioners and scholars across the globe.

List of Contributors

Christopher J. Marrocco and Ruth L. Bush
Scott and White Hospital, Texas A & M College of Medicine, Temple, TX, USA

Reza Mofidi
James Cook University Hospital, Middlesbrough

Stuart A. Suttie
University of Dundee, Dundee, United Kingdom

Ricky Harminder Bhogal and Richard Downing
University of Birmingham & Worcestershire Royal Hospital, United Kingdom

Cheong J. Lee and Mark D. Morasch
Northwestern University, United States of America

Andrew Gonzalez
University of Illinois at Chicago, Chicago, Illinois, United States of America

Sossio Perrotta
Department of Cardiothoracic Surgery, Sahlgrenska University Hospital, Gothenburg, Sweden

Salvatore Lentini
Department of Cardiothoracic Surgery, University Hospital "G Martino", University of Messina, Messina, Italy

Júlia Čanádyová and Aleš Mokráček
Department of Cardiac Surgery, Regional Hospital České Budějovice, Czech Republic

John A. Kalef-Ezra
University of Ioannina, Medical School, Greece

Yusuke Asakura
Department of Anesthesiology, Nagoya, Japan

Hideki Takagi
Department of Orthopedic Surgery, Nagoya Kyoritsu Hospital, Nagoya, Japan

Sergio Santana Porbén
Nutritional Support Group, "Hermanos Ameijeiras" Clinical surgical Hospital, La Habana, Cuba

Andriy O. Samokhin and Dieter Brömme
University of British Columbia, Vancouver, Canada

Index

A

Abdominal Aortic Aneurysm, 2-5, 8-17, 20-31, 34-47, 68-79, 92-94, 136-137, 166-167, 170-171, 173-175, 188-190, 192, 204-205, 209-215, 219-224

Abdominal Ultrasonography, 2, 27

Acute Renal Failure, 50-55, 62-63, 68-69, 88-89

Anatomy, 4-5, 8-9, 12-13, 20-23, 36-37, 48-49, 56-57, 62-67, 81-87, 116-117, 120-123, 134, 176-177, 188-189

Aneurismal Disease, 3, 78

Aneurysm Diameter, 28-29, 32-33, 44-45

Aneurysm Expansion, 36-39, 42-45

Aneurysm Growth Rate, 38-39

Aneurysm Morphology, 36-37, 68-69

Aneurysm Rupture, 2, 8-9, 16-21, 27, 30-31, 40-45, 56-59, 62-65

Aortic Arch, 46-47, 54-55, 70-75, 96-97, 106-107, 110-111, 214-215

Aortic Clamping, 50-55, 58-59, 70-73

Aortic Disease, 1, 3, 26, 40-41, 60-61, 78-79, 172, 191

Aortic Dissection, 102-103, 108-109, 112-113, 132-133

Aortic Necks, 56-57

Aortic Root Dilatation, 106-109, 114-115

Aortic Valve Replacement, 81, 96-97, 102-103, 106-115, 130-134

Aortoplasty, 80, 95-115

Ascending Aorta Redilatation, 106-107

C

Cardiac Surgery, 38-39, 42-43, 100-101, 106-107, 114-115, 132-133

Cardio-vascular Disease, 36-37

Cardiopulmonary Bypass, 46-47, 56-57, 106-107

Cerebrospinal Fluid, 52-53, 72-73

D

Dermal Atrophy, 140-143

Dermal Necrosis, 140-141

Device Migration, 30-31, 34-35, 64-65

Distal Aortic Perfusion, 52-55

Dose Area Product, 138-139, 144-145

Dose Fractionation, 140-141, 148-149

E

Endoleaks, 30-31, 50-51, 56-57, 60-61, 64-65, 86-87, 168-169

Endotension, 3, 64-67, 72-73, 78

Endothelial Cells, 36-37, 142-143, 192, 209-213, 223-224

Endovascular Repair, 6-19, 22-26, 30-37, 42-43, 50-51, 66-77, 79, 81-84, 86, 88-94, 134, 137-138, 140, 142, 144, 146, 148, 150, 152, 154, 156, 158, 160, 162, 164, 166-171, 188-190

F

Fluoroscopy, 58-61, 138-139, 144-146, 148-155, 158-163, 166-169

G

Gestation Period, 144-145, 158-161

H

Hazard Ratio, 12-13, 16-17, 36-37

High Density Lipoproteins, 36-37

Hypothermia, 52-53, 92-93

I

Imaging Utilization, 14-15

Intercostal Artery, 54-57

International Atomic Energy Agency, 140-141, 166-167

Irradiation, 138-146, 148-151, 154-155, 166-171

K

Keratosis, 142-143

L

Laparoscopy, 56-57, 70-71

Left Heart Bypass, 52-55, 70-71

Life Expectancy, 8-11, 22-23, 138-139

Lipid Profiles, 206-207

M

Macrophages, 36-37, 192, 209-217, 219-220, 223-224

Medical Co-morbidities, 30-31, 36-37

Mental Retardation, 144-145

Monocytes, 36-37, 212-215,223-224

Morbidity, 3, 6-7, 10-13, 18-21,30-39, 42-43, 48-57, 60-63,66-67, 78, 81-83, 88-91, 104-107, 134

Mortality, 2-25, 27-45, 48-69, 72-75, 78, 81-85, 88-94, 100-101, 104-109, 114-115, 132-134, 137, 146, 148-149, 174-175, 188-190, 204-207

Myocardial Infraction, 54-55

N

Nonagenarians, 10-11, 24-25

O

Octogenarians, 8-11, 24-25, 36-37

Open Surgery, 8-9, 12-13, 20-21, 24-25, 42-43, 52-53, 56-57, 60-63, 66-69, 81-83, 88-94, 134

Open Versus Endovascular Repair, 34-35, 66-67, 74-75, 90-91

Organogenesis, 144-145

P

Paraplegia, 54-57, 62-63, 68-73, 174-175

Post-thoracotomy Pain, 54-57

Postoperative Complications, 16-17, 36-37, 82-83, 204-205

Prenatal Irradiation, 144-145

Progenitor Cells, 140-141

Prosthetic Material, 52-53

Protective Effect, 38-39, 54-55

Q

Quality Of Life, 6-7, 12-13, 16-19, 22-23, 34-37, 52-53, 62-67, 174-175

R

Radiation Dose, 144-145, 148-149, 162-171

Radiological Imaging, 48-49, 56-57

Randomisation, 28-29, 34-35

Randomized Clinical Trials, 12-13, 18-19, 24-25, 66-67

Redilatation, 96-97, 100-109, 112-113

Reintervention Rate, 12-13, 36-37

Resource Utilization, 14-15, 24-25, 42-43

Retrospective Analysis, 14-15, 66-67

Right Lateral Decubitus Position, 52-53, 56-57

Ruptured Aneurysm, 8-11, 92-93

S

Sinotubular Junction, 102-103, 106-111, 116-123, 130-131

Smooth Muscle Cells, 36-37, 192, 209-217, 221-224

Society For Vascular Surgery, 4-5, 60-61, 70-71, 92-93, 204-205

Statin Therapy, 36-39, 42-43

Systole, 106-107, 130-131

T

Thoracic Aorta, 48-49, 52-53, 60-61, 64-65, 74-77, 98-99, 102-103, 110-111

Thoracic Surgery, 54-55, 70-75

Thoracoscope, 56-57

Tubular Graft, 62-63, 102-103, 106-109, 124, 126, 128-129

U

Ultrasound Surveillance, 2, 6-7, 18-19, 27, 32-33, 40-41

V

Vessel Wall, 36-37, 96-97

www.ingramcontent.com/pod-product-compliance
Lightning Source LLC
LaVergne TN
LVHW080610210926
848485LV00003B/131

* 9 7 8 1 6 3 9 2 7 8 9 2 3 *